NLN Guide to Undergraduate RN Education

5th Edition

Pub. No. PBTRAD977378

**NLN Center for Research
in Nursing Education and Community Health**

National League for Nursing · New York

Contents

Section 2

Baccalaureate Degree Programs by State 153

Section 3
Diploma Programs by State 245

Section 4

Baccalaureate Degree Programs Designed Exclusively for RNs by State

Introduction

People choose nursing as a career for many reasons. Perhaps you have had some exposure to nursing through a family member or friend who was ill and you saw firsthand how nurses cared for people in hospitals or their homes. Or you may have known nurses and heard stories of their experiences with people in health care. You may be someone who likes the independence of working and living in different parts of the country, or you may want the option to choose to work with people of different ages and cultures. Whatever your reasons, the exciting diversity and choices available in nursing will always make it an attractive profession.

This book will serve as a guide to provide pertinent information about nursing and nursing educational programs leading to registered nurse (RN) licensure. It will answer some of the questions you may have if you are considering nursing as a career. The book is divided into the following parts:

- The first part describes the profession of nursing, including educational requirements and various professional roles of the nurse.

- The second part is a directory of schools of nursing in the country. The schools that have National League for Nursing accreditation are indicated individually. This revised edition includes a list of schools that offer BSN programs for non-RNs with degrees in other fields.

- The third part includes a glossary of terms commonly used in nursing.

We hope that you find this guide useful in planning your RN education.

Delroy Louden, PhD
Executive Director
Center for Research in Nursing Education
and Community Health

NLN CENTER FOR RESEARCH IN NURSING EDUCATION AND COMMUNITY HEALTH

NLN Research has expanded its focus and activities and is now the NLN Center for Research in Nursing Education and Community Health. The Center serves as a linking resource for nursing education and practice, research initiatives, community health care delivery, and information. For example, the Center will serve as a repository of nursing education statistics and will maintain and expand NLN's national data bank, conduct research, and publish results of surveys and studies.

Since 1953, NLN Research has been maintaining and updating a comprehensive data bank on all state-approved nursing education programs. NLN's Annual Survey is conducted using a sophisticated research design and rigorous data collection methodology. Every year, with the cooperation of each state board of nursing, NLN Research surveys the more than 3,000 nursing education programs in operation within the United States.

In addition, the Center has expanded into community-based research that is data driven and population-focused. Many of these special initiatives are collaborative, joining the Center with partners from new arenas ranging from small communities to sister organizations across the globe.

Three councils are affiliated with the Center for Research: Council for Community Health Services, Council for Nursing Informatics, and Council for Research in Nursing Education. These councils are active members of the Center, participating in manuscript preparation, maintaining expertise in developing technologies, and providing leadership in nursing education and community health.

The NLN Center for Research in Nursing Education and Community Health is also exploring new opportunities to create a dialogue with members of the research community. To accomplish this, the Center has initiated the following programs:

Seminars—NLN has brought together intimate groups of major thinkers to discuss contemporary issues and set direction for policy, planning, and implementation. NLN's First Annual Research Institute held in August, 1995 focused on community-based nursing and public health.

Training—NLN welcomes pre- and post-doctoral students from the fields of nursing, sociology, psychology, and epidemiology. In addition, faculty visit on an ongoing basis from around the world. Recent scholars have come from universities in both the United States and the United Kingdom.

NLN engages in international collaborative work through memorandum of understanding. Recently, we have signed a memorandum of understanding with the Nursing Council of Spain in which NLN provides research training in nursing education and health policy issues.

Internships—NLN offers internships to provide meaningful research experiences that will foster the development of the next generation of health researchers. The interns have access to NLN Research's database, or they may use data which they have collected, to provide them with hands-on experience in statistical analysis.

Monograph Series—The Center has launched a monograph series that explores topics related to the rapidly changing health care system, research methodology, and nursing's roles in community partnerships. The first of the series is produced by the Council for Community Health Services and entitled "Home Health Outcomes and Resource Utilization: Integrating Today's Critical Priorities."

For further information about other publications and activities available through the NLN Center for Research in Nursing Education and Community Health, call 800-669-9656, option 1, or use our internet address: nlninform@nln.org.

How to Use This Book

Description

If you are not familiar with nursing, you may want to read the first section of this book, which describes the profession and career of nursing. If you are primarily interested in applying to specific schools, you may want to refer to the school section immediately.

The section on schools is divided into four areas:

Associate Degree Programs

Baccalaureate Degree Programs

Diploma Programs

Baccalaureate Degree Programs Designed Exclusively for RNs

Each school section is then organized alphabetically by state and includes specific information on the nursing program. All the schools contained in this book are state approved and the majority are accredited by the National League for Nursing. **The information is based on data which was collected by the NLN in November 1996, so any changes made after this time will not be reflected in this publication. Please note that under the school listings, the dash indicates that the information was not available or the school requested that the data not be published.**

The glossary is a handy reference which will inform you of the various terms used in the nursing profession.

NURSING AS CAREER

Nursing as a career is both an intellectual and interpersonal challenge. Professional nurses integrate knowledge of the physical sciences, nursing theory, and sophisticated technology with an ability to care for and nurture people of all ages and cultural backgrounds.

Nursing as a profession offers a variety of choices in career options and mobility. Registered nurses are given the opportunity to choose to work in various health care settings. As a nurse you will be prepared to work with ill patients in hospitals and patient homes, as well as healthy patients and families in primary health care settings. The diversity of opportunities for practice include, but are not limited to, hospital patient care units, student health, home health, occupational health, and nursing centers. Nursing offers life-long career opportunities and immeasurable personal satisfaction. As a registered nurse you become the coordinator of patient care, case provider, coordinator of services, researcher, and health educator for the patient, family, and significant others, all of which are highly valued roles. Today there are 2 million nurses in the United States, and the need for nurses will continue to increase within the next decade. As the U.S. health care delivery system undergoes rapid changes, nurses will have opportunities to practice in new and innovative settings and roles. Nursing is a profession which will continue to grow and expand in order to meet the many health needs of an increasingly diverse population. The profession needs bright, qualified applicants. If you enjoy working with people and welcome a challenge, then nursing is a profession for you to consider.

What Is a Registered Nurse (RN)?

Registered nurses are licensed, independent health care providers legally responsible for their own practice. To be eligible for licensure a person must have graduated from a school of nursing, met the requirements of the State Board of Nursing, and successfully passed the registered nurse licensing exam.

What Is the Difference between a Registered Nurse and a Licensed Practical Nurse (LPN)?

The differences between a registered nurse and a licensed practical nurse are in the education, responsibility, and the opportunity for career advancement of the RN and the LPN. Licensed practical nurse programs are generally 12 to 18 months of study and the majority of programs are in technical and vocational schools. The course of study in practical nurse programs is not as difficult as in registered nurse programs. If you are thinking of becoming a nurse and you have some difficulty with school work, particularly science courses, a practical nurse program may be best for you. It is also less costly than other RN programs.

After graduation, a practical nurse takes a state licensing exam in order to qualify for practice. LPNs work under the direct supervision of RNs.

HOW TO BECOME A NURSE

If you want to become a registered nurse, you need to start planning in high school. All nursing schools require a high school degree with course work in math, English, history, and the physical sciences such as biology and chemistry.

Seek out a high school counselor who will be able to provide you with detailed information so you can concentrate on the courses you need for acceptance to a nursing program.

WHICH PROGRAM TO CHOOSE: DIPLOMA, ASSOCIATE, OR BACCALAUREATE DEGREE?

There are three different types of basic nursing programs you may choose from: diploma, associate degree, and baccalaureate degree. Combined they total 1,508 nursing programs across the United States. There are 876 associate degree programs, 523 baccalaureate degree programs, and 109 diploma programs. The programs vary in the courses they offer, length of study, and cost. Some questions for the potential student to consider in choosing a program are:

"What are my financial resources?"

"What are my academic capabilities?"

"What are my long term goals as a nurse?"

Although graduates from all three programs are qualified to take the licensing exam, employment and career advancement will vary depending on the basic program you attend.

NATIONAL LEAGUE FOR NURSING CENTER FOR CAREER ADVANCEMENT

The National League for Nursing has established The NLN Center for Career Advancement in order to further assist you with your career plans. Individuals interested in a nursing career or RNs who want to advance in their career can request reliable information or advice on nursing programs through this network. A customized computer search can be performed to match your needs to specific programs through the NLN's national data base. The Center offers exclusive informational resources designed to help you shape your career objectives. Call the **NLN Center for Career Advancement at 800/669-9656, ext. 160** for a brochure or more information.

DIPLOMA PROGRAMS

Diploma programs are hospital based and take between 2–3 years to complete. Graduates usually assume staff positions in hospitals. Advancement beyond a staff position is not likely without additional educational preparation.

Some diploma programs are affiliated with local community colleges and offer courses in conjunction with the colleges. If you want to obtain a degree, you will have to demonstrate by an examination or documentation that you are qualified. You may also apply to a school which has an articulation agreement with a college or university.

The cost of diploma programs are proportionately less than associate and baccalaureate programs.

ASSOCIATE DEGREE PROGRAMS

Associate Degree programs are two-year programs primarily affiliated with junior and community colleges. A small number are found in senior colleges and universities. Associate degree programs are shorter and less expensive than baccalaureate programs, and course work includes both liberal arts and nursing courses. Courses are also offered on a part-time or evening basis. Graduates with an associate degree are prepared to practice in structured care settings such as hospitals and nursing homes. They do not have the career advancement opportunities available to baccalaureate graduates. Presently, they constitute the largest group of graduating nurses.

Most baccalaureate programs provide articulation opportunities for associate degree graduates to obtain a baccalaureate degree through recognition of prior course work and mobility exams.

BACCALAUREATE PROGRAMS

Baccalaureate programs are programs affiliated with universities and senior colleges. The course of study is typically four years, with a nursing major in the last two years. Graduates of baccalaureate programs are employed in a variety of patient care settings including hospitals, community agencies, schools, and clinics.

Baccalaureate programs are the most costly in time and money; however, the investment results in long term professional mobility and recognition.

BACCALAUREATE PROGRAMS FOR RNs

Baccalaureate programs for RNs are programs designed solely for individuals already licensed as RNs, and require one or two years to complete. Presently, there are 149 such programs across the United States.

PROGRAM ACCREDITATION

Nursing programs must be approved by State Boards of Nursing for graduates to take the licensure exam. Many are also accredited by the National League for Nursing (NLN), the official accrediting agency for schools of nursing. Because this is a voluntary accreditation process, accreditation by the National League for Nursing assures the student that the school has met specific standards of academic excellence. Knowledge of whether a nursing program has NLN accreditation is important; certain scholarships or loans may not be available if the school does not have accreditation, and graduate programs limit enrollment to graduates of NLN-approved schools. Also, opportunities for military service as a nurse are restricted to graduates of NLN accredited programs.

Career Benefits in Nursing

Once you obtain your license to practice nursing, a variety of career choices may be open to you depending on your credentials and geographic location. In the past, the majority of new nurses were employed in hospitals. Now, more and more nurses are finding jobs in a variety of settings. For their initial positions many nurses choose to work at a hospital in which they have had experience as a student. Others find employment in long-term care facilities, community and public health clinics, and schools and physicians' offices. Position availability varies from region to region throughout the country.

In 1994, the national average salary for new registered nurses ranged from $25,000 to $35,000, depending upon the region where they were employed. The highest average salaries were in the Northeast, and the lowest average salaries were in the South and Midwest.

Major benefits of a nursing career are education and career advancement. Hospitals and other employers often encourage career mobility by providing tuition reimbursement for nurses who attend school. This is an excellent way for nurses to promote their careers and obtain advanced degrees.

WHAT IS ARTICULATION?

Articulation is a process in which a nurse who has one credential may advance to a higher level in nursing. There are a large number of schools which provide articulation programs for nurses who want to advance from a licensed practical nurse to a registered nurse and from a diploma to associate, bachelor's, or master's degree on either a full or part-time basis. You may start your nursing career with a diploma or associate degree and then, after working a few years, decide that you want to get a bachelor's or a master's degree.

Included in the school listing section of this book you will find some schools which specify an articulation from one program to another. The articulations vary from school to school, and you will need to ask specific questions about the program in the school of your choice. Registered nurses in articulated programs can earn liberal arts and nursing credits usually by taking courses or by demonstrating knowledge through examinations. Some states, including Iowa, Colorado, Maryland, California, Arkansas, and Maine have statewide models of articulation. This means that schools in these states have facilitated educational movement for students among and between institutions so as to minimize repetition of courses.

NON-NURSE COLLEGE GRADUATES

Often graduates of college with non-nursing degrees decide for a variety of reasons to make a career change to nursing. There are a number of colleges in the country which offer special programs for the non-nurse college graduate. If you are already a college graduate, you should consider these programs. They vary in length from one to two years and, depending on the length of the program, you may obtain a bachelor or master's degree. For specific information on these programs contact the National League for Nursing.

Nursing Specialties

Once you choose nursing as your career you will have the option of working in a variety of specialty areas with patients of different age groups and health conditions. The following is a list of specialty practice areas with a description of the type of nursing practice.

Community Nursing: Involves working with patients and families of all ages in a variety of settings: health departments, clinics, schools, and homes. The emphasis of care may be on health promotion, disease prevention, or care of the ill. Community health nurses know how to work with entire communites to solve complex problems.

Critical Care Nursing: Involves working with acutely ill patients, usually at a time of crisis. Critical care units are separated according to age and specialization of care. There are neonatal (newborn), pediatric, and a variety of adult critical care units. These nurses work with one, two or three patients who require intense, bedside care from a highly skilled provider. The nurse is a highly valued member of a team made up of physicians and other health care workers administering patient centered care.

Emergency Nursing: Involves working with a variety of patients requiring immediate, emergency treatment. Generally, hospitals in large urban areas have very busy emergency rooms, and the action intensifies on weekends and in the summer. Nurses who work in emergency rooms have to know how to set priorities and make quick, life-saving decisions.

Geriatric Nursing: This is a specialty in which nurses work with the elderly. The demand for qualified nurses in this area is increasing as the aging population expands in our society. Nurses working in this specialty work in a variety of settings including nursing homes, nursing centers and home health care settings.

Home Health Nursing: Involves working with patients and families in their homes and over extended periods of time. Patients today are discharged very quickly from hospitals and usually require close monitoring and care at home. The area of home health nursing has expanded over the past ten years and is very challenging. Nurses who work in this area usually prefer the independence, autonomy, and diversity of this type of setting. These nurses work closely with patients, families and significant others and spend a great deal of time teaching. Home health nurses allow patients to receive nursing care in the comfort of their own homes that used to be provided only in the hospital.

Medical Nursing: Involves working with patients who have both acute and chronic illnesses. Nurses working with medical patients need to have a broad-based knowledge of many treatment modalities, diagnostic tests, and complex nursing interventions. They may work with patients and families over a long period of time or for as long as the patient is in the hospital or needs care at home.

Obstetrical Nursing: Involves caring for pregnant women through labor and delivery. Nurses working in obstetrics have the opportunity to teach mothers and families at a very special time in their lives. Nurses have contact with patients for a short period of time.

Occupational Health Nursing: Involves working with people in their employment environment. Nurses administer emergency care, perform health exams, and provide counseling and teaching. Today, many companies have excellent health care facilities for their employees, and they emphasize preventive health care and teaching. In some settings nurses have to take a special credentialing exam to work in the area of occupational nursing.

Oncology Nursing: This very specialized area of nursing practice involves working with patients who are being treated for cancer. The settings vary, and nurses may work in out-patient clinics, hospitals, hospices or research areas. Nurses may choose to work with either children or adults but they also work very closely with families. In large medical centers, nurses have the opportunity to work in bone transplant units and with other experimental treatments. Nurses who specialize in oncology usually take a credentialing exam and become certified.

Operating Room Nursing: This is a highly specialized, technical area of nursing practice. Nurses working in the operating room practice in a very circumscribed, regulated environment. Today there are many technicians taking on the role formerly performed by the operating room nurse with the RN functioning as a supervisor or manager.

Pediatric Nursing: This area of nursing is for those who welcome the challenge of working with children and it can be extremely rewarding. Nurses working with children use a special combination of caring, which includes holding, hugging, and playing as well as administering sophisticated types of treatments. Pediatrics requires specialized knowledge and understanding of growth and development.

Psychiatric Nursing: This is an area of nursing very different from acute care nursing. Generally patients are not physically ill, and the role of the nurse relies on a strong understanding of interpersonal skills and communication. Working in this area of nursing requires self-understanding and a combination of objectivity and compassion towards the patient. Psychiatric nurses may work in a variety of settings including hospitals, homes and clinics.

Rehabilitation Nursing: This area of nursing requires a number of skills and characteristics including patience, tolerance and a sense of humor. Rehabilitation nurses work with patients who have debilitating and long-term disabilities and injuries. Very often the patients are young and just starting out in life when they sustain an injury which alters their lives. Nurses work closely with patients and families over long periods of time. This can be very challenging and requires resourcefulness and an ability to work as part of a team. Nurses can also be certified as specialists in rehabilitation nursing.

Career Opportunities Around the World

Nursing is a career which provides opportunities for world travel. As a nurse you can work and experience the world at the same time. There are a number of agencies which sponsor nurses to work abroad.

The military is the best known way for nurses to experience the challenge of working in foreign countries. The Armed Services, including the Army, Navy, and the Air Force, provide scholarship funds to applicants who are enrolled in baccalaureate programs.

The Peace Corps is another avenue to international nursing. Usually a two-year commitment has to be made after graduation from an NLN accredited school. The training and preparation for the Peace Corps is demanding, and not everyone who applies successfully completes it. The choice of the Peace Corps can be a challenging and rewarding experience.

Religious and international service organizations, including American Field Service, the International Red Cross, Catholic Charities, CARE, and Project Hope also provide opportunities for nursing throughout the world. Some require special preparation for the work they do in addition to nursing credentials.

Section 1
Associate Degree
Programs by State

Alabama

Alabama Southern Community College
—Monroeville—

Full-Time Enrollments:	87	Evening Classes:	No
Part-Time Enrollments:	—	Weekend Classes:	No
Affiliation:	Public	Distance Learning:	No

NLN ACCREDITATION: No

Articulation: LPN to Associate

For Further Information Contact:

Dr June Chandler, Chair
Alabama Southern Community College
PO Box 2000
Monroeville, AL 36461
(334) 575-3156

Bevill State Community College
—Sumiton—

Full-Time Enrollments:	255	Evening Classes:	No
Part-Time Enrollments:	—	Weekend Classes:	No
Affiliation:	Public	Distance Learning:	No

NLN ACCREDITATION: Yes

Articulation: Associate to Baccalaureate
LPN to Associate

For Further Information Contact:

Mrs Alice Roberts, Assistant Dean
Bevill State Community College
PO Drawer 800
Sumiton, AL 35148
(205) 648-3271

Bishop State Community College
—Mobile—

Full-Time Enrollments:	128	Evening Classes:	—
Part-Time Enrollments:	83	Weekend Classes:	—
Affiliation:	Public	Distance Learning:	—

NLN ACCREDITATION: Yes

Articulation: None

For Further Information Contact:

Ms Linda Shepherd, Director
Bishop State Community College
1365 Dr Martin Luther King Ave
Mobile, AL 36609-5898
(334) 690-6440

Central Alabama Community College
—Alexander City—

Full-Time Enrollments:	—	Evening Classes:	—
Part-Time Enrollments:	—	Weekend Classes:	—
Affiliation:	Public	Distance Learning:	—

NLN ACCREDITATION: No

Articulation: —

For Further Information Contact:

Dr Melenie Bolton, Director
Central Alabama Community College
PO Box 669
Alexander City, AL 35010
(205) 249-5716

Chattahoochee Valley State Community College
—Phenix City—

Full-Time Enrollments:	44	Evening Classes:	Yes
Part-Time Enrollments:	—	Weekend Classes:	Yes
Affiliation:	Public	Distance Learning:	No

NLN ACCREDITATION: Yes

Articulation: Associate to Baccalaureate

For Further Information Contact:

Mrs Dixie Peterson, Chair
Chattahoochee Valley State Community College
2602 College Dr
Phenix City, AL 36867
(334) 291-4925

Gadsden State Community College
—Gadsden—

Full-Time Enrollments:	159	Evening Classes:	No
Part-Time Enrollments:	—	Weekend Classes:	No
Affiliation:	Public	Distance Learning:	No

NLN ACCREDITATION: Yes

Articulation: None

For Further Information Contact:

Ms Linda L Davis, Director
Gadsden State Community College
PO Box 227
Gadsden, AL 35902
(205) 549-8321

George C Wallace State Community College
—Dothan—

Full-Time Enrollments:	216	Evening Classes:	No
Part-Time Enrollments:	7	Weekend Classes:	No
Affiliation:	Public	Distance Learning:	No

NLN ACCREDITATION: Yes

Articulation: Associate to Baccalaureate
LPN to Associate

For Further Information Contact:

Dr Belinda Downing, Chair
George C Wallace State Community College
Route 6 Box 62
Dothan, AL 36303
(334) 983-3521

George C Wallace State Community College
—Hanceville—

Full-Time Enrollments:	52	Evening Classes:	—
Part-Time Enrollments:	200	Weekend Classes:	—
Affiliation:	Public	Distance Learning:	—

NLN ACCREDITATION: Yes

Articulation: None

For Further Information Contact:

Ms Denise Elliott, Director
George C Wallace State Community College
PO Box 2000
Hanceville, AL 35077
(205) 352-6403

George C Wallace State Community College
—Selma—

Full-Time Enrollments:	124	Evening Classes:	No
Part-Time Enrollments:	52	Weekend Classes:	No
Affiliation:	Public	Distance Learning:	No

NLN ACCREDITATION: Yes

Articulation: Associate to Baccalaureate
LPN to Associate

For Further Information Contact:

Mrs Becky Casey, Director
George C Wallace State Community College
PO Drawer 1049
Selma, AL 36701
(334) 875-2634

Ida V Moffett School-Samford University
—Birmingham—

Full-Time Enrollments:	97	Evening Classes:	Yes
Part-Time Enrollments:	63	Weekend Classes:	Yes
Affiliation:	Religious	Distance Learning:	Yes

NLN ACCREDITATION: Yes

Articulation: Associate to Baccalaureate
Diploma to Associate
LPN to Associate

For Further Information Contact:

Dr Marian K Baur, Dean
Ida V Moffett School-Samford University
Birmingham, AL 35229
(205) 870-2861

Jefferson Davis State Jr College
—Brewton—

Full-Time Enrollments:	59	Evening Classes:	—
Part-Time Enrollments:	—	Weekend Classes:	—
Affiliation:	Public	Distance Learning:	—

NLN ACCREDITATION: Yes

Articulation: None

For Further Information Contact:

Mrs Norma M Hammac, Director
Jefferson Davis State Jr College
220 Alco Drive
Brewton, AL 36426
(334) 867-4832

No longer thar [handwritten]

Jefferson State Community College
—Birmingham—

Full-Time Enrollments:	121	Evening Classes:	No
Part-Time Enrollments:	—	Weekend Classes:	No
Affiliation:	Public	Distance Learning:	No

NLN ACCREDITATION: Yes

Articulation: None

For Further Information Contact:

Mrs Anita Norton, Chair
Jefferson State Community College
2601 Carson Rd
Birmingham, AL 35215
(205) 856-1200

John C Calhoun State Community College
—Decatur—

Full-Time Enrollments:	112	Evening Classes:	No
Part-Time Enrollments:	66	Weekend Classes:	No
Affiliation:	Public	Distance Learning:	No

NLN ACCREDITATION: Yes

Articulation: Associate to Baccalaureate
LPN to Associate

For Further Information Contact:

Mrs Jane Floyd, Chair
John C Calhoun State Community College
PO Box 2216
Decatur, AL 35602
(205) 306-2808

Northeast Alabama Community College
—Rainsville—

Full-Time Enrollments:	29	Evening Classes:	No
Part-Time Enrollments:	102	Weekend Classes:	No
Affiliation:	Public	Distance Learning:	No

NLN ACCREDITATION: Yes

Articulation: Associate to Baccalaureate

For Further Information Contact:

Dr Cindy M Jones, Director
Northeast Alabama Community College
PO Box 159
Rainsville, AL 35986
(205) 228-6001

Northwest Shoals Community College
—Phil Campbell—

Full-Time Enrollments:	177	Evening Classes:	Yes
Part-Time Enrollments:	—	Weekend Classes:	No
Affiliation:	Public	Distance Learning:	No

NLN ACCREDITATION: Yes

Articulation: None

For Further Information Contact:

Mrs Anita Rhodes, Chair
Northwest Shoals Community College
2080 College Rd
Phil Campbell, AL 35581
(205) 331-6251

Oakwood College
—Huntsville—

Full-Time Enrollments:	47	Evening Classes:	No
Part-Time Enrollments:	7	Weekend Classes:	No
Affiliation:	Religious	Distance Learning:	No

NLN ACCREDITATION: No

Articulation: Associate to Baccalaureate
LPN to Associate

For Further Information Contact:

Mrs Selena P Simons, Chair
Oakwood College
Oakwood Rd, NW
Huntsville, AL 35896
(205) 726-7287

Shelton State Community College
—Tuscaloosa—

Full-Time Enrollments:	110	Evening Classes:	No
Part-Time Enrollments:	—	Weekend Classes:	No
Affiliation:	Public	Distance Learning:	No

NLN ACCREDITATION: Yes

Articulation: LPN to Associate

For Further Information Contact:

Mrs Gladys Hill, Director
Shelton State Community College
202 Skyland Blvd
Tuscaloosa, AL 35405
(205) 391-2265

Southern Union State Community College
—Valley—

Full-Time Enrollments:	258	Evening Classes:	No
Part-Time Enrollments:	2	Weekend Classes:	No
Affiliation:	Public	Distance Learning:	No

NLN ACCREDITATION: Yes

Articulation: Associate to Baccalaureate
LPN to Associate

For Further Information Contact:

Mrs Regina Beaird, Chair
Southern Union State Community College
321 Fob James Dr
Valley, AL 36854
(334) 756-4151

T A Lawson State Community College
—Birmingham—

Full-Time Enrollments:	99	Evening Classes:	No
Part-Time Enrollments:	—	Weekend Classes:	No
Affiliation:	Public	Distance Learning:	No

NLN ACCREDITATION: Yes

Articulation: Associate to Baccalaureate

For Further Information Contact:

Dr Sheila Marable, Acting Chair
T A Lawson State Community College
3060 Wilson Rd
Birmingham, AL 35221
(205) 925-2515

Troy State University
—Montgomery—

Full-Time Enrollments:	106	Evening Classes:	—
Part-Time Enrollments:	199	Weekend Classes:	—
Affiliation:	Public	Distance Learning:	Yes

NLN ACCREDITATION: Yes

Articulation: Associate to Baccalaureate

For Further Information Contact:

Dr Sandra Greniewicki, Dean
Troy State University
305 South Ripley St
Montgomery, AL 36104
(334) 834-2320

UAB-Walker College
—Jasper—

Full-Time Enrollments:	23	Evening Classes:	No
Part-Time Enrollments:	70	Weekend Classes:	No
Affiliation:	Public	Distance Learning:	No

NLN ACCREDITATION: Yes

Articulation: None

For Further Information Contact:

Dr Malissa Williams, Chair
UAB-Walker College
1411 Indiana Ave
Jasper, AL 35501
(205) 759-1541

University of Mobile
—Mobile—

Full-Time Enrollments:	53	Evening Classes:	No
Part-Time Enrollments:	94	Weekend Classes:	No
Affiliation:	Religious	Distance Learning:	No

NLN ACCREDITATION: Yes

Articulation: None

For Further Information Contact:

Dr Rosemary Adams, Dean
University of Mobile
PO Box 13220
Mobile, AL 36663-0220
(334) 675-5990

University of West Alabama
—Livingston—

Full-Time Enrollments:	125	Evening Classes:	No
Part-Time Enrollments:	—	Weekend Classes:	No
Affiliation:	Public	Distance Learning:	No

NLN ACCREDITATION: Yes

Articulation: Associate to Baccalaureate

For Further Information Contact:

Mrs Sylvia B Homan, Chair
University of West Alabama
Station 28
Livingston, AL 35470
(205) 652-9661

Alaska

University of Alaska, Anchorage
—Anchorage—

Full-Time Enrollments:	10	Evening Classes:	Yes
Part-Time Enrollments:	48	Weekend Classes:	No
Affiliation:	Public	Distance Learning:	—

NLN ACCREDITATION: Yes

Articulation: Associate to Baccalaureate

For Further Information Contact:

Dr Tina Delapp, Interim Director
University of Alaska, Anchorage
3211 Providence Dr
Anchorage, AK 99508-8030
(907) 786-4550

American Samoa

American Samoa Community College
—Pago Pago—

Full-Time Enrollments: —   Evening Classes: —
Part-Time Enrollments: —   Weekend Classes: —
Affiliation: Public   Distance Learning: —

NLN ACCREDITATION: No

Articulation: None

For Further Information Contact:

Miss Loata Sipili, Chair
American Samoa Community College
Mapusaga
Pago Pago, AM 96799
(684) 699-9155 Ext 51

Arizona

Arizona Western College
—Yuma—

Full-Time Enrollments: 77   Evening Classes: —
Part-Time Enrollments: —   Weekend Classes: —
Affiliation: Public   Distance Learning: —

NLN ACCREDITATION: Yes

Articulation: None

For Further Information Contact:

Ms Judy Jondahl, Director
Arizona Western College
PO Box 929
Yuma, AZ 85364
(520) 344-7559

Central Arizona College-Signal Peak Campus
—Coolidge—

Full-Time Enrollments: 5   Evening Classes: —
Part-Time Enrollments: 59   Weekend Classes: —
Affiliation: Public   Distance Learning: —

NLN ACCREDITATION: Yes

Articulation: None

For Further Information Contact:

Dr Eleanor Strang, Director
Central Arizona College-Signal Peak Campus
8470 N Overfield Rd
Coolidge, AZ 85228
(602) 426-4330

Cochise College
—Douglas—

Full-Time Enrollments: 108   Evening Classes: No
Part-Time Enrollments: —   Weekend Classes: No
Affiliation: Public   Distance Learning: Yes

NLN ACCREDITATION: Yes

Articulation: Associate to Baccalaureate

For Further Information Contact:

Mrs Susan Barnes, Coordinator
Cochise College
Douglas, AZ 85607
(520) 364-0216

Eastern Arizona College
—Thatcher—

Full-Time Enrollments: 20   Evening Classes: —
Part-Time Enrollments: —   Weekend Classes: —
Affiliation: Private   Distance Learning: —

NLN ACCREDITATION: No

Articulation: None

For Further Information Contact:

Ms Mayuree Sozanski, Director
Eastern Arizona College
Thatcher, AZ 85552
(520) 428-8396

Gateway Community College
—Phoenix—

Full-Time Enrollments: 58   Evening Classes: Yes
Part-Time Enrollments: 57   Weekend Classes: Yes
Affiliation: Public   Distance Learning: No

NLN ACCREDITATION: Yes

Articulation: LPN to Associate

For Further Information Contact:

Ms Meta Seltzer, Director
Gateway Community College
108 N 40th St
Phoenix, AZ 85034
(602) 392-5094

Glendale Community College
—Glendale—

Full-Time Enrollments: 85   Evening Classes: No
Part-Time Enrollments: 55   Weekend Classes: No
Affiliation: Public   Distance Learning: No

NLN ACCREDITATION: Yes

Articulation: None

For Further Information Contact:

Ms Ann Marthaler, Chair
Glendale Community College
6000 W Olive Ave
Glendale, AZ 85302
(602) 435-3205

Mesa Community College
—Mesa—

Full-Time Enrollments:	246	Evening Classes:	Yes
Part-Time Enrollments:	—	Weekend Classes:	—
Affiliation:	Public	Distance Learning:	—

NLN ACCREDITATION: Yes

Articulation: Associate to Baccalaureate
LPN to Associate

For Further Information Contact:

Ms Claire Keyworth, Chair
Mesa Community College
1833 W Southern Ave
Mesa, AZ 85202
(602) 461-7113

Mohave Community College
—Kingman—

Full-Time Enrollments:	60	Evening Classes:	No
Part-Time Enrollments:	36	Weekend Classes:	No
Affiliation:	Public	Distance Learning:	No

NLN ACCREDITATION: No

Articulation: None

For Further Information Contact:

Ms Lynn Young, Assoc Dean
Mohave Community College
1971 Jagerson Ave
Kingman, AZ 86401
(520) 757-0862

Northland Pioneer College
—Halbrook—

Full-Time Enrollments:	57	Evening Classes:	No
Part-Time Enrollments:	—	Weekend Classes:	No
Affiliation:	Public	Distance Learning:	Yes

NLN ACCREDITATION: No

Articulation: Associate to Baccalaureate

For Further Information Contact:

Mrs Karen Jones, Director
Northland Pioneer College
PO Box 610
Halbrook, AZ 86025-0610
(520) 537-2976

Phoenix College
—Phoenix—

Full-Time Enrollments:	115	Evening Classes:	No
Part-Time Enrollments:	—	Weekend Classes:	No
Affiliation:	Public	Distance Learning:	No

NLN ACCREDITATION: Yes

Articulation: Associate to Baccalaureate
LPN to Associate

For Further Information Contact:

Dr Daniel Tetting, Chair
Phoenix College
1202 W Thomas Rd
Phoenix, AZ 85013
(602) 285-7128

Pima Community College West
—Tucson—

Full-Time Enrollments:	237	Evening Classes:	No
Part-Time Enrollments:	—	Weekend Classes:	No
Affiliation:	Public	Distance Learning:	No

NLN ACCREDITATION: Yes

Articulation: Associate to Baccalaureate

For Further Information Contact:

Mrs Joan C Gilbert, Director
Pima Community College West
2202 Ankland Rd
Tucson, AZ 85709
(602) 884-6661

Scottsdale Community College
—Scottsdale—

Full-Time Enrollments:	—	Evening Classes:	—
Part-Time Enrollments:	—	Weekend Classes:	—
Affiliation:	Public	Distance Learning:	—

NLN ACCREDITATION: Yes

Articulation: —

For Further Information Contact:

Ms Nellie Nelson, Chair
Scottsdale Community College
Pima and Chapparral Rd
Scottsdale, AZ 85256-2699
(602) 423-6225

Yavapai College
—Prescott—

Full-Time Enrollments:	80	**Evening Classes:**	Yes
Part-Time Enrollments:	36	**Weekend Classes:**	Yes
Affiliation:	Public	**Distance Learning:**	Yes

NLN ACCREDITATION: Yes

Articulation: Associate to Baccalaureate

For Further Information Contact:

Dr Lynn Nugent, Chair
Yavapai College
1100 E Sheldon
Prescott, AZ 86301
(520) 445-7300

Arkansas

Arkansas State University
—State University—

Full-Time Enrollments:	182	**Evening Classes:**	No
Part-Time Enrollments:	—	**Weekend Classes:**	No
Affiliation:	Public	**Distance Learning:**	Yes

NLN ACCREDITATION: Yes

Articulation: Associate to Baccalaureate
LPN to Baccalaureate
LPN to Associate

For Further Information Contact:

Dr Elizabeth Stokes, Interim Chair
Arkansas State University
PO Box 69
State University, AR 72467-0069
(501) 972-3074

East Arkansas Community College
—Forrest City—

Full-Time Enrollments:	78	**Evening Classes:**	Yes
Part-Time Enrollments:	—	**Weekend Classes:**	Yes
Affiliation:	Public	**Distance Learning:**	Yes

NLN ACCREDITATION: Yes

Articulation: Associate to Baccalaureate

For Further Information Contact:

Ms Joanna Christiansen, Director
East Arkansas Community College
1700 Newcastle Rd
Forrest City, AR 72335-9598
(501) 633-4480

Garland County Community College
—Hot Springs—

Full-Time Enrollments:	85	**Evening Classes:**	Yes
Part-Time Enrollments:	37	**Weekend Classes:**	Yes
Affiliation:	Public	**Distance Learning:**	No

NLN ACCREDITATION: Yes

Articulation: LPN to Associate

For Further Information Contact:

Dr Deborah Gibson, Chair
Garland County Community College
101 College Dr
Hot Springs, AR 71913-9174
(501) 767-9371

Mississippi County Community College
—Blytheville—

Full-Time Enrollments:	27	**Evening Classes:**	No
Part-Time Enrollments:	51	**Weekend Classes:**	No
Affiliation:	Public	**Distance Learning:**	No

NLN ACCREDITATION: Yes

Articulation: Associate to Baccalaureate

For Further Information Contact:

Mrs Sharon Fulling, Assistant Dean
Mississippi County Community College
PO Box 1109
Blytheville, AR 72315
(501) 762-1020

North Arkansas Community Technical College
—Harrison—

Full-Time Enrollments:	33	**Evening Classes:**	No
Part-Time Enrollments:	44	**Weekend Classes:**	No
Affiliation:	Public	**Distance Learning:**	No

NLN ACCREDITATION: Yes

Articulation: Associate to Baccalaureate
LPN to Associate

For Further Information Contact:

Mrs Elizabeth Robinson, Chair
North Arkansas Community Technical College
Pioneer Ridge
Harrison, AR 72601
(501) 743-3000

North Arkansas Community Technical College
—Batesville—

Full-Time Enrollments:	20	Evening Classes:	No
Part-Time Enrollments:	—	Weekend Classes:	No
Affiliation:	Public	Distance Learning:	No

NLN ACCREDITATION: Yes

Articulation: LPN to Associate

For Further Information Contact:

Mrs Deborah Jarrett, Director
North Arkansas Community Technical College
PO Box 2404
Batesville, AR 72503
(501) 793-4919

Northwest Arkansas Community College
—Bentonville—

Full-Time Enrollments:	68	Evening Classes:	Yes
Part-Time Enrollments:	—	Weekend Classes:	—
Affiliation:	Public	Distance Learning:	—

NLN ACCREDITATION: No

Articulation: LPN to Associate

For Further Information Contact:

Ms Ann Garrigues, Director
Northwest Arkansas Community College
One College Dr
Bentonville, AR 72712
(501) 619-4150

Phillips Community College of the University Arkansas
—Helena—

Full-Time Enrollments:	90	Evening Classes:	—
Part-Time Enrollments:	—	Weekend Classes:	—
Affiliation:	Public	Distance Learning:	Yes

NLN ACCREDITATION: Yes

Articulation: Associate to Baccalaureate

For Further Information Contact:

Mrs Mary Goza, Dean
Phillips Community College of the University Arkansas
PO Box 785
Helena, AR 72342-0785
(501) 338-6474

Southern Arkansas University
—Magnolia—

Full-Time Enrollments:	135	Evening Classes:	No
Part-Time Enrollments:	—	Weekend Classes:	No
Affiliation:	Public	Distance Learning:	No

NLN ACCREDITATION: Yes

Articulation: Associate to Baccalaureate
LPN to Associate

For Further Information Contact:

Dr Josephine Kahler, Chair
Southern Arkansas University
PO Box 1406
Magnolia, AR 71753
(501) 235-4330

University of Arkansas at Little Rock
—Little Rock—

Full-Time Enrollments:	45	Evening Classes:	Yes
Part-Time Enrollments:	131	Weekend Classes:	No
Affiliation:	Public	Distance Learning:	No

NLN ACCREDITATION: Yes

Articulation: LPN to Associate

For Further Information Contact:

Mrs C U Bradham, Interim Chair
University of Arkansas at Little Rock
2801 S Univ Ave
Little Rock, AR 72204
(501) 569-8081

Westark Community College
—Fort Smith—

Full-Time Enrollments:	211	Evening Classes:	No
Part-Time Enrollments:	—	Weekend Classes:	Yes
Affiliation:	Public	Distance Learning:	No

NLN ACCREDITATION: Yes

Articulation: LPN to Associate

For Further Information Contact:

Mrs Mary J Keel, Director
Westark Community College
PO Box 3649
Fort Smith, AR 72913
(501) 785-7361

California

Allan Hancock College
—Santa Maria—

Full-Time Enrollments: —   Evening Classes: —
Part-Time Enrollments: —   Weekend Classes: —
Affiliation: Public   Distance Learning: —

NLN ACCREDITATION: No

Articulation: None

For Further Information Contact:

Ms Ellen White, Director
Allan Hancock College
800 South College Dr
Santa Maria, CA 93454
(805) 922-6966

American River College
—Sacramento—

Full-Time Enrollments: 120   Evening Classes: Yes
Part-Time Enrollments: —   Weekend Classes: No
Affiliation: Public   Distance Learning: No

NLN ACCREDITATION: No

Articulation: Associate to Baccalaureate
Diploma to Associate
LPN to Associate

For Further Information Contact:

Dr Lucille Rybka, Director
American River College
4700 College Oak Dr
Sacramento, CA 95841
(916) 484-8335

Antelope Valley College
—Lancaster—

Full-Time Enrollments: 181   Evening Classes: No
Part-Time Enrollments: —   Weekend Classes: No
Affiliation: Public   Distance Learning: No

NLN ACCREDITATION: No

Articulation: Associate to Baccalaureate

For Further Information Contact:

Dr Vivian Thornton, Dean
Antelope Valley College
3041 W Avenue K
Lancaster, CA 93536-5426
(805) 943-3241

Bakersfield College
—Bakersfield—

Full-Time Enrollments: —   Evening Classes: —
Part-Time Enrollments: —   Weekend Classes: —
Affiliation: Public   Distance Learning: —

NLN ACCREDITATION: No

Articulation: —

For Further Information Contact:

Ms Sheran DeLeon, Director
Bakersfield College
1801 Panorama Dr
Bakersfield, CA 93305
(805) 395-4281

Butte College
—Oroville—

Full-Time Enrollments: 23   Evening Classes: —
Part-Time Enrollments: —   Weekend Classes: —
Affiliation: Public   Distance Learning: —

NLN ACCREDITATION: No

Articulation: None

For Further Information Contact:

Ms Linda Clark, Chair
Butte College
3536 Butte Campus Dr
Oroville, CA 95965
(916) 895-2329

Cabrillo College
—Aptos—

Full-Time Enrollments: 75   Evening Classes: No
Part-Time Enrollments: —   Weekend Classes: No
Affiliation: Public   Distance Learning: No

NLN ACCREDITATION: No

Articulation: Associate to Baccalaureate
LPN to Associate

For Further Information Contact:

Mrs Joan Frommhagen, Director
Cabrillo College
6500 Soquel Dr
Aptos, CA 95003
(408) 479-6280

Cerritos College
—Norwalk—

Full-Time Enrollments:	161	Evening Classes:	—
Part-Time Enrollments:	—	Weekend Classes:	—
Affiliation:	Public	Distance Learning:	—

NLN ACCREDITATION: Yes

Articulation: None

For Further Information Contact:

Dr Henrietta Baramki, Director
Cerritos College
11110 E Alondra Blvd
Norwalk, CA 90650
(310) 860-2451

Chabot College
—Hayward—

Full-Time Enrollments:	75	Evening Classes:	No
Part-Time Enrollments:	1	Weekend Classes:	No
Affiliation:	Public	Distance Learning:	Yes

NLN ACCREDITATION: No

Articulation: Associate to Baccalaureate
LPN to Associate

For Further Information Contact:

Dr Nancy Cowan, Director
Chabot College
25555 Hesperian Blvd
Hayward, CA 94545
(510) 786-6871

Chaffey College
—Rancho Cucamonga—

Full-Time Enrollments:	102	Evening Classes:	No
Part-Time Enrollments:	—	Weekend Classes:	No
Affiliation:	Public	Distance Learning:	No

NLN ACCREDITATION: Yes

Articulation: None

For Further Information Contact:

Mrs Marcha Talton, Director
Chaffey College
5885 Haven Ave
Rancho Cucamonga, CA 91707
(909) 941-2694

City College of San Francisco
—San Francisco—

Full-Time Enrollments:	—	Evening Classes:	—
Part-Time Enrollments:	—	Weekend Classes:	—
Affiliation:	Public	Distance Learning:	—

NLN ACCREDITATION: No

Articulation: None

For Further Information Contact:

Mrs Cecile Dawydiak, Chair
City College of San Francisco
50 Phelan Ave
San Francisco, CA 94112
(415) 239-3218

College of Marin
—Kentfield—

Full-Time Enrollments:	88	Evening Classes:	No
Part-Time Enrollments:	—	Weekend Classes:	No
Affiliation:	Public	Distance Learning:	No

NLN ACCREDITATION: Yes

Articulation: Associate to Baccalaureate

For Further Information Contact:

Mrs Rosalind Hartman, Director
College of Marin
835 College Ave
Kentfield, CA 94904
(415) 485-9326

College of San Mateo
—San Mateo—

Full-Time Enrollments:	72	Evening Classes:	No
Part-Time Enrollments:	—	Weekend Classes:	No
Affiliation:	Public	Distance Learning:	No

NLN ACCREDITATION: No

Articulation: Associate to Baccalaureate

For Further Information Contact:

Ms Ruth A McCracken, Director
College of San Mateo
1700 W Hillsdale Blvd
San Mateo, CA 94402
(415) 574-6219

College of the Canyons
—Santa Clarita—

Full-Time Enrollments: 60   Evening Classes: Yes
Part-Time Enrollments: —   Weekend Classes: Yes
Affiliation: Public   Distance Learning: —

NLN ACCREDITATION: No

Articulation: Associate to Baccalaureate

For Further Information Contact:

Dr Kathleen Welch, Director
College of the Canyons
26455 N Rockwell Canyon Rd
Santa Clarita, CA 91355
(805) 259-7800

College of the Desert
—Palm Desert—

Full-Time Enrollments: 128   Evening Classes: Yes
Part-Time Enrollments: —   Weekend Classes: No
Affiliation: Public   Distance Learning: Yes

NLN ACCREDITATION: Yes

Articulation: Diploma to Associate
LPN to Associate

For Further Information Contact:

Mrs Celia Hartley, Chair
College of the Desert
43-500 Monterey
Palm Desert, CA 92234
(619) 773-2578

College of the Redwoods
—Eureka—

Full-Time Enrollments: 82   Evening Classes: No
Part-Time Enrollments: —   Weekend Classes: No
Affiliation: Public   Distance Learning: Yes

NLN ACCREDITATION: No

Articulation: Associate to Baccalaureate
LPN to Associate

For Further Information Contact:

Mrs Kathleen Patterson, Director
College of the Redwoods
7351 Tompkins Hill Rd
Eureka, CA 95501
(707) 445-6873

College of the Sequoias
—Visalia—

Full-Time Enrollments: 114   Evening Classes: No
Part-Time Enrollments: —   Weekend Classes: No
Affiliation: Public   Distance Learning: No

NLN ACCREDITATION: No

Articulation: LPN to Associate

For Further Information Contact:

Dr Lynn H Mirviss, Associate Dean
College of the Sequoias
915 S Mooney Blvd
Visalia, CA 93277
(209) 730-3732

Compton College
—Compton—

Full-Time Enrollments: 74   Evening Classes: —
Part-Time Enrollments: —   Weekend Classes: —
Affiliation: Public   Distance Learning: —

NLN ACCREDITATION: No

Articulation: None

For Further Information Contact:

Ms Mary Montgomery, Director
Compton College
1111 E Artesia Blvd
Compton, CA 90221
(310) 637-2660

Contra Costa College
—San Pablo—

Full-Time Enrollments: 87   Evening Classes: No
Part-Time Enrollments: —   Weekend Classes: No
Affiliation: Public   Distance Learning: No

NLN ACCREDITATION: No

Articulation: LPN to Associate

For Further Information Contact:

Mrs Lynda Schweid, Assistant Dean
Contra Costa College
2600 Mission Bell Dr
San Pablo, CA 94806
(510) 235-7800

Cuesta College
—San Luis Obispo—

Full-Time Enrollments:	88	Evening Classes:	Yes
Part-Time Enrollments:	—	Weekend Classes:	No
Affiliation:	Public	Distance Learning:	—

NLN ACCREDITATION: No

Articulation: Associate to Baccalaureate

For Further Information Contact:

Dr Mary Parker, Director
Cuesta College
PO Box 8106
San Luis Obispo, CA 93405-8106
(805) 546-3241

Cypress College
—Cypress—

Full-Time Enrollments:	143	Evening Classes:	Yes
Part-Time Enrollments:	—	Weekend Classes:	No
Affiliation:	Public	Distance Learning:	No

NLN ACCREDITATION: No

Articulation: Associate to Baccalaureate
Diploma to Associate
LPN to Associate

For Further Information Contact:

Ms Andrea L Hannon, Director
Cypress College
9200 Valley View
Cypress, CA 90630
(714) 826-2220

De Anza College
—Cupertino—

Full-Time Enrollments:	132	Evening Classes:	—
Part-Time Enrollments:	—	Weekend Classes:	—
Affiliation:	Public	Distance Learning:	—

NLN ACCREDITATION: No

Articulation: None

For Further Information Contact:

Ms Georgeanne Adamy, Acting Head
De Anza College
21250 Stevens Creek Blvd
Cupertino, CA 95014
(408) 864-8908

East Los Angeles College
—Monterey Park—

Full-Time Enrollments:	97	Evening Classes:	—
Part-Time Enrollments:	63	Weekend Classes:	—
Affiliation:	Public	Distance Learning:	—

NLN ACCREDITATION: No

Articulation: None

For Further Information Contact:

Ms Lurelean Gaines, Chair
East Los Angeles College
1301 Cesar Chavez Ave
Monterey Park, CA 91754-6099
(213) 265-8896

El Camino College
—Torrance—

Full-Time Enrollments:	172	Evening Classes:	No
Part-Time Enrollments:	17	Weekend Classes:	No
Affiliation:	Public	Distance Learning:	No

NLN ACCREDITATION: Yes

Articulation: Associate to Baccalaureate
RN to MSN

For Further Information Contact:

Dr Katherine Townsend, Director
El Camino College
16007 Crenshaw Blvd
Torrance, CA 90506
(310) 660-3282

Evergreen Valley College
—San Jose—

Full-Time Enrollments:	110	Evening Classes:	Yes
Part-Time Enrollments:	—	Weekend Classes:	No
Affiliation:	Public	Distance Learning:	No

NLN ACCREDITATION: Yes

Articulation: Associate to Baccalaureate
LPN to Associate

For Further Information Contact:

Miss LaZelle Westbrook, Director
Evergreen Valley College
3095 Yerba Buena Rd
San Jose, CA 95135
(408) 270-6448

Fresno City College
—Fresno—

Full-Time Enrollments:	133	**Evening Classes:**	No
Part-Time Enrollments:	—	**Weekend Classes:**	No
Affiliation:	Public	**Distance Learning:**	No

NLN ACCREDITATION: No

Articulation: LPN to Associate

For Further Information Contact:

Dr Carolyn Drake, Director
Fresno City College
1101 E Univ Ave
Fresno, CA 93741
(209) 244-2604

Gavilan College
—Gilroy—

Full-Time Enrollments:	20	**Evening Classes:**	Yes
Part-Time Enrollments:	—	**Weekend Classes:**	—
Affiliation:	Public	**Distance Learning:**	—

NLN ACCREDITATION: No

Articulation: Associate to Baccalaureate
LPN to Associate

For Further Information Contact:

Ms K Bedell, Director
Gavilan College
5055 Santa Teresa Blvd
Gilroy, CA 95020
(408) 848-4883

Glendale Community College
—Glendale—

Full-Time Enrollments:	55	**Evening Classes:**	No
Part-Time Enrollments:	1	**Weekend Classes:**	No
Affiliation:	Public	**Distance Learning:**	No

NLN ACCREDITATION: No

Articulation: LPN to Associate

For Further Information Contact:

Dr Sharon Hall, Assoc Dean
Glendale Community College
1500 N Verdugo Blvd
Glendale, CA 91208
(818) 249-1005

Golden West College
—Huntington Beach—

Full-Time Enrollments:	167	**Evening Classes:**	No
Part-Time Enrollments:	—	**Weekend Classes:**	No
Affiliation:	Public	**Distance Learning:**	No

NLN ACCREDITATION: Yes

Articulation: Diploma to Associate
LPN to Associate

For Further Information Contact:

Ms Linda Stevens, Dean
Golden West College
15744 Golden West St
Huntington Beach, CA 92647
(714) 895-8163

Grossmont College
—El Cajon—

Full-Time Enrollments:	147	**Evening Classes:**	No
Part-Time Enrollments:	—	**Weekend Classes:**	No
Affiliation:	Public	**Distance Learning:**	No

NLN ACCREDITATION: Yes

Articulation: Diploma to Associate
LPN to Associate

For Further Information Contact:

Mrs Ann Burgess, Director
Grossmont College
8800 Grossmont College Dr
El Cajon, CA 92020
(619) 465-1700

Hartnell College
—Salinas—

Full-Time Enrollments:	59	**Evening Classes:**	—
Part-Time Enrollments:	—	**Weekend Classes:**	—
Affiliation:	Public	**Distance Learning:**	—

NLN ACCREDITATION: No

Articulation: None

For Further Information Contact:

Chris Eaton, Acting Director
Hartnell College
156 Homestead Ave
Salinas, CA 93901
(408) 755-6771

Imperial Valley College
—Imperial—

Full-Time Enrollments:	73	Evening Classes:	No
Part-Time Enrollments:	—	Weekend Classes:	No
Affiliation:	Public	Distance Learning:	Yes

NLN ACCREDITATION: No

Articulation: LPN to Associate

For Further Information Contact:

Dr Betty Marks, Director
Imperial Valley College
PO Box 158
Imperial, CA 92251
(760) 352-8320

Long Beach City College
—Long Beach—

Full-Time Enrollments:	209	Evening Classes:	No
Part-Time Enrollments:	—	Weekend Classes:	No
Affiliation:	Public	Distance Learning:	No

NLN ACCREDITATION: Yes

Articulation: Associate to Baccalaureate
LPN to Associate

For Further Information Contact:

Dr Marilyn Balint, Director
Long Beach City College
4901 E Carson St
Long Beach, CA 90808
(310) 938-4533

Los Angeles County Medical Center School of Nursing
—Los Angeles—

Full-Time Enrollments:	86	Evening Classes:	No
Part-Time Enrollments:	84	Weekend Classes:	No
Affiliation:	Public	Distance Learning:	No

NLN ACCREDITATION: No

Articulation: None

For Further Information Contact:

Mrs Sharon Hilton, Dean
Los Angeles County Medical Center School of Nursing
1200 N State St Muir Hall 114
Los Angeles, CA 90033
(213) 226-6301

Los Angeles Harbor College
—Wilmington—

Full-Time Enrollments:	159	Evening Classes:	No
Part-Time Enrollments:	—	Weekend Classes:	No
Affiliation:	Public	Distance Learning:	No

NLN ACCREDITATION: No

Articulation: Associate to Baccalaureate
LPN to Associate

For Further Information Contact:

Ms Wendy Hollis, Chair
Los Angeles Harbor College
1111 Figueroa Pl
Wilmington, CA 90744-2397
(310) 522-8200

Los Angeles Pierce College
—Woodland Hills—

Full-Time Enrollments:	130	Evening Classes:	No
Part-Time Enrollments:	18	Weekend Classes:	No
Affiliation:	Public	Distance Learning:	No

NLN ACCREDITATION: Yes

Articulation: LPN to Associate

For Further Information Contact:

Ms Carole Delgado, Director
Los Angeles Pierce College
6201 Winnetka Ave
Woodland Hills, CA 91371
(818) 719-6477

Los Angeles Southwest College
—Los Angeles—

Full-Time Enrollments:	139	Evening Classes:	—
Part-Time Enrollments:	—	Weekend Classes:	—
Affiliation:	Public	Distance Learning:	—

NLN ACCREDITATION: No

Articulation: None

For Further Information Contact:

Mrs Vivian Lott, Director
Los Angeles Southwest College
1600 West Imperial Hwy
Los Angeles, CA 90047
(213) 241-5225

Los Angeles Trade Technical College
—Los Angeles—

Full-Time Enrollments:	117	Evening Classes:	No
Part-Time Enrollments:	—	Weekend Classes:	No
Affiliation:	Public	Distance Learning:	No

NLN ACCREDITATION: Yes

Articulation: Associate to Baccalaureate

For Further Information Contact:

Ms Gladys N Smith, Associate Dean
Los Angeles Trade Technical College
400 W Washington Blvd
Los Angeles, CA 90015
(213) 744-9450

Los Angeles Valley College
—Van Nuys—

Full-Time Enrollments:	158	Evening Classes:	No
Part-Time Enrollments:	—	Weekend Classes:	No
Affiliation:	Public	Distance Learning:	No

NLN ACCREDITATION: Yes

Articulation: Associate to Baccalaureate
LPN to Associate

For Further Information Contact:

Ms Gina Aguirre, Chair
Los Angeles Valley College
5800 Fulton Ave
Van Nuys, CA 91401
(818) 781-1200

Los Medanos College
—Pittsburg—

Full-Time Enrollments:	80	Evening Classes:	No
Part-Time Enrollments:	—	Weekend Classes:	No
Affiliation:	Public	Distance Learning:	No

NLN ACCREDITATION: No

Articulation: Associate to Baccalaureate
LPN to Associate

For Further Information Contact:

Ms Veronica Flagg, Assistant Dean
Los Medanos College
2700 E Leland Rd
Pittsburg, CA 94565
(510) 439-2185

Maric College Medical Career
—San Diego—

Full-Time Enrollments:	169	Evening Classes:	No
Part-Time Enrollments:	—	Weekend Classes:	No
Affiliation:	Private	Distance Learning:	No

NLN ACCREDITATION: No

Articulation: Associate to Baccalaureate

For Further Information Contact:

Dr Beverly Peterson, Director
Maric College Medical Career
3666 Kearny
San Diego, CA 92123
(619) 654-3650

Merced College
—Merced—

Full-Time Enrollments:	47	Evening Classes:	No
Part-Time Enrollments:	—	Weekend Classes:	No
Affiliation:	Public	Distance Learning:	No

NLN ACCREDITATION: No

Articulation: Associate to Baccalaureate
LPN to Associate

For Further Information Contact:

Ms Mary Ann Duncan, Director
Merced College
3600 M St
Merced, CA 95348
(209) 384-6133

Merritt College
—Oakland—

Full-Time Enrollments:	48	Evening Classes:	No
Part-Time Enrollments:	30	Weekend Classes:	No
Affiliation:	Public	Distance Learning:	No

NLN ACCREDITATION: No

Articulation: Associate to Baccalaureate

For Further Information Contact:

Mrs Sandra Takakura, Director
Merritt College
12500 Campus Dr D116
Oakland, CA 94619
(510) 436-2422

Modesto Jr College-Health Occupation Department
—Modesto—

Full-Time Enrollments:	—	Evening Classes:	—
Part-Time Enrollments:	—	Weekend Classes:	—
Affiliation:	Public	Distance Learning:	—

NLN ACCREDITATION: No

Articulation: None

For Further Information Contact:

Bonnie Costello, Director
Modesto Jr College-Health Occupation Department
435 College Ave
Modesto, CA 95350-9977
(209) 575-6362

Monterey Peninsula College
—Monterey—

Full-Time Enrollments:	98	Evening Classes:	Yes
Part-Time Enrollments:	—	Weekend Classes:	No
Affiliation:	Public	Distance Learning:	No

NLN ACCREDITATION: Yes

Articulation: Associate to Baccalaureate
LPN to Associate

For Further Information Contact:

Ms Debra Schulte, Director
Monterey Peninsula College
980 Fremont
Monterey, CA 93940
(408) 646-4258

Moorpark College
—Moorpark—

Full-Time Enrollments:	64	Evening Classes:	No
Part-Time Enrollments:	42	Weekend Classes:	No
Affiliation:	Public	Distance Learning:	No

NLN ACCREDITATION: Yes

Articulation: Associate to Baccalaureate

For Further Information Contact:

Mrs Brenda R Shubert, Coordinator
Moorpark College
7075 Campus Rd
Moorpark, CA 93021
(805) 378-1433

Mt San Antonio College
—Walnut—

Full-Time Enrollments:	120	Evening Classes:	No
Part-Time Enrollments:	—	Weekend Classes:	No
Affiliation:	Public	Distance Learning:	No

NLN ACCREDITATION: No

Articulation: None

For Further Information Contact:

Mr Mike Gilliam, Director
Mt San Antonio College
1100 Grand Ave
Walnut, CA 91789
(909) 594-5611

Mt San Jacinto College
—Menifer—

Full-Time Enrollments:	21	Evening Classes:	Yes
Part-Time Enrollments:	—	Weekend Classes:	—
Affiliation:	Public	Distance Learning:	—

NLN ACCREDITATION: Yes

Articulation: None

For Further Information Contact:

Ms Nancy Stark Napolitano, Director
Mt San Jacinto College
23287 La Piedra Rd
Menifer, CA 92584
(909) 672-6752

Mt St Mary's College-Doheny Campus
—Los Angeles—

Full-Time Enrollments:	—	Evening Classes:	—
Part-Time Enrollments:	—	Weekend Classes:	—
Affiliation:	Religious	Distance Learning:	—

NLN ACCREDITATION: No

Articulation: None

For Further Information Contact:

Ms Miyo Minato, Director
Mt St Mary's College-Doheny Campus
10 Chester Pl
Los Angeles, CA 90007
(213) 746-0450

Napa Valley College
—Napa—

Full-Time Enrollments:	94	**Evening Classes:**	No
Part-Time Enrollments:	—	**Weekend Classes:**	No
Affiliation:	Public	**Distance Learning:**	No

NLN ACCREDITATION: No

Articulation: Associate to Baccalaureate

For Further Information Contact:

Ms Joan Von Grabow, Assistant Dean
Napa Valley College
2277 Napa Vallejo Hwy
Napa, CA 94558
(707) 253-3120

Ohlone College
—Fremont—

Full-Time Enrollments:	89	**Evening Classes:**	No
Part-Time Enrollments:	—	**Weekend Classes:**	No
Affiliation:	Public	**Distance Learning:**	No

NLN ACCREDITATION: Yes

Articulation: Associate to Baccalaureate
LPN to Associate

For Further Information Contact:

Ms Sharlene Limon, Dean
Ohlone College
43600 Mission Blvd
Fremont, CA 94539-5884
(510) 659-6030

Pacific Union College
—Angwin—

Full-Time Enrollments:	127	**Evening Classes:**	—
Part-Time Enrollments:	—	**Weekend Classes:**	—
Affiliation:	Religious	**Distance Learning:**	—

NLN ACCREDITATION: Yes

Articulation: Associate to Baccalaureate
LPN to Associate

For Further Information Contact:

Dr Julia Pearce, Chair
Pacific Union College
1720 Cesar Chavez Ave
Angwin, CA 94508
(707) 965-7262

Palomar College
—San Marcos—

Full-Time Enrollments:	126	**Evening Classes:**	Yes
Part-Time Enrollments:	—	**Weekend Classes:**	No
Affiliation:	Public	**Distance Learning:**	No

NLN ACCREDITATION: Yes

Articulation: Associate to Baccalaureate

For Further Information Contact:

Ms Susan Griffin, Chair
Palomar College
1140 W Mission
San Marcos, CA 92069
(619) 744-1150

Pasadena City College
—Pasadena—

Full-Time Enrollments:	192	**Evening Classes:**	No
Part-Time Enrollments:	—	**Weekend Classes:**	No
Affiliation:	Public	**Distance Learning:**	No

NLN ACCREDITATION: Yes

Articulation: LPN to Associate

For Further Information Contact:

Ms Mary Wynn, Interim Dean
Pasadena City College
1570 E Colorado Blvd
Pasadena, CA 91106
(818) 585-7326

Rancho Santiago College
—Santa Ana—

Full-Time Enrollments:	136	**Evening Classes:**	No
Part-Time Enrollments:	—	**Weekend Classes:**	No
Affiliation:	Public	**Distance Learning:**	No

NLN ACCREDITATION: Yes

Articulation: Associate to Baccalaureate
LPN to Associate

For Further Information Contact:

Mrs Carol Comeau, Director
Rancho Santiago College
1530 West 17th St
Santa Ana, CA 92706
(714) 564-6825

Rio Hondo College
—Whittier—

Full-Time Enrollments:	96	Evening Classes:	No
Part-Time Enrollments:	—	Weekend Classes:	No
Affiliation:	Public	Distance Learning:	No

NLN ACCREDITATION: No

Articulation: Associate to Baccalaureate
LPN to Associate

For Further Information Contact:

Mrs Marcia McCormick, Director
Rio Hondo College
3600 Workman Mill Rd
Whittier, CA 90601
(310) 692-0921

Riverside Community College
—Riverside—

Full-Time Enrollments:	201	Evening Classes:	Yes
Part-Time Enrollments:	—	Weekend Classes:	No
Affiliation:	Public	Distance Learning:	No

NLN ACCREDITATION: Yes

Articulation: LPN to Associate

For Further Information Contact:

Dr Carolyn S Kross, Director
Riverside Community College
4800 Magnolia Ave
Riverside, CA 92506
(909) 222-8408

Sacramento City College
—Sacramento—

Full-Time Enrollments:	114	Evening Classes:	No
Part-Time Enrollments:	—	Weekend Classes:	No
Affiliation:	Public	Distance Learning:	No

NLN ACCREDITATION: No

Articulation: Associate to Baccalaureate
Diploma to Associate
LPN to Associate

For Further Information Contact:

Mrs Diane Welch, Director
Sacramento City College
3835 Freeport Blvd
Sacramento, CA 95822
(916) 558-2271

Saddleback College
—Mission Viejo—

Full-Time Enrollments:	120	Evening Classes:	Yes
Part-Time Enrollments:	78	Weekend Classes:	No
Affiliation:	Public	Distance Learning:	No

NLN ACCREDITATION: Yes

Articulation: Associate to Baccalaureate
Diploma to Associate
LPN to Associate

For Further Information Contact:

Mrs Dixie L Bullock, Dean
Saddleback College
28000 Marguerite Pkwy
Mission Viejo, CA 92692
(714) 582-4700

San Bernardino Valley College
—San Bernardino—

Full-Time Enrollments:	166	Evening Classes:	Yes
Part-Time Enrollments:	—	Weekend Classes:	Yes
Affiliation:	Public	Distance Learning:	—

NLN ACCREDITATION: Yes

Articulation: Associate to Baccalaureate
LPN to Associate

For Further Information Contact:

Mrs Arlene H Johnson, Dean
San Bernardino Valley College
701 S Mt Vernon Ave
San Bernardino, CA 91024
(909) 888-6511

San Diego City College
—San Diego—

Full-Time Enrollments:	99	Evening Classes:	No
Part-Time Enrollments:	—	Weekend Classes:	No
Affiliation:	Public	Distance Learning:	No

NLN ACCREDITATION: No

Articulation: Associate to Baccalaureate

For Further Information Contact:

Ms Jo-Ann L Rossitto, Dean
San Diego City College
1313 12th Ave
San Diego, CA 92101
(619) 230-2439

San Joaquin Delta College
—Stockton—

Full-Time Enrollments:	97	Evening Classes:	No
Part-Time Enrollments:	61	Weekend Classes:	No
Affiliation:	Public	Distance Learning:	No

NLN ACCREDITATION: Yes

Articulation: Associate to Baccalaureate
LPN to Associate

For Further Information Contact:

Ms Virginia Antaran, Director
San Joaquin Delta College
5151 Pacific Ave
Stockton, CA 95207
(209) 474-5516

Santa Barbara City College
—Santa Barbara—

Full-Time Enrollments:	120	Evening Classes:	No
Part-Time Enrollments:	—	Weekend Classes:	No
Affiliation:	Public	Distance Learning:	No

NLN ACCREDITATION: Yes

Articulation: Associate to Baccalaureate
LPN to Associate

For Further Information Contact:

Mrs Claudia Mitchell, Director
Santa Barbara City College
721 Cliff Dr
Santa Barbara, CA 93109
(805) 965-0581

Santa Monica College
—Santa Monica—

Full-Time Enrollments:	120	Evening Classes:	No
Part-Time Enrollments:	—	Weekend Classes:	No
Affiliation:	Public	Distance Learning:	No

NLN ACCREDITATION: Yes

Articulation: Associate to Baccalaureate
LPN to Associate

For Further Information Contact:

Ms Marilyn Humphrey, Director
Santa Monica College
1900 Pico Blvd
Santa Monica, CA 90405
(310) 452-9363

Santa Rosa Jr College
—Santa Rosa—

Full-Time Enrollments:	117	Evening Classes:	No
Part-Time Enrollments:	—	Weekend Classes:	No
Affiliation:	Public	Distance Learning:	No

NLN ACCREDITATION: No

Articulation: Associate to Baccalaureate
LPN to Associate

For Further Information Contact:

Ms Marian O'Laughlin, Director
Santa Rosa Jr College
1501 Mendocino Ave
Santa Rosa, CA 95401
(707) 527-4271

Shasta College
—Redding—

Full-Time Enrollments:	100	Evening Classes:	No
Part-Time Enrollments:	—	Weekend Classes:	No
Affiliation:	Public	Distance Learning:	Yes

NLN ACCREDITATION: No

Articulation: LPN to Associate

For Further Information Contact:

Ms Georgianne M Dinkel, Director
Shasta College
11555 Old Oregon Trail
Redding, CA 96049
(916) 225-4725

Sierra College
—Rocklin—

Full-Time Enrollments:	50	Evening Classes:	—
Part-Time Enrollments:	39	Weekend Classes:	—
Affiliation:	Public	Distance Learning:	—

NLN ACCREDITATION: No

Articulation: None

For Further Information Contact:

Ms Margaret White, Assistant Dean
Sierra College
5000 Rocklin Rd
Rocklin, CA 95677
(916) 781-0556

Solano Community College
—Suisun—

Full-Time Enrollments:	93	Evening Classes:	No
Part-Time Enrollments:	—	Weekend Classes:	No
Affiliation:	Public	Distance Learning:	No

NLN ACCREDITATION: No

Articulation: Associate to Baccalaureate
LPN to Associate

For Further Information Contact:

Dr Elaine Norinsky, Div Dean
Solano Community College
4000 Suisun Valley Rd
Suisun, CA 94585
(707) 864-7108

Southwestern College
—Chula Vista—

Full-Time Enrollments:	70	Evening Classes:	No
Part-Time Enrollments:	—	Weekend Classes:	No
Affiliation:	Public	Distance Learning:	No

NLN ACCREDITATION: Yes

Articulation: None

For Further Information Contact:

Mrs Charlotte Erdahl, Dean
Southwestern College
900 Otay Lakes Rd
Chula Vista, CA 92010
(619) 421-0376

Ventura College
—Ventura—

Full-Time Enrollments:	93	Evening Classes:	—
Part-Time Enrollments:	60	Weekend Classes:	—
Affiliation:	Public	Distance Learning:	—

NLN ACCREDITATION: No

Articulation: None

For Further Information Contact:

Mrs Joan Beem, Director
Ventura College
4667 Telegraph Rd
Ventura, CA 93003
(805) 654-6342

Victor Valley College
—Victorville—

Full-Time Enrollments:	—	Evening Classes:	No
Part-Time Enrollments:	157	Weekend Classes:	No
Affiliation:	Public	Distance Learning:	No

NLN ACCREDITATION: Yes

Articulation: Associate to Baccalaureate

For Further Information Contact:

Mrs Diane Cline, Dean
Victor Valley College
18422 Bear Valley Rd
Victorville, CA 92392
(619) 245-4271

Yuba College
—Marysville—

Full-Time Enrollments:	78	Evening Classes:	No
Part-Time Enrollments:	—	Weekend Classes:	No
Affiliation:	Public	Distance Learning:	Yes

NLN ACCREDITATION: No

Articulation: Associate to Baccalaureate
LPN to Associate

For Further Information Contact:

Ms Margot J Loschke, Director
Yuba College
2088 N Beale Rd
Marysville, CA 95901
(916) 741-6785

Colorado

Arapahoe Community College
—Littleton—

Full-Time Enrollments:	109	Evening Classes:	Yes
Part-Time Enrollments:	1	Weekend Classes:	No
Affiliation:	Public	Distance Learning:	No

NLN ACCREDITATION: No

Articulation: LPN to Associate

For Further Information Contact:

Ms Linda Stroup, Director
Arapahoe Community College
5900 South Santa Fe Dr
Littleton, CO 80120
(303) 797-5890

Community College of Denver
—Denver—

Full-Time Enrollments:	100	Evening Classes:	No	
Part-Time Enrollments:	65	Weekend Classes:	No	
Affiliation:	Public	Distance Learning:	No	

NLN ACCREDITATION: No

Articulation: Associate to Baccalaureate
LPN to Associate

For Further Information Contact:

Mrs Vicki Earnest, Coordinator
Community College of Denver
1111 W Colfax
Denver, CO 80217-3363
(303) 556-3842

Front Range Community College
—Fort Collins—

Full-Time Enrollments:	—	Evening Classes:	No	
Part-Time Enrollments:	82	Weekend Classes:	No	
Affiliation:	Public	Distance Learning:	No	

NLN ACCREDITATION: No

Articulation: LPN to Associate

For Further Information Contact:

Mrs Audrey Bopp, Coordinator
Front Range Community College
4616 South Sheilds
Fort Collins, CO 80526
(970) 226-2500

Front Range Community College
—Westminster—

Full-Time Enrollments:	197	Evening Classes:	No	
Part-Time Enrollments:	8	Weekend Classes:	No	
Affiliation:	Public	Distance Learning:	No	

NLN ACCREDITATION: No

Articulation: Associate to Baccalaureate
LPN to Associate

For Further Information Contact:

Mrs Alma Mueller, Director
Front Range Community College
3645 W 112th Ave
Westminster, CO 80030
(303) 466-8811

Morgan Community College-Northeastern Jr College
—Fort Morgan—

Full-Time Enrollments:	22	Evening Classes:	No	
Part-Time Enrollments:	—	Weekend Classes:	No	
Affiliation:	Public	Distance Learning:	No	

NLN ACCREDITATION: No

Articulation: LPN to Associate

For Further Information Contact:

Mrs Darla Brennemann, Coordinator
Morgan Community College-Northeastern Jr College
17800 Road 20
Fort Morgan, CO 80701
(970) 867-3081

Otero Junior College
—La Junta—

Full-Time Enrollments:	48	Evening Classes:	—	
Part-Time Enrollments:	2	Weekend Classes:	—	
Affiliation:	Public	Distance Learning:	—	

NLN ACCREDITATION: Yes

Articulation: None

For Further Information Contact:

Mrs Denise Root, Director
Otero Junior College
La Junta, CO 81050
(719) 384-6899

Pikes Peak Community College
—Colorado Springs—

Full-Time Enrollments:	93	Evening Classes:	Yes	
Part-Time Enrollments:	—	Weekend Classes:	No	
Affiliation:	Public	Distance Learning:	No	

NLN ACCREDITATION: No

Articulation: LPN to Associate

For Further Information Contact:

Ms Sandra Zettel-Clark, Chair
Pikes Peak Community College
5675 S Academy Blvd
Colorado Springs, CO 80906
(719) 540-7413

Pueblo Community College (2 Branches)
—Pueblo—

Full-Time Enrollments:	51	Evening Classes:	—
Part-Time Enrollments:	—	Weekend Classes:	—
Affiliation:	Public	Distance Learning:	—

NLN ACCREDITATION: Yes

Articulation: None

For Further Information Contact:

Dr Sharon Van Sell, Director
Pueblo Community College (2 Branches)
415 Harrison
Pueblo, CO 81004-1499
(719) 549-3409

Trinidad State Jr College
—Trinidad—

Full-Time Enrollments:	—	Evening Classes:	—
Part-Time Enrollments:	—	Weekend Classes:	—
Affiliation:	Public	Distance Learning:	—

NLN ACCREDITATION: Yes

Articulation: None

For Further Information Contact:

Ms Judie Stickel, Coordinator
Trinidad State Jr College
600 Prospect St Box 150
Trinidad, CO 81082
(719) 846-5524

Connecticut

Capital Community Technical College
—Hartford—

Full-Time Enrollments:	4	Evening Classes:	No
Part-Time Enrollments:	223	Weekend Classes:	No
Affiliation:	Public	Distance Learning:	No

NLN ACCREDITATION: Yes

Articulation: Associate to Baccalaureate
LPN to Associate

For Further Information Contact:

Mrs Judith Patrizzi, Director
Capital Community Technical College
61 Woodland St
Hartford, CT 06105
(860) 520-7835

Naugatuck Valley Community Technical College
—Waterbury—

Full-Time Enrollments:	8	Evening Classes:	No
Part-Time Enrollments:	151	Weekend Classes:	No
Affiliation:	Public	Distance Learning:	No

NLN ACCREDITATION: Yes

Articulation: Associate to Baccalaureate
LPN to Associate

For Further Information Contact:

Dr Patricia Bouffard, Director
Naugatuck Valley Community Technical College
750 Chase Pkwy
Waterbury, CT 06708
(203) 575-8057

Norwalk Community Technical College
—Norwalk—

Full-Time Enrollments:	11	Evening Classes:	No
Part-Time Enrollments:	88	Weekend Classes:	No
Affiliation:	Public	Distance Learning:	No

NLN ACCREDITATION: Yes

Articulation: Associate to Baccalaureate
LPN to Associate

For Further Information Contact:

Ms Mary Schuler, Director
Norwalk Community Technical College
188 Richards Ave
Norwalk, CT 06854-1655
(203) 857-7122

St Vincent's College
—Bridgeport—

Full-Time Enrollments:	69	Evening Classes:	Yes
Part-Time Enrollments:	142	Weekend Classes:	Yes
Affiliation:	Religious	Distance Learning:	No

NLN ACCREDITATION: Yes

Articulation: Associate to Baccalaureate
LPN to Associate

For Further Information Contact:

Ms Joanne Wolfertz, Chair
St Vincent's College
2800 Main St
Bridgeport, CT 06606
(203) 576-5578

Three Rivers Community Technical College
—Norwich—

Full-Time Enrollments:	16	Evening Classes:	No
Part-Time Enrollments:	81	Weekend Classes:	No
Affiliation:	Public	Distance Learning:	No

NLN ACCREDITATION: Yes

Articulation: None

For Further Information Contact:

Ms Christine Crawford, Director
Three Rivers Community Technical College
Mahan Dr
Norwich, CT 06360
(203) 886-1931

Wilcox College of Nursing
—Middletown—

Full-Time Enrollments:	2	Evening Classes:	Yes
Part-Time Enrollments:	95	Weekend Classes:	No
Affiliation:	Private	Distance Learning:	No

NLN ACCREDITATION: Yes

Articulation: Associate to Baccalaureate

For Further Information Contact:

Mrs Kathleen Stolzenberger, President
Wilcox College of Nursing
28 Crescent St
Middletown, CT 06457
(860) 344-6402

Delaware

Delaware Technical & Community College
—Dover—

Full-Time Enrollments:	16	Evening Classes:	Yes
Part-Time Enrollments:	—	Weekend Classes:	Yes
Affiliation:	Public	Distance Learning:	Yes

NLN ACCREDITATION: No

Articulation: LPN to Associate

For Further Information Contact:

Mrs Ruth Yanos, Chair
Delaware Technical & Community College
Terry Campus
Dover, DE 19901
(302) 739-5444

Delaware Technical & Community College-S Campus
—Georgetown—

Full-Time Enrollments:	42	Evening Classes:	Yes
Part-Time Enrollments:	51	Weekend Classes:	No
Affiliation:	Public	Distance Learning:	No

NLN ACCREDITATION: Yes

Articulation: Associate to Baccalaureate
LPN to Associate

For Further Information Contact:

Mrs Judith Caldwell, Chair
Delaware Technical & Community College-S Campus
PO Box 610
Georgetown, DE 19947
(302) 856-5400

Delaware Technical & Community College-Stanton Branch
—Newark—

Full-Time Enrollments:	191	Evening Classes:	Yes
Part-Time Enrollments:	—	Weekend Classes:	Yes
Affiliation:	Public	Distance Learning:	Yes

NLN ACCREDITATION: Yes

Articulation: Associate to Baccalaureate
LPN to Associate

For Further Information Contact:

Mrs Nancy Snyder, Chair
Delaware Technical & Community College-Stanton Branch
400 Christiana-Stanton Rd
Newark, DE 19702
(302) 454-3948

Wesley College
—Dover—

Full-Time Enrollments:	54	Evening Classes:	No
Part-Time Enrollments:	45	Weekend Classes:	No
Affiliation:	Religious	Distance Learning:	No

NLN ACCREDITATION: Yes

Articulation: LPN to Associate
RN to MSN

For Further Information Contact:

Dr Lucille Gambardella, Chair
Wesley College
Div Of Nsg
Dover, DE 19901
(302) 736-2482

District of Columbia

University of District of Columbia
—Washington—

Full-Time Enrollments:	70	Evening Classes:	No
Part-Time Enrollments:	5	Weekend Classes:	No
Affiliation:	Public	Distance Learning:	No

NLN ACCREDITATION: Yes

Articulation: Associate to Baccalaureate
LPN to Associate

For Further Information Contact:

Dr Hazel Marshall, Interim Director
University of District of Columbia
4200 Conn Ave, NW, Bldg 44
Washington, DC 20008
(202) 274-5957

Florida

Brevard Community College
—Cocoa—

Full-Time Enrollments:	141	Evening Classes:	Yes
Part-Time Enrollments:	—	Weekend Classes:	Yes
Affiliation:	Public	Distance Learning:	—

NLN ACCREDITATION: No

Articulation: Associate to Baccalaureate
LPN to Associate

For Further Information Contact:

Mrs Jene M Holland, Chair
Brevard Community College
1519 Clearlake Rd
Cocoa, FL 32922
(407) 632-1111

Broward Community College (3 Campuses)
—Ft Lauderdale—

Full-Time Enrollments:	731	Evening Classes:	Yes
Part-Time Enrollments:	—	Weekend Classes:	No
Affiliation:	Public	Distance Learning:	Yes

NLN ACCREDITATION: Yes

Articulation: Diploma to Associate
LPN to Associate

For Further Information Contact:

Mrs Diane Whitehead, Dept Head
Broward Community College (3 Campuses)
3501 SW Davie Rd Bldg 9
Ft Lauderdale, FL 33314
(954) 475-6921

Central Florida Community College
—Ocala—

Full-Time Enrollments:	117	Evening Classes:	No
Part-Time Enrollments:	54	Weekend Classes:	No
Affiliation:	Public	Distance Learning:	No

NLN ACCREDITATION: Yes

Articulation: LPN to Associate

For Further Information Contact:

Dr G Lapham-Alcorn, Associate Dean
Central Florida Community College
3001 S W College Rd
Ocala, FL 34474
(904) 237-2111

Chipola Jr College
—Marianna—

Full-Time Enrollments:	66	Evening Classes:	No
Part-Time Enrollments:	—	Weekend Classes:	No
Affiliation:	Public	Distance Learning:	No

NLN ACCREDITATION: No

Articulation: Associate to Baccalaureate
LPN to Associate

For Further Information Contact:

Mrs Kathy Wheeler, Coordinator
Chipola Jr College
3094 Indian Circle
Marianna, FL 32446
(904) 526-2761

Daytona Beach Community College
—Daytona Beach—

Full-Time Enrollments:	306	Evening Classes:	Yes
Part-Time Enrollments:	—	Weekend Classes:	No
Affiliation:	Public	Distance Learning:	No

NLN ACCREDITATION: Yes

Articulation: Associate to Baccalaureate
LPN to Associate

For Further Information Contact:

Dr Donna Brandmeyer, Chair
Daytona Beach Community College
1200 International Speed Way
Daytona Beach, FL 32120
(904) 255-8131

Edison Community College
—Fort Myers—

Full-Time Enrollments:	84	Evening Classes:	Yes
Part-Time Enrollments:	120	Weekend Classes:	—
Affiliation:	Public	Distance Learning:	Yes

NLN ACCREDITATION: Yes

Articulation: LPN to Associate

For Further Information Contact:

Dr Shirley Ruder, Director
Edison Community College
8099 College Pkwy NW
Fort Myers, FL 33919-3566
(941) 489-9239

Florida Community College
—Jacksonville—

Full-Time Enrollments:	357	Evening Classes:	Yes
Part-Time Enrollments:	—	Weekend Classes:	Yes
Affiliation:	Public	Distance Learning:	No

NLN ACCREDITATION: Yes

Articulation: LPN to Associate

For Further Information Contact:

Mrs Donna Perry, Chair
Florida Community College
4501 Capper Rd N Campus
Jacksonville, FL 32218-4499
(904) 766-6581

Florida Hospital College of Health Sciences
—Orlando—

Full-Time Enrollments:	94	Evening Classes:	No
Part-Time Enrollments:	—	Weekend Classes:	No
Affiliation:	Religious	Distance Learning:	No

NLN ACCREDITATION: No

Articulation: Associate to Baccalaureate

For Further Information Contact:

Mrs Cheryl Galusha, Chair
Florida Hospital College of Health Sciences
795 Lake Estelle Dr
Orlando, FL 32803
(407) 897-5600

Florida Keys Community College
—Key West—

Full-Time Enrollments:	65	Evening Classes:	Yes
Part-Time Enrollments:	—	Weekend Classes:	No
Affiliation:	Public	Distance Learning:	No

NLN ACCREDITATION: No

Articulation: Associate to Baccalaureate

For Further Information Contact:

Ms Coleen Dooley, Director
Florida Keys Community College
5901 W Jr College Rd
Key West, FL 33040
(305) 296-9081

Gulf Coast Community College
—Panama City—

Full-Time Enrollments:	—	Evening Classes:	Yes
Part-Time Enrollments:	151	Weekend Classes:	No
Affiliation:	Public	Distance Learning:	Yes

NLN ACCREDITATION: Yes

Articulation: Associate to Baccalaureate
LPN to Associate

For Further Information Contact:

Ms Anna Marie Baugh, Coordinator
Gulf Coast Community College
5230 W Hwy 98
Panama City, FL 32401-1058
(904) 769-1551

Hillsborough Community College-Dale Mabry Campus
—Tampa—

Full-Time Enrollments:	350	Evening Classes:	No
Part-Time Enrollments:	—	Weekend Classes:	No
Affiliation:	Public	Distance Learning:	No

NLN ACCREDITATION: Yes

Articulation: Associate to Baccalaureate
LPN to Associate

For Further Information Contact:

Dr Robert Chunn, Dean
Hillsborough Community College-Dale Mabry Campus
4100 Tampa Bay Blvd
Tampa, FL 33630
(813) 253-7255

Indian River Community College
—Fort Pierce—

Full-Time Enrollments:	222	Evening Classes:	No
Part-Time Enrollments:	—	Weekend Classes:	No
Affiliation:	Public	Distance Learning:	No

NLN ACCREDITATION: Yes

Articulation: LPN to Associate

For Further Information Contact:

Ms Jane Cebelak, Director
Indian River Community College
3209 Virginia Ave
Fort Pierce, FL 34981-5599
(561) 462-4778

Lake City Community College
—Lake City—

Full-Time Enrollments:	7	Evening Classes:	No
Part-Time Enrollments:	93	Weekend Classes:	No
Affiliation:	Public	Distance Learning:	No

NLN ACCREDITATION: Yes

Articulation: LPN to Associate

For Further Information Contact:

Mrs Lane Dekle, Coordinator
Lake City Community College
Route 19 Box 1030
Lake City, FL 32025
(904) 752-1822

Lake-Sumter Community College
—Leesburg—

Full-Time Enrollments:	56	Evening Classes:	Yes
Part-Time Enrollments:	—	Weekend Classes:	No
Affiliation:	Public	Distance Learning:	Yes

NLN ACCREDITATION: No

Articulation: Associate to Baccalaureate
LPN to Associate

For Further Information Contact:

Mrs Susan Pennacchia, Director
Lake-Sumter Community College
9501 US Hwy 441
Leesburg, FL 34788-8751
(352) 365-3519

Manatee Community College
—Bradenton—

Full-Time Enrollments:	217	Evening Classes:	Yes
Part-Time Enrollments:	—	Weekend Classes:	No
Affiliation:	Public	Distance Learning:	No

NLN ACCREDITATION: Yes

Articulation: LPN to Associate

For Further Information Contact:

Dr Carol A Singer, Director
Manatee Community College
5840 26th St West
Bradenton, FL 34206
(941) 755-1511

Miami-Dade Community College-Medical Center Campus
—Miami—

Full-Time Enrollments:	546	Evening Classes:	Yes
Part-Time Enrollments:	118	Weekend Classes:	Yes
Affiliation:	Public	Distance Learning:	No

NLN ACCREDITATION: Yes

Articulation: Associate to Baccalaureate
Diploma to Associate

For Further Information Contact:

Dr Susan Kah, Exec Dean
Miami-Dade Community College-Medical Center
Campus
950 NW 20 St
Miami, FL 33127
(305) 237-4100

Palm Beach Community College
—Lake Worth—

Full-Time Enrollments:	442	Evening Classes:	Yes
Part-Time Enrollments:	—	Weekend Classes:	No
Affiliation:	Public	Distance Learning:	No

NLN ACCREDITATION: Yes

Articulation: Associate to Baccalaureate
LPN to Associate

For Further Information Contact:

Mrs Selma Ann Verse, Coordinator
Palm Beach Community College
4200 Congress Ave
Lake Worth, FL 33461-4796
(561) 439-8092

Pasco-Hernando Community College (3 Campuses)
—New Port Richey—

Full-Time Enrollments:	173	Evening Classes:	No
Part-Time Enrollments:	—	Weekend Classes:	No
Affiliation:	Public	Distance Learning:	No

NLN ACCREDITATION: Yes

Articulation: LPN to Associate

For Further Information Contact:

Ms Karen Richardson, Director
Pasco-Hernando Community College (3 Campuses)
10239 Ridge Rd
New Port Richey, FL 34654
(813) 847-2727

Pensacola Jr College
—Pensacola—

Full-Time Enrollments:	195	Evening Classes:	—
Part-Time Enrollments:	125	Weekend Classes:	—
Affiliation:	Public	Distance Learning:	—

NLN ACCREDITATION: No

Articulation: None

For Further Information Contact:

Dr Joan Connell, Dept Head
Pensacola Jr College
5555 W Hwy 98
Pensacola, FL 32507
(904) 484-2254

Polk Community College
—Winter Haven—

Full-Time Enrollments:	250	Evening Classes:	Yes
Part-Time Enrollments:	—	Weekend Classes:	No
Affiliation:	Public	Distance Learning:	Yes

NLN ACCREDITATION: Yes

Articulation: Associate to Baccalaureate

For Further Information Contact:

Mrs Sharon Davis, Director
Polk Community College
999 Ave "H" NE
Winter Haven, FL 33881
(941) 297-1036

Santa Fe Community College
—Gainesville—

Full-Time Enrollments:	116	Evening Classes:	No
Part-Time Enrollments:	92	Weekend Classes:	No
Affiliation:	Public	Distance Learning:	No

NLN ACCREDITATION: Yes

Articulation: LPN to Associate

For Further Information Contact:

Ms Rita Sutherland, Director
Santa Fe Community College
3000 NW 83rd St Box 1530
Gainesville, FL 32606
(352) 395-5700

Seminole Community College
—Sanford—

Full-Time Enrollments:	123	Evening Classes:	—
Part-Time Enrollments:	—	Weekend Classes:	—
Affiliation:	Public	Distance Learning:	—

NLN ACCREDITATION: Yes

Articulation: Associate to Baccalaureate
LPN to Associate

For Further Information Contact:

Mrs Laura Aromando, Chair
Seminole Community College
100 Weldon Blvd
Sanford, FL 32773
(407) 323-1450

South Florida Community College
—Avon Park—

Full-Time Enrollments:	37	Evening Classes:	—
Part-Time Enrollments:	—	Weekend Classes:	—
Affiliation:	Public	Distance Learning:	—

NLN ACCREDITATION: No

Articulation: None

For Further Information Contact:

Dr Mary Ann Fritz, Chair
South Florida Community College
600 West College Dr
Avon Park, FL 33825
(813) 453-6661

St Petersburg Jr College Health
—St Petersburg—

Full-Time Enrollments:	420	Evening Classes:	Yes
Part-Time Enrollments:	—	Weekend Classes:	No
Affiliation:	Public	Distance Learning:	No

NLN ACCREDITATION: Yes

Articulation: Associate to Baccalaureate
LPN to Associate

For Further Information Contact:

Dr Jodi Parks Doyle, Director
St Petersburg Jr College Health
PO Box 13489
St Petersburg, FL 33733
(813) 341-3618

Tallahassee Community College
—Tallahassee—

Full-Time Enrollments:	78	Evening Classes:	No
Part-Time Enrollments:	—	Weekend Classes:	No
Affiliation:	Public	Distance Learning:	No

NLN ACCREDITATION: No

Articulation: Associate to Baccalaureate
LPN to Associate

For Further Information Contact:

Dr Patricia Muar, Chair
Tallahassee Community College
444 Appleyard Dr
Tallahassee, FL 32304
(904) 488-9200

Valencia Community College
—Orlando—

Full-Time Enrollments:	123	Evening Classes:	No
Part-Time Enrollments:	80	Weekend Classes:	No
Affiliation:	Public	Distance Learning:	No

NLN ACCREDITATION: Yes

Articulation: Associate to Baccalaureate
LPN to Associate

For Further Information Contact:

Mrs Anne Miller, Director
Valencia Community College
1800 S Kirkman Rd
Orlando, FL 32811
(407) 299-5000

Georgia

Abraham Baldwin Agriculture College
—Tifton—

Full-Time Enrollments:	175	Evening Classes:	Yes
Part-Time Enrollments:	18	Weekend Classes:	No
Affiliation:	Public	Distance Learning:	Yes

NLN ACCREDITATION: Yes

Articulation: Associate to Baccalaureate
LPN to Associate

For Further Information Contact:

Ms R Joy Conger, Chair
Abraham Baldwin Agriculture College
PO Box 52 ABAC Station
Tifton, GA 31793-4401
(912) 386-3262

Armstrong Atlantic State University
—Savannah—

Full-Time Enrollments:	40	Evening Classes:	Yes
Part-Time Enrollments:	77	Weekend Classes:	No
Affiliation:	Public	Distance Learning:	Yes

NLN ACCREDITATION: Yes

Articulation: Associate to Baccalaureate

For Further Information Contact:

Dr Deanna Cross, Coordinator
Armstrong Atlantic State University
Savannah, GA 31419-1997
(912) 927-5311

Athens Area Technical Institute
—Athens—

Full-Time Enrollments:	33	Evening Classes:	Yes
Part-Time Enrollments:	36	Weekend Classes:	No
Affiliation:	Public	Distance Learning:	Yes

NLN ACCREDITATION: Yes

Articulation: LPN to Associate

For Further Information Contact:

Dr Gloria Linden Buck, Director
Athens Area Technical Institute
800 US Highway 29 North
Athens, GA 30601-1500
(706) 355-5037

Augusta State University
—Augusta—

Full-Time Enrollments:	7	Evening Classes:	No
Part-Time Enrollments:	86	Weekend Classes:	No
Affiliation:	Public	Distance Learning:	No

NLN ACCREDITATION: Yes

Articulation: Associate to Baccalaureate

For Further Information Contact:

Dr Letha Lierman, Chair
Augusta State University
2500 Walton Way
Augusta, GA 30904-2200
(706) 737-1725

Clayton College & State University
—Morrow—

Full-Time Enrollments:	—	Evening Classes:	Yes
Part-Time Enrollments:	118	Weekend Classes:	Yes
Affiliation:	Public	Distance Learning:	Yes

NLN ACCREDITATION: Yes

Articulation: Associate to Baccalaureate

For Further Information Contact:

Dr Linda Samson, Dean
Clayton College & State University
PO Box 285
Morrow, GA 30260
(770) 961-3430

Coastal Georgia Community College
—Brunswick—

Full-Time Enrollments:	134	Evening Classes:	—
Part-Time Enrollments:	—	Weekend Classes:	—
Affiliation:	Public	Distance Learning:	—

NLN ACCREDITATION: Yes

Articulation: None

For Further Information Contact:

Dr Diane Y Smith, Dept Head
Coastal Georgia Community College
Brunswick, GA 31520
(912) 262-7357

Columbus State University
—Columbus—

Full-Time Enrollments:	50	Evening Classes:	No
Part-Time Enrollments:	22	Weekend Classes:	No
Affiliation:	Public	Distance Learning:	No

NLN ACCREDITATION: Yes

Articulation: Associate to Baccalaureate
Diploma to Baccalaureate

For Further Information Contact:

Mrs Peggy Batastini, Director
Columbus State University
4225 University Ave
Columbus, GA 31907-5645
(706) 568-2053

Dalton College
—Dalton—

Full-Time Enrollments:	24	Evening Classes:	No
Part-Time Enrollments:	82	Weekend Classes:	No
Affiliation:	Public	Distance Learning:	No

NLN ACCREDITATION: Yes

Articulation: Associate to Baccalaureate

For Further Information Contact:

Mrs Trudy Swilling, Chair
Dalton College
213 North College Dr
Dalton, GA 30720-3797
(706) 272-4440

Darton College
—Albany—

Full-Time Enrollments:	67	Evening Classes:	Yes
Part-Time Enrollments:	173	Weekend Classes:	—
Affiliation:	Public	Distance Learning:	—

NLN ACCREDITATION: Yes

Articulation: Associate to Baccalaureate

For Further Information Contact:

Mrs Betty A Page, Chair
Darton College
2400 Gillionville Rd
Albany, GA 31707
(912) 430-6820

DeKalb College
—Clarkston—

Full-Time Enrollments:	—	Evening Classes:	—
Part-Time Enrollments:	—	Weekend Classes:	—
Affiliation:	Public	Distance Learning:	—

NLN ACCREDITATION: Yes

Articulation: None

For Further Information Contact:

Ms Anne Tidmore, Dept Head
DeKalb College
555 N Indian Creek Dr
Clarkston, GA 30021
(404) 299-4177

Floyd College
—Rome—

Full-Time Enrollments:	106	Evening Classes:	Yes
Part-Time Enrollments:	58	Weekend Classes:	No
Affiliation:	Public	Distance Learning:	No

NLN ACCREDITATION: Yes

Articulation: LPN to Associate

For Further Information Contact:

Mrs Belen D Nora, Chair
Floyd College
PO Box 1864
Rome, GA 30161
(706) 295-6321

Georgia Southwestern University
—Americus—

Full-Time Enrollments:	78	Evening Classes:	Yes
Part-Time Enrollments:	37	Weekend Classes:	No
Affiliation:	Public	Distance Learning:	No

NLN ACCREDITATION: Yes

Articulation: Associate to Baccalaureate
LPN to Associate

For Further Information Contact:

Dr Martha Buhler, Acting Dean
Georgia Southwestern University
Americus, GA 31709
(912) 931-2275

Gordon College
—Barnesville—

Full-Time Enrollments:	182	Evening Classes:	Yes
Part-Time Enrollments:	—	Weekend Classes:	No
Affiliation:	Public	Distance Learning:	—

NLN ACCREDITATION: Yes

Articulation: LPN to Associate

For Further Information Contact:

Dr Judith Malachowski, Chair
Gordon College
Barnesville, GA 30204
(770) 358-5085

Kennesaw University
—Marietta—

Full-Time Enrollments:	20	Evening Classes:	No
Part-Time Enrollments:	46	Weekend Classes:	No
Affiliation:	Public	Distance Learning:	No

NLN ACCREDITATION: Yes

Articulation: LPN to Associate

No longer there

For Further Information Contact:

Dr Vanice Roberts, Chair
Kennesaw University
PO Box 444
Marietta, GA 30061
(770) 423-6064

Macon College
—Macon—

Full-Time Enrollments:	—	Evening Classes:	Yes
Part-Time Enrollments:	238	Weekend Classes:	—
Affiliation:	Public	Distance Learning:	—

NLN ACCREDITATION: Yes

Articulation: LPN to Associate

For Further Information Contact:

Dr Diane M Craine, Chair
Macon College
100 College Station Dr
Macon, GA 31206-5144
(912) 471-2761

Middle Georgia College
—Cochran—

Full-Time Enrollments: 126   Evening Classes: No
Part-Time Enrollments: 10   Weekend Classes: No
Affiliation: Public   Distance Learning: —

NLN ACCREDITATION: Yes

Articulation: Associate to Baccalaureate
LPN to Associate

For Further Information Contact:

Jo Anne Jackson, Director
Middle Georgia College
Cochran, GA 31014
(912) 934-3057

North Georgia College & State University
—Dahlonega—

Full-Time Enrollments: 43   Evening Classes: No
Part-Time Enrollments: 91   Weekend Classes: No
Affiliation: Public   Distance Learning: Yes

NLN ACCREDITATION: Yes

Articulation: Associate to Baccalaureate
Diploma to Baccalaureate
LPN to Associate

For Further Information Contact:

Dr Linda Roberts-Betsch, Dept Head
North Georgia College & State University
RT 60
Dahlonega, GA 30597
(706) 864-1934

South Georgia College
—Douglas—

Full-Time Enrollments: 50   Evening Classes: No
Part-Time Enrollments: 160   Weekend Classes: No
Affiliation: Public   Distance Learning: No

NLN ACCREDITATION: Yes

Articulation: LPN to Associate

For Further Information Contact:

Ms Carol Hurst, Chair
South Georgia College
Douglas, GA 31533-5098
(912) 383-4203

State University of West Georgia
—Carrollton—

Full-Time Enrollments: 44   Evening Classes: No
Part-Time Enrollments: 27   Weekend Classes: No
Affiliation: Public   Distance Learning: No

NLN ACCREDITATION: Yes

Articulation: None

For Further Information Contact:

Dr Jeanette C Bernhardt, Chair
State University of West Georgia
Carrollton, GA 30118-4500
(770) 836-6552

Hawaii

Hawaii Community College
—Hilo—

Full-Time Enrollments: —   Evening Classes: —
Part-Time Enrollments: —   Weekend Classes: —
Affiliation: Public   Distance Learning: —

NLN ACCREDITATION: No

Articulation: —

For Further Information Contact:

Dr Elizabeth Ojala, Director
Hawaii Community College
523 W Lanikaula St
Hilo, HI 96720-4091
(808) 933-3560

Kapiolani Community College-University of Hawaii
—Honolulu—

Full-Time Enrollments: —   Evening Classes: —
Part-Time Enrollments: —   Weekend Classes: —
Affiliation: Public   Distance Learning: —

NLN ACCREDITATION: Yes

Articulation: None

For Further Information Contact:

Mrs Joan Matsukawa, Chair
Kapiolani Community College-University of Hawaii
4303 Diamond Head Rd
Honolulu, HI 96813
(808) 734-9455

Kauai Community College-University of Hawaii
—Lihue—

Full-Time Enrollments:	16	Evening Classes:	No
Part-Time Enrollments:	8	Weekend Classes:	No
Affiliation:	Public	Distance Learning:	No

NLN ACCREDITATION: Yes

Articulation: Associate to Baccalaureate

For Further Information Contact:

Mr Richard Carmichael, Director
Kauai Community College-University of Hawaii
3-1901 Kaumualii Hwy
Lihue, HI 96766
(808) 242-1250

Maui Community College
—Kahului Maui—

Full-Time Enrollments:	65	Evening Classes:	—
Part-Time Enrollments:	—	Weekend Classes:	—
Affiliation:	Public	Distance Learning:	—

NLN ACCREDITATION: Yes

Articulation: None

For Further Information Contact:

Mrs Nancy Johnson, Chair
Maui Community College
310 Kaahumanu Ave
Kahului Maui, HI 96732
(808) 244-9181

Idaho

Boise State University
—Boise—

Full-Time Enrollments:	99	Evening Classes:	No
Part-Time Enrollments:	—	Weekend Classes:	No
Affiliation:	Public	Distance Learning:	Yes

NLN ACCREDITATION: Yes

Articulation: Associate to Baccalaureate
LPN to Associate

For Further Information Contact:

Dr Anne Payne, Chair
Boise State University
1910 Univ Dr
Boise, ID 83725
(208) 385-3600

College of Southern Idaho
—Twin Falls—

Full-Time Enrollments:	100	Evening Classes:	Yes
Part-Time Enrollments:	—	Weekend Classes:	Yes
Affiliation:	Public	Distance Learning:	Yes

NLN ACCREDITATION: Yes

Articulation: Associate to Baccalaureate
LPN to Associate

For Further Information Contact:

Dr Claudeen Buettner, Chair
College of Southern Idaho
PO Box 1238
Twin Falls, ID 83303-1238
(208) 733-9554

North Idaho College
—Coeur D'Alene—

Full-Time Enrollments:	86	Evening Classes:	No
Part-Time Enrollments:	—	Weekend Classes:	No
Affiliation:	Public	Distance Learning:	No

NLN ACCREDITATION: Yes

Articulation: Associate to Baccalaureate
LPN to Associate

For Further Information Contact:

Mrs H Joan Brogan, Director
North Idaho College
1000 West Garden
Coeur D'Alene, ID 83814
(208) 769-3480

Ricks College
—Rexburg—

Full-Time Enrollments:	128	Evening Classes:	No
Part-Time Enrollments:	—	Weekend Classes:	No
Affiliation:	Religious	Distance Learning:	No

NLN ACCREDITATION: Yes

Articulation: Associate to Baccalaureate

For Further Information Contact:

Mr Kim Van Wagoner, Chair
Ricks College
Clarke Bldg Rm 175
Rexburg, ID 83460-0620
(208) 356-1326

ASSOCIATE DEGREE

Illinois

Belleville Area College
—Belleville—

Full-Time Enrollments:	119	Evening Classes:	No
Part-Time Enrollments:	—	Weekend Classes:	No
Affiliation:	Public	Distance Learning:	No

NLN ACCREDITATION: Yes

Articulation: Associate to Baccalaureate

For Further Information Contact:

Ms Carol Eckert, Director
Belleville Area College
2500 Carlysle Rd
Belleville, IL 62221
(618) 235-2700

Black Hawk College
—Moline—

Full-Time Enrollments:	33	Evening Classes:	Yes
Part-Time Enrollments:	95	Weekend Classes:	No
Affiliation:	Public	Distance Learning:	Yes

NLN ACCREDITATION: Yes

Articulation: LPN to Associate

For Further Information Contact:

Mrs Carolyn Judge, Chair
Black Hawk College
6600 34th Ave
Moline, IL 61265
(309) 796-1311

Carl Sandburg College
—Galesburg—

Full-Time Enrollments:	66	Evening Classes:	No
Part-Time Enrollments:	—	Weekend Classes:	No
Affiliation:	Public	Distance Learning:	No

NLN ACCREDITATION: No

Articulation: LPN to Associate

For Further Information Contact:

Mrs Alice Enderlin, Coordinator
Carl Sandburg College
2232 S Lake Storey Rd
Galesburg, IL 61401
(309) 344-2518

College of Du Page
—Glen Ellyn—

Full-Time Enrollments:	53	Evening Classes:	Yes
Part-Time Enrollments:	117	Weekend Classes:	Yes
Affiliation:	Public	Distance Learning:	No

NLN ACCREDITATION: Yes

Articulation: Associate to Baccalaureate
                 LPN to Associate

For Further Information Contact:

Mrs Ellen Davel, Coordinator
College of Du Page
22nd & Lambert Rd
Glen Ellyn, IL 60137
(630) 942-2652

College of Lake County
—Grayslake—

Full-Time Enrollments:	20	Evening Classes:	Yes
Part-Time Enrollments:	151	Weekend Classes:	No
Affiliation:	Public	Distance Learning:	No

NLN ACCREDITATION: Yes

Articulation: Associate to Baccalaureate

For Further Information Contact:

Ms Delores M Swan, Director
College of Lake County
19351 W Washington St
Grayslake, IL 60030
(847) 223-6601

Elgin Community College
—Elgin—

Full-Time Enrollments:	116	Evening Classes:	No
Part-Time Enrollments:	75	Weekend Classes:	No
Affiliation:	Public	Distance Learning:	Yes

NLN ACCREDITATION: Yes

Articulation: Associate to Baccalaureate
                 LPN to Associate

For Further Information Contact:

Mrs Maryann Vaca, Associate Dean
Elgin Community College
1700 Spartan Dr
Elgin, IL 60123
(847) 697-7350

Heartland Community College
—Bloomington—

Full-Time Enrollments:	53	Evening Classes:	Yes
Part-Time Enrollments:	—	Weekend Classes:	No
Affiliation:	Public	Distance Learning:	No

NLN ACCREDITATION: No

Articulation: LPN to Associate

For Further Information Contact:

Ms Jacqueline Perley, Director
Heartland Community College
1226 Towanda Ave
Bloomington, IL 61701
(309) 827-0500

Highland Community College
—Freeport—

Full-Time Enrollments:	73	Evening Classes:	—
Part-Time Enrollments:	—	Weekend Classes:	—
Affiliation:	Public	Distance Learning:	—

NLN ACCREDITATION: No

Articulation: None

For Further Information Contact:

Mrs Alice Nied, Director
Highland Community College
2998 Pearl City Rd
Freeport, IL 61032
(815) 235-6121

Illinois Central College
—East Peoria—

Full-Time Enrollments:	6	Evening Classes:	No
Part-Time Enrollments:	123	Weekend Classes:	No
Affiliation:	Public	Distance Learning:	No

NLN ACCREDITATION: Yes

Articulation: LPN to Associate

For Further Information Contact:

Mrs Flora Knutson, Supv
Illinois Central College
1 College Dr
East Peoria, IL 61635
(309) 694-5011

Illinois Eastern Community Colleges
(3 Branches)
—Olney—

Full-Time Enrollments:	50	Evening Classes:	No
Part-Time Enrollments:	83	Weekend Classes:	No
Affiliation:	Public	Distance Learning:	No

NLN ACCREDITATION: Yes

Articulation: None

For Further Information Contact:

Dr Judy Johnson, Associate Dean
Illinois Eastern Community Colleges (3 Branches)
305 North West St
Olney, IL 62450
(618) 395-4351

Illinois Valley Community College
—Oglesby—

Full-Time Enrollments:	10	Evening Classes:	No
Part-Time Enrollments:	130	Weekend Classes:	No
Affiliation:	Public	Distance Learning:	No

NLN ACCREDITATION: Yes

Articulation: Associate to Baccalaureate
LPN to Associate

For Further Information Contact:

Mrs Bonnie Grusk, Director
Illinois Valley Community College
2578 E 350th Rd
Oglesby, IL 61348
(815) 224-2720

John Logan College
—Caterville—

Full-Time Enrollments:	36	Evening Classes:	Yes
Part-Time Enrollments:	36	Weekend Classes:	Yes
Affiliation:	Public	Distance Learning:	—

NLN ACCREDITATION: No

Articulation: Associate to Baccalaureate
LPN to Associate

For Further Information Contact:

Mrs Anne Williams, Director
John Logan College
RR#2
Caterville, IL 62918
(618) 985-3741

John Wood Community College
—Quincy—

Full-Time Enrollments:	28	Evening Classes:	Yes
Part-Time Enrollments:	25	Weekend Classes:	No
Affiliation:	Public	Distance Learning:	Yes

NLN ACCREDITATION: No

Articulation: Associate to Baccalaureate

For Further Information Contact:

Mrs Julie Barry, Director
John Wood Community College
150 South 48th St
Quincy, IL 62302
(217) 224-6500

Joliet Jr College-Nursing Education
—Joliet—

Full-Time Enrollments:	200	Evening Classes:	Yes
Part-Time Enrollments:	29	Weekend Classes:	Yes
Affiliation:	Public	Distance Learning:	No

NLN ACCREDITATION: Yes

Articulation: Associate to Baccalaureate
LPN to Associate

For Further Information Contact:

Ms Michaelene Nash, Chair
Joliet Jr College-Nursing Education
1216 Houbolt Rd
Joliet, IL 60436
(815) 729-9020

Kankakee Community College
—Kankakee—

Full-Time Enrollments:	67	Evening Classes:	—
Part-Time Enrollments:	43	Weekend Classes:	—
Affiliation:	Public	Distance Learning:	—

NLN ACCREDITATION: No

Articulation: None

For Further Information Contact:

Mrs Phyllis Nichols, Director
Kankakee Community College
Box 888 River Rd
Kankakee, IL 60901
(815) 933-0295

Kaskaskia College
—Centralia—

Full-Time Enrollments:	139	Evening Classes:	Yes
Part-Time Enrollments:	52	Weekend Classes:	Yes
Affiliation:	Public	Distance Learning:	Yes

NLN ACCREDITATION: Yes

Articulation: Associate to Baccalaureate
LPN to Associate

For Further Information Contact:

Mrs Marylou Whitten, Director
Kaskaskia College
27210 College Rd
Centralia, IL 62801
(618) 532-1981

Kennedy-King College-Chicago City Colleges
—Chicago—

Full-Time Enrollments:	190	Evening Classes:	—
Part-Time Enrollments:	—	Weekend Classes:	—
Affiliation:	Public	Distance Learning:	—

NLN ACCREDITATION: Yes

Articulation: None

For Further Information Contact:

Dr Barbara Norman, Chair
Kennedy-King College-Chicago City Colleges
6800 S Wentworth Ave
Chicago, IL 60621
(312) 602-5222

Kishwaukee College
—Malta—

Full-Time Enrollments:	—	Evening Classes:	—
Part-Time Enrollments:	—	Weekend Classes:	—
Affiliation:	Public	Distance Learning:	—

NLN ACCREDITATION: No

Articulation: None

For Further Information Contact:

Ms Heather Peters, Director
Kishwaukee College
21193 Malta Rd
Malta, IL 60150
(815) 825-2086

Lake Land College
—Matton—

Full-Time Enrollments:	6	Evening Classes:	No
Part-Time Enrollments:	59	Weekend Classes:	No
Affiliation:	Public	Distance Learning:	No

NLN ACCREDITATION: Yes

Articulation: LPN to Associate

For Further Information Contact:

Kathleen M Doehring, Director
Lake Land College
5001 Lake Land Blvd
Matton, IL 61938
(217) 235-3131

Lewis and Clark Community College
—Godfrey—

Full-Time Enrollments:	123	Evening Classes:	No
Part-Time Enrollments:	32	Weekend Classes:	No
Affiliation:	Public	Distance Learning:	No

NLN ACCREDITATION: Yes

Articulation: Associate to Baccalaureate
LPN to Associate

For Further Information Contact:

Dr Linda Harner, Coordinator
Lewis and Clark Community College
5800 Godfrey Rd
Godfrey, IL 62002
(618) 466-3411

Lincoln Land Community College
—Springfield—

Full-Time Enrollments:	154	Evening Classes:	Yes
Part-Time Enrollments:	—	Weekend Classes:	No
Affiliation:	Public	Distance Learning:	No

NLN ACCREDITATION: Yes

Articulation: Associate to Baccalaureate
LPN to Associate

For Further Information Contact:

Mrs Joan C Lewis, Chair
Lincoln Land Community College
Shepherd Rd
Springfield, IL 62794
(217) 786-2436

Malcolm X College-Chicago City Colleges
—Chicago—

Full-Time Enrollments:	106	Evening Classes:	No
Part-Time Enrollments:	—	Weekend Classes:	No
Affiliation:	Public	Distance Learning:	No

NLN ACCREDITATION: No

Articulation: None

For Further Information Contact:

Mrs Shirley Howard, Chair
Malcolm X College-Chicago City Colleges
1900 W Van Buren
Chicago, IL 60612
(312) 850-7000

Moraine Valley Community College
—Palos Hills—

Full-Time Enrollments:	91	Evening Classes:	No
Part-Time Enrollments:	57	Weekend Classes:	No
Affiliation:	Public	Distance Learning:	No

NLN ACCREDITATION: Yes

Articulation: LPN to Associate

For Further Information Contact:

Mrs Margaret Moe, Chair
Moraine Valley Community College
10900 S 88th Ave
Palos Hills, IL 60465
(708) 974-5708

Morton College
—Cicero—

Full-Time Enrollments:	91	Evening Classes:	No
Part-Time Enrollments:	—	Weekend Classes:	Yes
Affiliation:	Public	Distance Learning:	No

NLN ACCREDITATION: No

Articulation: Associate to Baccalaureate

For Further Information Contact:

Mrs Aline Tupa, Coordinator
Morton College
3801 S Central
Cicero, IL 60650
(708) 656-8000

Oakton Community College Nursing Program
—Des Plaines—

Full-Time Enrollments:	143	Evening Classes:	Yes
Part-Time Enrollments:	—	Weekend Classes:	Yes
Affiliation:	Public	Distance Learning:	—

NLN ACCREDITATION: Yes

Articulation: Associate to Baccalaureate
LPN to Associate

For Further Information Contact:

Ms Marilou A Wasseluk, Chair
Oakton Community College Nursing Program
1600 East Golf Rd
Des Plaines, IL 60016
(847) 635-1720

Olive-Harvey College-Chicago City Colleges
—Chicago—

Full-Time Enrollments:	100	Evening Classes:	No
Part-Time Enrollments:	—	Weekend Classes:	No
Affiliation:	Public	Distance Learning:	No

NLN ACCREDITATION: No

Articulation: None

For Further Information Contact:

Dr Rosarica Naron, Chair
Olive-Harvey College-Chicago City Colleges
10001 S Woodlawn Ave
Chicago, IL 60628
(773) 291-3700

Parkland College
—Champaign—

Full-Time Enrollments:	301	Evening Classes:	Yes
Part-Time Enrollments:	—	Weekend Classes:	Yes
Affiliation:	Public	Distance Learning:	No

NLN ACCREDITATION: Yes

Articulation: LPN to Associate

For Further Information Contact:

Dr Sharon Gerth, Chair
Parkland College
2400 W Bradley
Champaign, IL 61821
(217) 351-2480

Prairie State College
—Chicago Heights—

Full-Time Enrollments:	146	Evening Classes:	Yes
Part-Time Enrollments:	—	Weekend Classes:	Yes
Affiliation:	Public	Distance Learning:	Yes

NLN ACCREDITATION: Yes

Articulation: Associate to Baccalaureate

For Further Information Contact:

Ms Patricia L Hunter, Chair
Prairie State College
202 S Halsted St
Chicago Heights, IL 60411
(708) 709-3529

Rent Lake College
—Ina—

Full-Time Enrollments:	—	Evening Classes:	—
Part-Time Enrollments:	—	Weekend Classes:	—
Affiliation:	Public	Distance Learning:	—

NLN ACCREDITATION:

Articulation: None

For Further Information Contact:

Mrs Wilanna Patton, Chair
Rent Lake College
Rt 1
Ina, IL 62846
(618) 437-5321

Richard J Daley College-Chicago City Colleges
—Chicago—

Full-Time Enrollments:	58	Evening Classes:	No
Part-Time Enrollments:	60	Weekend Classes:	No
Affiliation:	Public	Distance Learning:	No

NLN ACCREDITATION: Yes

Articulation: Associate to Baccalaureate
LPN to Associate

For Further Information Contact:

Prof Teresita Manzano, Director
Richard J Daley College-Chicago City Colleges
7500 S Pulaski Rd
Chicago, IL 60652
(773) 838-7684

Richland Community College
—Decatur—

Full-Time Enrollments:	20	Evening Classes:	Yes
Part-Time Enrollments:	49	Weekend Classes:	—
Affiliation:	Public	Distance Learning:	—

NLN ACCREDITATION: Yes

Articulation: None

For Further Information Contact:

Dr Lois Hamilton, Dean
Richland Community College
One College Park
Decatur, IL 62521
(217) 875-7200

Rock Valley College
—Rockford—

Full-Time Enrollments:	4	Evening Classes:	—
Part-Time Enrollments:	80	Weekend Classes:	—
Affiliation:	Public	Distance Learning:	—

NLN ACCREDITATION: No

Articulation: None

For Further Information Contact:

Ms Iva Schumude, Director
Rock Valley College
3301 N Mulford Rd
Rockford, IL 61114
(815) 654-4409

Sauk Valley Community College
—Dixon—

Full-Time Enrollments:	36	Evening Classes:	No
Part-Time Enrollments:	—	Weekend Classes:	No
Affiliation:	Public	Distance Learning:	No

NLN ACCREDITATION: No

Articulation: LPN to Associate

For Further Information Contact:

Ms Rosemary Johnson, Director
Sauk Valley Community College
173 Illinois Route #2
Dixon, IL 61021
(815) 288-5511

Shawnee Community College
—Ullin—

Full-Time Enrollments:	—	Evening Classes:	—
Part-Time Enrollments:	—	Weekend Classes:	—
Affiliation:	Private	Distance Learning:	—

NLN ACCREDITATION: No

Articulation: None

For Further Information Contact:

Dr Jeannine Hayduk, Director
Shawnee Community College
Route 1 Box 53
Ullin, IL 62992
(618) 634-2242

South Suburban College
—South Holland—

Full-Time Enrollments:	—	Evening Classes:	—
Part-Time Enrollments:	—	Weekend Classes:	—
Affiliation:	Public	Distance Learning:	—

NLN ACCREDITATION: Yes

Articulation: —

For Further Information Contact:

Mrs Judith Coglianese, Exec Director
South Suburban College
15800 S State
South Holland, IL 60473
(708) 596-2000

Southeastern Illinois College
—Harrisburgh—

Full-Time Enrollments:	—	Evening Classes:	—
Part-Time Enrollments:	—	Weekend Classes:	—
Affiliation:	Public	Distance Learning:	—

NLN ACCREDITATION: Yes

Articulation: None

For Further Information Contact:

Ms Nancy Buttry, Director
Southeastern Illinois College
3575 College Rd
Harrisburgh, IL 62946
(618) 252-6376

Spoon River College
—Canton—

Full-Time Enrollments: 20
Part-Time Enrollments: —
Affiliation: Public

Evening Classes: No
Weekend Classes: No
Distance Learning: No

NLN ACCREDITATION: No

Articulation: Associate to Baccalaureate
LPN to Baccalaureate

For Further Information Contact:

Ms Beverly Breitfield, Associate Dean
Spoon River College
23235 N County 22
Canton, IL 61520
(309) 647-4645

Trinity College of Nursing
—Moline—

Full-Time Enrollments: 56
Part-Time Enrollments: 45
Affiliation: Private

Evening Classes: Yes
Weekend Classes: No
Distance Learning: Yes

NLN ACCREDITATION:

Articulation: None

For Further Information Contact:

Ms Jo Ellen Sharer, President
Trinity College of Nursing
501 10th Ave
Moline, IL 61265
(309) 757-2910

Triton College
—River Grove—

Full-Time Enrollments: 248
Part-Time Enrollments: —
Affiliation: Public

Evening Classes: Yes
Weekend Classes: Yes
Distance Learning: No

NLN ACCREDITATION: Yes

Articulation: Associate to Baccalaureate

For Further Information Contact:

Mrs Joan Libner, Chair
Triton College
2000 5th Ave
River Grove, IL 60171
(708) 456-0300

Truman College-Chicago City Colleges
—Chicago—

Full-Time Enrollments: 159
Part-Time Enrollments: —
Affiliation: Public

Evening Classes: No
Weekend Classes: No
Distance Learning: No

NLN ACCREDITATION: Yes

Articulation: Associate to Baccalaureate

For Further Information Contact:

Ms Jean Weimer, Chair
Truman College-Chicago City Colleges
1145 W Wilson Ave
Chicago, IL 60640
(773) 878-1700

Waubonsee Community College
—Sugar Grove—

Full-Time Enrollments: 118
Part-Time Enrollments: —
Affiliation: Public

Evening Classes: No
Weekend Classes: No
Distance Learning: No

NLN ACCREDITATION: No

Articulation: None

For Further Information Contact:

Ms Joan M Flanagan, Associate Dean
Waubonsee Community College
Route 47 at Harter Rd
Sugar Grove, IL 60554
(630) 466-4811

William Rainey Harper College
—Palatine—

Full-Time Enrollments: 64
Part-Time Enrollments: 165
Affiliation: Public

Evening Classes: No
Weekend Classes: Yes
Distance Learning: No

NLN ACCREDITATION: Yes

Articulation: Associate to Baccalaureate
LPN to Associate

For Further Information Contact:

Ms Judith R Dincher, Director
William Rainey Harper College
1200 West Algonquin Rd
Palatine, IL 60067
(847) 925-6533

Indiana

Ball State University
—Muncie—

Full-Time Enrollments:	41	Evening Classes:	Yes
Part-Time Enrollments:	3	Weekend Classes:	No
Affiliation:	Public	Distance Learning:	Yes

NLN ACCREDITATION: Yes

Articulation: Associate to Baccalaureate
RN to MSN

For Further Information Contact:

Mrs Linda Siktberg, Associate Director
Ball State University
2000 Univ Ave
Muncie, IN 47306
(317) 285-5571

Bethel College
—Mishawaka—

Full-Time Enrollments:	50	Evening Classes:	No
Part-Time Enrollments:	31	Weekend Classes:	No
Affiliation:	Religious	Distance Learning:	No

NLN ACCREDITATION: Yes

Articulation: Associate to Baccalaureate

For Further Information Contact:

Dr Ruth Davidhizar, Dean
Bethel College
1001 West Mckinley Ave
Mishawaka, IN 46545
(219) 259-8511

IUPU Fort Wayne/Parkview Hospital
—Fort Wayne—

Full-Time Enrollments:	80	Evening Classes:	Yes
Part-Time Enrollments:	171	Weekend Classes:	Yes
Affiliation:	Public	Distance Learning:	Yes

NLN ACCREDITATION: Yes

Articulation: Associate to Baccalaureate
LPN to Associate

For Further Information Contact:

Dr Elaine W Cowen, Chair
IUPU Fort Wayne/Parkview Hospital
2101 Coliseum Blvd E
Fort Wayne, IN 46805
(219) 481-6816

IVY State College
—Indianapolis—

Full-Time Enrollments:	83	Evening Classes:	Yes
Part-Time Enrollments:	—	Weekend Classes:	Yes
Affiliation:	Public	Distance Learning:	Yes

NLN ACCREDITATION: Yes

Articulation: LPN to Associate

For Further Information Contact:

Mrs Janet Kramer, Chair
IVY State College
One West 26th St
Indianapolis, IN 46206-1763
(317) 927-7177

IVY Technical State College
—Lafayette—

Full-Time Enrollments:	70	Evening Classes:	Yes
Part-Time Enrollments:	—	Weekend Classes:	Yes
Affiliation:	Public	Distance Learning:	No

NLN ACCREDITATION: Yes

Articulation: Associate to Baccalaureate
LPN to Associate

For Further Information Contact:

Mrs Karen Dolk, Chair
IVY Technical State College
3101 S Creasy Lane Box 6299
Lafayette, IN 47903
(317) 772-9192

Indiana State University
—Terre Haute—

Full-Time Enrollments:	200	Evening Classes:	Yes
Part-Time Enrollments:	141	Weekend Classes:	Yes
Affiliation:	Public	Distance Learning:	No

NLN ACCREDITATION: Yes

Articulation: Associate to Baccalaureate

For Further Information Contact:

Dr Ann Tomey, Dean
Indiana State University
Terre Haute, IN 47809
(812) 237-2323

Indiana University
—Indianapolis—

Full-Time Enrollments:	58	Evening Classes:	No
Part-Time Enrollments:	185	Weekend Classes:	No
Affiliation:	Public	Distance Learning:	No

NLN ACCREDITATION: Yes

Articulation: Associate to Baccalaureate
LPN to Associate
RN to MSN

For Further Information Contact:

Dr Angela McBride, Univ Dean
Indiana University
1111 Middle Dr
Indianapolis, IN 46223-5107
(317) 274-1486

Indiana University East
—Richmond—

Full-Time Enrollments:	20	Evening Classes:	Yes
Part-Time Enrollments:	51	Weekend Classes:	Yes
Affiliation:	Public	Distance Learning:	Yes

NLN ACCREDITATION: Yes

Articulation: Associate to Baccalaureate
Diploma to Baccalaureate
LPN to Associate

For Further Information Contact:

Dr Joanne Rains, Dean
Indiana University East
2325 Chester Blvd
Richmond, IN 47374
(317) 973-8205

Indiana University Kokomo
—Kokomo—

Full-Time Enrollments:	16	Evening Classes:	Yes
Part-Time Enrollments:	102	Weekend Classes:	—
Affiliation:	Public	Distance Learning:	—

NLN ACCREDITATION: Yes

Articulation: Associate to Baccalaureate
LPN to Associate

For Further Information Contact:

Dr Penny Cass, Dean
Indiana University Kokomo
2300 S Washington St Box 9003
Kokomo, IN 46904-9003
(317) 455-9288

Indiana University Northwest
—Gary—

Full-Time Enrollments:	50	Evening Classes:	Yes
Part-Time Enrollments:	107	Weekend Classes:	Yes
Affiliation:	Public	Distance Learning:	Yes

NLN ACCREDITATION: Yes

Articulation: Associate to Baccalaureate
Diploma to Baccalaureate
LPN to Associate

For Further Information Contact:

Dr Doris R Blaney, Dean
Indiana University Northwest
3400 Broadway
Gary, IN 46408
(219) 980-6603

Indiana University South Bend
—South Bend—

Full-Time Enrollments:	38	Evening Classes:	Yes
Part-Time Enrollments:	19	Weekend Classes:	Yes
Affiliation:	Public	Distance Learning:	Yes

NLN ACCREDITATION: Yes

Articulation: None

For Further Information Contact:

Dr Marian Pettengill, Dean
Indiana University South Bend
1700 Mishawaka PO Box 7111
South Bend, IN 46634
(219) 237-4282

Indiana Vocational Technical College
—Evansville—

Full-Time Enrollments:	72	Evening Classes:	No
Part-Time Enrollments:	—	Weekend Classes:	No
Affiliation:	Public	Distance Learning:	No

NLN ACCREDITATION: Yes

Articulation: Associate to Baccalaureate

For Further Information Contact:

Ms Judith McCutchan, Chair
Indiana Vocational Technical College
3501 First Ave
Evansville, IN 47710
(812) 429-1383

Indiana Vocational Technical College
Region 10
—Bloomington—

Full-Time Enrollments:	59	Evening Classes:	Yes
Part-Time Enrollments:	—	Weekend Classes:	No
Affiliation:	Public	Distance Learning:	No

NLN ACCREDITATION: No

Articulation: Associate to Baccalaureate
LPN to Associate

For Further Information Contact:

Dr Edith Collins, Chair
Indiana Vocational Technical College Region 10
3116 Canterbury Court
Bloomington, IN 47404
(812) 332-1559

Indiana Vocational Technical College
Region 1
—Gary—

Full-Time Enrollments:	46	Evening Classes:	No
Part-Time Enrollments:	—	Weekend Classes:	Yes
Affiliation:	Public	Distance Learning:	No

NLN ACCREDITATION: No

Articulation: LPN to Associate

For Further Information Contact:

Mrs Socorro Roman, Chair
Indiana Vocational Technical College Region 1
1440 East 35th Ave
Gary, IN 46409
(219) 981-1111

Indiana Vocational Technical College
Region 11
—Madison—

Full-Time Enrollments:	29	Evening Classes:	No
Part-Time Enrollments:	—	Weekend Classes:	No
Affiliation:	Public	Distance Learning:	No

NLN ACCREDITATION: No

Articulation: Associate to Baccalaureate

For Further Information Contact:

Ms Gene Ann Shapinsky, Chair
Indiana Vocational Technical College Region 11
Highway 62 & Ivy Tech Dr
Madison, IN 47250
(812) 265-2580

Indiana Vocational Technical College
Region 9
—Richmond—

Full-Time Enrollments:	27	Evening Classes:	No
Part-Time Enrollments:	—	Weekend Classes:	No
Affiliation:	Public	Distance Learning:	No

NLN ACCREDITATION: Yes

Articulation: None

For Further Information Contact:

Mrs Jillene Anderson, Chair
Indiana Vocational Technical College Region 9
2325 Chester Blvd
Richmond, IN 47374
(317) 983-3210

Indiana Vocational Technical College
Region 13
—Sellerburg—

Full-Time Enrollments:	96	Evening Classes:	—
Part-Time Enrollments:	—	Weekend Classes:	—
Affiliation:	Public	Distance Learning:	—

NLN ACCREDITATION: No

Articulation: None

For Further Information Contact:

Mrs Donna Reeves, Chair
Indiana Vocational Technical College Region 13
8204 Highway 311
Sellerburg, IN 47172
(812) 246-3301

Indiana Vocational Technical College
Region 2
—South Bend—

Full-Time Enrollments:	53	Evening Classes:	Yes
Part-Time Enrollments:	10	Weekend Classes:	Yes
Affiliation:	Public	Distance Learning:	Yes

NLN ACCREDITATION: Yes

Articulation: LPN to Associate

For Further Information Contact:

Mrs Susan Sypniewski, Chair
Indiana Vocational Technical College Region 2
1538 W Sample St
South Bend, IN 46619
(219) 289-7001

Lutheran College
—Fort Wayne—

Full-Time Enrollments:	125	Evening Classes:	Yes
Part-Time Enrollments:	192	Weekend Classes:	—
Affiliation:	Religious	Distance Learning:	—

NLN ACCREDITATION: Yes

Articulation: None

For Further Information Contact:

Ms Vicky Kirkton, Associate Dean
Lutheran College
3024 Fairfield Ave
Fort Wayne, IN 46807-1697
(219) 458-2451

Marian College
—Indianapolis—

Full-Time Enrollments:	27	Evening Classes:	Yes
Part-Time Enrollments:	61	Weekend Classes:	Yes
Affiliation:	Religious	Distance Learning:	No

NLN ACCREDITATION: Yes

Articulation: Associate to Baccalaureate
Diploma to Baccalaureate
LPN to Associate

For Further Information Contact:

Dr Esther O'Dea, Chair
Marian College
3200 Cold Spring Rd
Indianapolis, IN 46222
(317) 929-0331

Purdue University-Calumet Campus
—Hammond—

Full-Time Enrollments:	188	Evening Classes:	Yes
Part-Time Enrollments:	47	Weekend Classes:	No
Affiliation:	Public	Distance Learning:	Yes

NLN ACCREDITATION: Yes

Articulation: LPN to Associate

For Further Information Contact:

Ms Gloria Smokvina, Dept Head
Purdue University-Calumet Campus
2233 171st St
Hammond, IN 46323
(219) 989-2813

Purdue University-North Central Campus
—Westville—

Full-Time Enrollments:	156	Evening Classes:	Yes
Part-Time Enrollments:	45	Weekend Classes:	No
Affiliation:	Public	Distance Learning:	Yes

NLN ACCREDITATION: Yes

Articulation: LPN to Associate

For Further Information Contact:

Mrs Marilyn Asteriadis, Chair
Purdue University-North Central Campus
1401 S US 421
Westville, IN 46391-9528
(219) 872-0527

University of Indianapolis
—Indianapolis—

Full-Time Enrollments:	7	Evening Classes:	No
Part-Time Enrollments:	68	Weekend Classes:	No
Affiliation:	Religious	Distance Learning:	No

NLN ACCREDITATION: Yes

Articulation: None

For Further Information Contact:

Mrs Susan Kuhn, Coordinator
University of Indianapolis
1400 E Hanna Ave
Indianapolis, IN 46227
(317) 788-3206

University of Southern Indiana School of Nursing
—Evansville—

Full-Time Enrollments:	—	Evening Classes:	—
Part-Time Enrollments:	—	Weekend Classes:	—
Affiliation:	Public	Distance Learning:	—

NLN ACCREDITATION: No

Articulation: None

For Further Information Contact:

Dr Nadine A Coudret, Dean
University of Southern Indiana School of Nursing
8600 University Blvd
Evansville, IN 47712-3534
(812) 428-7256

Vincennes University
—Vincennes—

Full-Time Enrollments:	156	Evening Classes:	Yes
Part-Time Enrollments:	59	Weekend Classes:	No
Affiliation:	Public	Distance Learning:	No

NLN ACCREDITATION: Yes

Articulation: Associate to Baccalaureate

For Further Information Contact:

Mrs Julie Herrold, Chair
Vincennes University
Vincennes, IN 47591
(812) 885-4413

Iowa

Des Moines Area Community College-Ankeny Campus
—Ankeny—

Full-Time Enrollments:	60	Evening Classes:	Yes
Part-Time Enrollments:	20	Weekend Classes:	Yes
Affiliation:	Public	Distance Learning:	Yes

NLN ACCREDITATION: Yes

Articulation: Associate to Baccalaureate
LPN to Associate

For Further Information Contact:

Ms Susan Wager, Director
Des Moines Area Community College-Ankeny Campus
2006 Ankeny Blvd Bldg 9
Ankeny, IA 50021
(515) 964-6316

Des Moines Area Community College-Boone Campus
—Boone—

Full-Time Enrollments:	33	Evening Classes:	Yes
Part-Time Enrollments:	5	Weekend Classes:	Yes
Affiliation:	Public	Distance Learning:	Yes

NLN ACCREDITATION: Yes

Articulation: Associate to Baccalaureate
LPN to Associate

For Further Information Contact:

Ms Susan Wager, Director
Des Moines Area Community College-Boone Campus
1125 Hancock Dr
Boone, IA 50036
(515) 432-7203

Des Moines Area Community College-Carroll Campus
—Carroll—

Full-Time Enrollments:	—	Evening Classes:	Yes
Part-Time Enrollments:	5	Weekend Classes:	Yes
Affiliation:	Public	Distance Learning:	Yes

NLN ACCREDITATION: Yes

Articulation: Associate to Baccalaureate
LPN to Associate

For Further Information Contact:

Ms Susan Wager, Director
Des Moines Area Community College-Carroll Campus
906 North Grant Rd
Carroll, IA 51401
(515) 244-4226

Eastern Iowa Community College-Clinton Community College
—Clinton—

Full-Time Enrollments:	15	Evening Classes:	—
Part-Time Enrollments:	—	Weekend Classes:	—
Affiliation:	Public	Distance Learning:	—

NLN ACCREDITATION: No

Articulation: None

For Further Information Contact:

Ms Nancy E Knutstrom, Coordinator
Eastern Iowa Community College-Clinton Community College
1000 Lincoln Blvd
Clinton, IA 52732-6299
(319) 242-6841

Eastern Iowa Community College-Scott Community College
—Bettendorf—

Full-Time Enrollments:	79	Evening Classes:	—
Part-Time Enrollments:	52	Weekend Classes:	—
Affiliation:	Public	Distance Learning:	—

NLN ACCREDITATION: No

Articulation: None

For Further Information Contact:

Ms Nancy E Knutstrom, Coordinator
Eastern Iowa Community College-Scott Community College
500 Belmont Rd
Bettendorf, IA 52722-6804
(319) 359-7531

ASSOCIATE DEGREE

Ellsworth Community College/Iowa Valley CC Dist
—Iowa Falls—

Full-Time Enrollments:	16	Evening Classes:	Yes
Part-Time Enrollments:	1	Weekend Classes:	No
Affiliation:	Public	Distance Learning:	No

NLN ACCREDITATION: No

Articulation: Associate to Baccalaureate
LPN to Associate

For Further Information Contact:

Mrs Mavis A Hunt, Coordinator
Ellsworth Community College/Iowa Valley CC Dist
1100 College Ave
Iowa Falls, IA 50126
(515) 648-4611

Hawkeye Community College
—Waterloo—

Full-Time Enrollments:	30	Evening Classes:	—
Part-Time Enrollments:	28	Weekend Classes:	—
Affiliation:	Public	Distance Learning:	—

NLN ACCREDITATION: No

Articulation: None

For Further Information Contact:

Mrs Brenda Berry, Coordinator
Hawkeye Community College
1501 E Orange Rd Box 8015
Waterloo, IA 50704-8015
(319) 296-2320

Indian Hills Community College
—Ottumwa—

Full-Time Enrollments:	—	Evening Classes:	—
Part-Time Enrollments:	—	Weekend Classes:	—
Affiliation:	Public	Distance Learning:	—

NLN ACCREDITATION: No

Articulation: None

For Further Information Contact:

Ms M Ann Aulwes, Dept Chair
Indian Hills Community College
525 Grandview
Ottumwa, IA 52501
(515) 683-5165

Iowa Central Community College-Fort Dodge
—Fort Dodge—

Full-Time Enrollments:	91	Evening Classes:	Yes
Part-Time Enrollments:	53	Weekend Classes:	No
Affiliation:	Public	Distance Learning:	Yes

NLN ACCREDITATION: Yes

Articulation: Associate to Baccalaureate
LPN to Associate

For Further Information Contact:

Mrs Brenda Gleason, Director
Iowa Central Community College-Fort Dodge
330 Avenue M
Fort Dodge, IA 50501
(515) 576-0099

Iowa Central Community College-Storm Lake
—Storm Lake—

Full-Time Enrollments:	13	Evening Classes:	Yes
Part-Time Enrollments:	12	Weekend Classes:	Yes
Affiliation:	Public	Distance Learning:	Yes

NLN ACCREDITATION: No

Articulation: LPN to Associate

For Further Information Contact:

Mrs Brenda Gleason, Director
Iowa Central Community College-Storm Lake
916 N Russell St
Storm Lake, IA 50588
(515) 576-7201

Iowa Central Community College-Webster City
—Webster City—

Full-Time Enrollments:	18	Evening Classes:	Yes
Part-Time Enrollments:	27	Weekend Classes:	Yes
Affiliation:	Public	Distance Learning:	Yes

NLN ACCREDITATION: No

Articulation: Associate to Baccalaureate
LPN to Associate

For Further Information Contact:

Mrs Diane Sorensen, Coordinator
Iowa Central Community College-Webster City
1725 Beach St
Webster City, IA 50595
(515) 576-7201

Iowa Lakes Community College
—Emmetsburg—

Full-Time Enrollments: 73   Evening Classes: Yes
Part-Time Enrollments: —   Weekend Classes: Yes
Affiliation: Public   Distance Learning: Yes

NLN ACCREDITATION: No

Articulation: Associate to Baccalaureate
LPN to Associate

For Further Information Contact:

Mrs Judi Donahue, Director
Iowa Lakes Community College
3200 College Dr
Emmetsburg, IA 50536
(712) 852-3554

Iowa Valley Community College Dist
—Marshalltown—

Full-Time Enrollments: 30   Evening Classes: Yes
Part-Time Enrollments: —   Weekend Classes: No
Affiliation: Public   Distance Learning: No

NLN ACCREDITATION: No

Articulation: Associate to Baccalaureate
LPN to Associate

For Further Information Contact:

Mrs Mavis A Hunt, Coordinator
Iowa Valley Community College Dist
3700 S Center St
Marshalltown, IA 50158
(515) 752-7106

Iowa Western Community College
—Council Bluffs—

Full-Time Enrollments: 67   Evening Classes: Yes
Part-Time Enrollments: —   Weekend Classes: Yes
Affiliation: Public   Distance Learning: Yes

NLN ACCREDITATION: No

Articulation: Associate to Baccalaureate
LPN to Associate

For Further Information Contact:

Mrs Karen Sojka, Associate Dean
Iowa Western Community College
2700 College Rd Box 4C
Council Bluffs, IA 51502
(712) 325-3200

Kirkwood Community College
—Cedar Rapids—

Full-Time Enrollments: 172   Evening Classes: —
Part-Time Enrollments: 110   Weekend Classes: —
Affiliation: Public   Distance Learning: —

NLN ACCREDITATION: No

Articulation: None

For Further Information Contact:

Ms Ann M Woodward, Coordinator
Kirkwood Community College
6301 Kirkwood Blvd Box 2068
Cedar Rapids, IA 52406
(319) 398-5630

Mercy College Health Science
—Des Moines—

Full-Time Enrollments: 33   Evening Classes: No
Part-Time Enrollments: 26   Weekend Classes: No
Affiliation: Private   Distance Learning: No

NLN ACCREDITATION: No

Articulation: Associate to Baccalaureate
Diploma to Baccalaureate

For Further Information Contact:

Ms Helen Roberts, Assistant Dean
Mercy College Health Science
928 6th Ave
Des Moines, IA 50314
(512) 362-6614

North Iowa Area Community College
—Mason City—

Full-Time Enrollments: 85   Evening Classes: Yes
Part-Time Enrollments: 19   Weekend Classes: No
Affiliation: Public   Distance Learning: No

NLN ACCREDITATION: Yes

Articulation: Associate to Baccalaureate

For Further Information Contact:

Mrs Donna J Orton, Interim Chair
North Iowa Area Community College
500 College Dr
Mason City, IA 50401
(515) 422-4215

Northeast Iowa Community College
—Calmar—

Full-Time Enrollments: 82
Part-Time Enrollments: —
Affiliation: Public

Evening Classes: Yes
Weekend Classes: —
Distance Learning: —

NLN ACCREDITATION: No

Articulation: None

For Further Information Contact:

Mrs Melinda Hanson, Chair
Northeast Iowa Community College
Box 400 Hwy 150 South
Calmar, IA 52132
(319) 562-3263

Northeast Iowa Community College
—Peosta—

Full-Time Enrollments: —
Part-Time Enrollments: —
Affiliation: Public

Evening Classes: —
Weekend Classes: —
Distance Learning: —

NLN ACCREDITATION: No

Articulation: None

For Further Information Contact:

Ms Geraldine Althoff, Director
Northeast Iowa Community College
10250 Sundown Rd
Peosta, IA 52068
(319) 556-5110 Ext 209

Southeastern Community College
—Keokuk—

Full-Time Enrollments: 33
Part-Time Enrollments: 1
Affiliation: Public

Evening Classes: No
Weekend Classes: No
Distance Learning: No

NLN ACCREDITATION: No

Articulation: Associate to Baccalaureate
LPN to Associate

For Further Information Contact:

Mrs Anita M Stineman, Admin
Southeastern Community College
335 Messenger Rd PO Box 6007
Keokuk, IA 52632
(319) 752-2731

Southeastern Community College
—West Burlington—

Full-Time Enrollments: 58
Part-Time Enrollments: 2
Affiliation: Public

Evening Classes: Yes
Weekend Classes: No
Distance Learning: No

NLN ACCREDITATION: No

Articulation: Associate to Baccalaureate
LPN to Associate

For Further Information Contact:

Mrs Anita Stineman, Admin
Southeastern Community College
1015 S Gear Ave
West Burlington, IA 52655
(319) 752-2731

Southwestern Community College (2 Campuses)
—Creston—

Full-Time Enrollments: 67
Part-Time Enrollments: —
Affiliation: Public

Evening Classes: Yes
Weekend Classes: No
Distance Learning: Yes

NLN ACCREDITATION: No

Articulation: Associate to Baccalaureate

For Further Information Contact:

Mrs Loretta A Eckels, Chair
Southwestern Community College (2 Campuses)
1501 Townline Rd
Creston, IA 50801
(515) 782-7081

St Luke's College of Nursing and Health Sciences
—Sioux City—

Full-Time Enrollments: 36
Part-Time Enrollments: 10
Affiliation: Private

Evening Classes: No
Weekend Classes: No
Distance Learning: No

NLN ACCREDITATION: No

Articulation: Associate to Baccalaureate

For Further Information Contact:

Mrs Regene Osborne, President
St Luke's College of Nursing and Health Sciences
2720 Stone Park Blvd
Sioux City, IA 51104
(712) 279-3172

Western Iowa Technical Community College
—Sheldon—

Full-Time Enrollments:	—	Evening Classes:	—
Part-Time Enrollments:	—	Weekend Classes:	—
Affiliation:	Public	Distance Learning:	—

NLN ACCREDITATION: Yes

Articulation: None

For Further Information Contact:

Mrs Gloria Stewart, Dept Head
Western Iowa Technical Community College
Highway 18 West
Sheldon, IA 51201
(712) 274-6350

Western Iowa Technical Community College
—Sioux City—

Full-Time Enrollments:	—	Evening Classes:	—
Part-Time Enrollments:	—	Weekend Classes:	—
Affiliation:	Public	Distance Learning:	—

NLN ACCREDITATION: Yes

Articulation: None

For Further Information Contact:

Mrs Gloria M Stewart, Dept Head
Western Iowa Technical Community College
4647 Stone Ave
Sioux City, IA 51105
(712) 274-6321

Kansas

Barton County Community College
—Great Bend—

Full-Time Enrollments:	40	Evening Classes:	No
Part-Time Enrollments:	—	Weekend Classes:	No
Affiliation:	Public	Distance Learning:	No

NLN ACCREDITATION: Yes

Articulation: LPN to Associate

For Further Information Contact:

Ms Karla P Homan, Director
Barton County Community College
Great Bend, KS 67530
(316) 792-2701

Butler County Community College
—El Dorado—

Full-Time Enrollments:	174	Evening Classes:	No
Part-Time Enrollments:	—	Weekend Classes:	No
Affiliation:	Public	Distance Learning:	No

NLN ACCREDITATION: Yes

Articulation: LPN to Associate

For Further Information Contact:

Ms Patricia Bayles, Dean
Butler County Community College
901 S Haverhill Rd
El Dorado, KS 67042
(316) 322-3140

Cloud County Community College
—Beloit—

Full-Time Enrollments:	36	Evening Classes:	No
Part-Time Enrollments:	—	Weekend Classes:	No
Affiliation:	Public	Distance Learning:	No

NLN ACCREDITATION: Yes

Articulation: LPN to Associate

For Further Information Contact:

Mrs Vera Streit, Coordinator
Cloud County Community College
PO Box 507
Beloit, KS 67420
(913) 738-2259

Colby Community College
—Colby—

Full-Time Enrollments:	30	Evening Classes:	No
Part-Time Enrollments:	—	Weekend Classes:	No
Affiliation:	Public	Distance Learning:	No

NLN ACCREDITATION: Yes

Articulation: LPN to Associate

For Further Information Contact:

Mrs Anita Horinek, Director
Colby Community College
1255 S Range
Colby, KS 67701
(913) 462-3984

Dodge City Community College
—Dodge City—

Full-Time Enrollments:	17	Evening Classes:	No
Part-Time Enrollments:	12	Weekend Classes:	No
Affiliation:	Public	Distance Learning:	Yes

NLN ACCREDITATION: Yes

Articulation: None

For Further Information Contact:

Mrs Linda K Sanko, Director
Dodge City Community College
2501 14th Ave
Dodge City, KS 67801
(316) 225-1321

Fort Scott Community College
—Fort Scott—

Full-Time Enrollments:	41	Evening Classes:	No
Part-Time Enrollments:	32	Weekend Classes:	No
Affiliation:	Public	Distance Learning:	No

NLN ACCREDITATION: Yes

Articulation: Associate to Baccalaureate
LPN to Associate

For Further Information Contact:

Mrs Caroline Helton, Director
Fort Scott Community College
2108 S Horton
Fort Scott, KS 66701
(316) 223-2700

Garden City Community College
—Garden City—

Full-Time Enrollments:	70	Evening Classes:	No
Part-Time Enrollments:	—	Weekend Classes:	No
Affiliation:	Public	Distance Learning:	No

NLN ACCREDITATION: Yes

Articulation: LPN to Associate

For Further Information Contact:

Dr Evelyn Bowman, Director
Garden City Community College
801 Campus Dr
Garden City, KS 67846
(316) 276-7611

Hesston College
—Hesston—

Full-Time Enrollments:	62	Evening Classes:	No
Part-Time Enrollments:	15	Weekend Classes:	No
Affiliation:	Religious	Distance Learning:	No

NLN ACCREDITATION: Yes

Articulation: LPN to Associate

For Further Information Contact:

Ms Bonnie Sowers, Director
Hesston College
PO Box 3000
Hesston, KS 67062
(316) 327-8313

Hutchinson Community College
—Hutchinson—

Full-Time Enrollments:	28	Evening Classes:	Yes
Part-Time Enrollments:	36	Weekend Classes:	Yes
Affiliation:	Public	Distance Learning:	No

NLN ACCREDITATION: Yes

Articulation: LPN to Associate

For Further Information Contact:

Mrs Debra Dudrey, Director
Hutchinson Community College
1300 N Plum St
Hutchinson, KS 67501
(316) 665-4930

Johnson County Community College
—Overland Park—

Full-Time Enrollments:	85	Evening Classes:	No
Part-Time Enrollments:	19	Weekend Classes:	No
Affiliation:	Public	Distance Learning:	Yes

NLN ACCREDITATION: Yes

Articulation: Associate to Baccalaureate
LPN to Associate

For Further Information Contact:

Miss Jeanne Walsh, Director
Johnson County Community College
College Blvd at Quivira Rd
Overland Park, KS 66210
(913) 469-8500

Kansas City Kansas Community College
—Kansas City—

Full-Time Enrollments: 23 Evening Classes: No
Part-Time Enrollments: 147 Weekend Classes: No
Affiliation: Public Distance Learning: No

NLN ACCREDITATION: Yes

Articulation: LPN to Associate

For Further Information Contact:

Mrs Shirley Wendel, Dean
Kansas City Kansas Community College
7250 State Ave
Kansas City, KS 66112
(913) 334-1100

Kansas Newman College
—Wichita—

Full-Time Enrollments: 39 Evening Classes: No
Part-Time Enrollments: 25 Weekend Classes: No
Affiliation: Religious Distance Learning: No

NLN ACCREDITATION: Yes

Articulation: Associate to Baccalaureate
Diploma to Baccalaureate
LPN to Associate

closed 1998

For Further Information Contact:

Dr Joan Felts, Chair
Kansas Newman College
3100 McCormick Ave
Wichita, KS 67213
(316) 942-4291

Kansas Wesleyan University
—Salina—

Full-Time Enrollments: 53 Evening Classes: No
Part-Time Enrollments: 26 Weekend Classes: No
Affiliation: Religious Distance Learning: No

NLN ACCREDITATION: Yes

Articulation: Associate to Baccalaureate
Diploma to Baccalaureate
LPN to Associate

For Further Information Contact:

Dr Patricia Kissell, Director
Kansas Wesleyan University
100 E Claflin
Salina, KS 67402-6196
(913) 827-5541 Ext 7212

Labette Community College
—Parsons—

Full-Time Enrollments: 4 Evening Classes: No
Part-Time Enrollments: 112 Weekend Classes: No
Affiliation: Public Distance Learning: No

NLN ACCREDITATION: Yes

Articulation: Associate to Baccalaureate
LPN to Associate

For Further Information Contact:

Dr Wanda Maxson-Ladage, Director
Labette Community College
200 S 14th St
Parsons, KS 67357
(316) 421-6700

Neosho County Community College
—Chanute—

Full-Time Enrollments: 120 Evening Classes: No
Part-Time Enrollments: — Weekend Classes: No
Affiliation: Public Distance Learning: No

NLN ACCREDITATION: Yes

Articulation: LPN to Associate

For Further Information Contact:

Mrs Leona Beezley, Director
Neosho County Community College
1000 South Allen
Chanute, KS 66720-2699
(316) 431-2820

North Central Kansas Technical College
—Beloit—

Full-Time Enrollments: 33 Evening Classes: —
Part-Time Enrollments: — Weekend Classes: —
Affiliation: Public Distance Learning: —

NLN ACCREDITATION: No

Articulation: None

For Further Information Contact:

Mrs Vero Streit, Coordinator
North Central Kansas Technical College
PO Box 507
Beloit, KS 67420
(913) 738-9025

Pratt Community College & Area Vocational School
—Pratt—

Full-Time Enrollments:	57	Evening Classes:	No
Part-Time Enrollments:	—	Weekend Classes:	No
Affiliation:	Public	Distance Learning:	No

NLN ACCREDITATION: Yes

Articulation: Associate to Baccalaureate
LPN to Associate

For Further Information Contact:

Ms Donna Bauer, Dean
Pratt Community College & Area Vocational School
348 NE SR 61
Pratt, KS 67124-8317
(316) 672-5641

Seward County Community College
—Liberal—

Full-Time Enrollments:	18	Evening Classes:	No
Part-Time Enrollments:	2	Weekend Classes:	No
Affiliation:	Public	Distance Learning:	No

NLN ACCREDITATION: Yes

Articulation: LPN to Associate

For Further Information Contact:

Mr Steve Hecox, Chair
Seward County Community College
Box 1137
Liberal, KS 67901
(316) 626-3026

Kentucky

Ashland Community College
—Ashland—

Full-Time Enrollments:	31	Evening Classes:	Yes
Part-Time Enrollments:	81	Weekend Classes:	Yes
Affiliation:	Public	Distance Learning:	—

NLN ACCREDITATION: No

Articulation: LPN to Associate

For Further Information Contact:

Ms Janie R Kitchen, Coordinator
Ashland Community College
1400 College Dr
Ashland, KY 41101
(606) 329-2999

Eastern Kentucky University
—Richmond—

Full-Time Enrollments:	104	Evening Classes:	No
Part-Time Enrollments:	138	Weekend Classes:	No
Affiliation:	Public	Distance Learning:	No

NLN ACCREDITATION: Yes

Articulation: Associate to Baccalaureate

For Further Information Contact:

Dr Pat H Jarczewski, Chair
Eastern Kentucky University
Richmond, KY 40475
(606) 622-1942

Elizabethtown Community College
—Elizabethtown—

Full-Time Enrollments:	37	Evening Classes:	No
Part-Time Enrollments:	94	Weekend Classes:	No
Affiliation:	Public	Distance Learning:	No

NLN ACCREDITATION: Yes

Articulation: Associate to Baccalaureate
LPN to Associate

For Further Information Contact:

Mrs Martha L Hill, Coordinator
Elizabethtown Community College
600 College St Rd
Elizabethtown, KY 42701-2402
(502) 769-2371

Hazard Community College (2 Campuses)
—Hazard—

Full-Time Enrollments:	—	Evening Classes:	—
Part-Time Enrollments:	—	Weekend Classes:	—
Affiliation:	Public	Distance Learning:	—

NLN ACCREDITATION: No

Articulation: None

For Further Information Contact:

Mrs Donna Combs, Coordinator
Hazard Community College (2 Campuses)
One Community College Dr
Hazard, KY 41701-2402
(606) 436-5721

Henderson Community College (2 Campuses)
—Henderson—

Full-Time Enrollments:	59	Evening Classes:	No
Part-Time Enrollments:	81	Weekend Classes:	No
Affiliation:	Public	Distance Learning:	No

NLN ACCREDITATION: Yes

Articulation: LPN to Associate

For Further Information Contact:

Dr Mary G Wilder, Coordinator
Henderson Community College (2 Campuses)
2660 South Green St
Henderson, KY 42420-4699
(502) 827-1867

Hopkinsville Community College
—Hopkinsville—

Full-Time Enrollments:	—	Evening Classes:	—
Part-Time Enrollments:	—	Weekend Classes:	—
Affiliation:	Public	Distance Learning:	—

NLN ACCREDITATION: No

Articulation: None

For Further Information Contact:

Ms Patricia Bush, Coordinator
Hopkinsville Community College
PO Box 2100
Hopkinsville, KY 42241
(502) 886-3921

Jefferson Community College
—Louisville—

Full-Time Enrollments:	—	Evening Classes:	—
Part-Time Enrollments:	—	Weekend Classes:	—
Affiliation:	Public	Distance Learning:	—

NLN ACCREDITATION: Yes

Articulation: None

For Further Information Contact:

Mrs Margie Charasika, Coordinator
Jefferson Community College
PO Box 1036 109 East Broadway
Louisville, KY 40202
(502) 584-0181

Kentucky State University
—Frankfort—

Full-Time Enrollments:	85	Evening Classes:	Yes
Part-Time Enrollments:	15	Weekend Classes:	No
Affiliation:	Public	Distance Learning:	No

NLN ACCREDITATION: Yes

Articulation: Associate to Baccalaureate
LPN to Associate

For Further Information Contact:

Mrs Patsy O Turner, Chair
Kentucky State University
East Main St
Frankfort, KY 40601
(502) 227-5957

Kentucky Wesleyan College
—Owensboro—

Full-Time Enrollments:	35	Evening Classes:	No
Part-Time Enrollments:	13	Weekend Classes:	No
Affiliation:	Religious	Distance Learning:	No

NLN ACCREDITATION: Yes

Articulation: None

For Further Information Contact:

Dr Elizabeth G Johnson, Chair
Kentucky Wesleyan College
3000 Frederica St Box 1039
Owensboro, KY 42302-1039
(502) 926-3111

Lexington Community College
—Lexington—

Full-Time Enrollments:	111	Evening Classes:	Yes
Part-Time Enrollments:	65	Weekend Classes:	No
Affiliation:	Public	Distance Learning:	No

NLN ACCREDITATION: Yes

Articulation: Associate to Baccalaureate
LPN to Associate

For Further Information Contact:

Ms Gail Carpenter, Coordinator
Lexington Community College
303 Oswald Bldg Cooper Dr
Lexington, KY 40506-0235
(606) 257-1029

ASSOCIATE DEGREE

Lincoln Memorial University
—Harrogate—

Full-Time Enrollments:	21	Evening Classes:	No
Part-Time Enrollments:	29	Weekend Classes:	No
Affiliation:	Private	Distance Learning:	No

NLN ACCREDITATION: Yes

Articulation: None

For Further Information Contact:

Mrs Elizabeth Yeary, Chair
Lincoln Memorial University
Box 1202
Harrogate, TN 37775
(615) 896-3611

Madisonville Community College
—Madisonville—

Full-Time Enrollments:	50	Evening Classes:	Yes
Part-Time Enrollments:	86	Weekend Classes:	No
Affiliation:	Public	Distance Learning:	No

NLN ACCREDITATION: Yes

Articulation: LPN to Associate

For Further Information Contact:

Mrs Linda Thomas, Coordinator
Madisonville Community College
2000 College Dr
Madisonville, KY 42431
(502) 821-2250

Maysville Community College
—Maysville—

Full-Time Enrollments:	21	Evening Classes:	Yes
Part-Time Enrollments:	43	Weekend Classes:	No
Affiliation:	Public	Distance Learning:	No

NLN ACCREDITATION: No

Articulation: Associate to Baccalaureate
LPN to Associate

For Further Information Contact:

Mrs Connie Lowe, Coordinator
Maysville Community College
1755 US 68
Maysville, KY 41056
(606) 759-7141

Midway College (2 Campuses)
—Midway—

Full-Time Enrollments:	72	Evening Classes:	—
Part-Time Enrollments:	47	Weekend Classes:	—
Affiliation:	Religious	Distance Learning:	—

NLN ACCREDITATION: Yes

Articulation: None

For Further Information Contact:

Mrs Patricia Emerson, Chair
Midway College (2 Campuses)
512 E Stephens St
Midway, KY 40347-1120
(606) 846-5337

Morehead State University
—Morehead—

Full-Time Enrollments:	69	Evening Classes:	No
Part-Time Enrollments:	10	Weekend Classes:	No
Affiliation:	Public	Distance Learning:	No

NLN ACCREDITATION: Yes

Articulation: None

For Further Information Contact:

Mrs Cheryl Clevenger, Coordinator
Morehead State University
214 A Lloyd Cassity
Morehead, KY 40351
(606) 783-2814

Northern Kentucky University
—Highland Heights—

Full-Time Enrollments:	137	Evening Classes:	No
Part-Time Enrollments:	50	Weekend Classes:	No
Affiliation:	Public	Distance Learning:	No

NLN ACCREDITATION: Yes

Articulation: Associate to Baccalaureate

For Further Information Contact:

Dr Mary Jeremy Buckman, Chair
Northern Kentucky University
Nunn Dr
Highland Heights, KY 41076
(606) 572-5248

Paducah Community College
—Paducah—

Full-Time Enrollments:	61	Evening Classes:	No
Part-Time Enrollments:	95	Weekend Classes:	No
Affiliation:	Public	Distance Learning:	No

NLN ACCREDITATION: Yes

Articulation: LPN to Associate

For Further Information Contact:

Mrs Tena Payne, Coordinator
Paducah Community College
Box 7380 Alben Barkley Dr
Paducah, KY 42002-7380
(502) 554-9200

Pikeville College
—Pikeville—

Full-Time Enrollments:	57	Evening Classes:	No
Part-Time Enrollments:	—	Weekend Classes:	No
Affiliation:	Private	Distance Learning:	No

NLN ACCREDITATION: No

Articulation: None

For Further Information Contact:

Ms Gayle Sunday, Chair
Pikeville College
Box 34
Pikeville, KY 41501-1194
(606) 432-9230

Prestonsburg Community College
—Prestonsburg—

Full-Time Enrollments:	40	Evening Classes:	No
Part-Time Enrollments:	29	Weekend Classes:	No
Affiliation:	Public	Distance Learning:	No

NLN ACCREDITATION: No

Articulation: LPN to Associate

For Further Information Contact:

Ms Lynn Weddle, Coordinator
Prestonsburg Community College
One Bert T Combs Dr
Prestonsburg, KY 41653-9502
(606) 886-3863

Somerset Community College
—Somerset—

Full-Time Enrollments:	58	Evening Classes:	No
Part-Time Enrollments:	25	Weekend Classes:	No
Affiliation:	Public	Distance Learning:	No

NLN ACCREDITATION: Yes

Articulation: LPN to Associate

For Further Information Contact:

Ms Linda Ballard, Coordinator
Somerset Community College
808 Monticello Rd
Somerset, KY 42501
(606) 679-8501

Southeast Community College
—Cumberland—

Full-Time Enrollments:	51	Evening Classes:	No
Part-Time Enrollments:	38	Weekend Classes:	No
Affiliation:	Public	Distance Learning:	No

NLN ACCREDITATION: Yes

Articulation: LPN to Associate

For Further Information Contact:

Mr Milton Borntrager, Coordinator
Southeast Community College
700 College Rd
Cumberland, KY 40823
(606) 589-2145

St Catherine College
—St Catherine—

Full-Time Enrollments:	34	Evening Classes:	Yes
Part-Time Enrollments:	—	Weekend Classes:	Yes
Affiliation:	Religious	Distance Learning:	No

NLN ACCREDITATION: No

Articulation: Associate to Baccalaureate

For Further Information Contact:

Dr Sara Jane Montgomery, Chair
St Catherine College
2735 Bardstown Rd
St Catherine, KY 46061
(606) 336-5082

Sue Bennett College
—London—

Full-Time Enrollments:	18	Evening Classes:	No
Part-Time Enrollments:	12	Weekend Classes:	No
Affiliation:	Religious	Distance Learning:	No

NLN ACCREDITATION: No

Articulation: None

For Further Information Contact:

Mrs Marlene Waller, Chair
Sue Bennett College
151 College St
London, KY 40741
(606) 864-2238

Western Kentucky University (Two Campuses)
—Bowling Green—

Full-Time Enrollments:	64	Evening Classes:	—
Part-Time Enrollments:	100	Weekend Classes:	—
Affiliation:	Public	Distance Learning:	—

NLN ACCREDITATION: Yes

Articulation: None

For Further Information Contact:

Dr Kay Carr, Interim Head
Western Kentucky University (Two Campuses)
Dept of Nursing
Bowling Green, KY 42101
(502) 745-3791

Louisiana

Delgado Community College/Charity School of Nursing
—New Orleans—

Full-Time Enrollments:	120	Evening Classes:	No
Part-Time Enrollments:	344	Weekend Classes:	No
Affiliation:	Public	Distance Learning:	No

NLN ACCREDITATION: Yes

Articulation: None

For Further Information Contact:

Ms Gayle Barrau, Dean
Delgado Community College/Charity School of Nursing
450 South Claiborne Ave
New Orleans, LA 70112
(504) 568-6466

Louisiana State University Medical Center
—New Orleans—

Full-Time Enrollments:	48	Evening Classes:	No
Part-Time Enrollments:	66	Weekend Classes:	No
Affiliation:	Public	Distance Learning:	No

NLN ACCREDITATION: Yes

Articulation: LPN to Associate

For Further Information Contact:

Dr Elizabeth Humphrey, Acting Dean
Louisiana State University Medical Center
1900 Gravier St
New Orleans, LA 70112-2262
(504) 568-4131

Louisiana State University at Alexandria
—Alexandria—

Full-Time Enrollments:	37	Evening Classes:	Yes
Part-Time Enrollments:	226	Weekend Classes:	—
Affiliation:	Public	Distance Learning:	—

NLN ACCREDITATION: Yes

Articulation: Associate to Baccalaureate
LPN to Associate

For Further Information Contact:

Ms Wanda Guidry, Dept Head
Louisiana State University at Alexandria
Alexandria, LA 71302
(318) 473-6461

Louisiana State University at Eunice
—Eunice—

Full-Time Enrollments:	14	Evening Classes:	No
Part-Time Enrollments:	101	Weekend Classes:	No
Affiliation:	Public	Distance Learning:	No

NLN ACCREDITATION: Yes

Articulation: LPN to Associate

For Further Information Contact:

Mrs Theresa deBeche, Dept Head
Louisiana State University at Eunice
PO Box 1129
Eunice, LA 70535
(318) 457-7311

Louisiana Tech University
—Ruston—

Full-Time Enrollments:	77	Evening Classes:	No
Part-Time Enrollments:	96	Weekend Classes:	No
Affiliation:	Public	Distance Learning:	No

NLN ACCREDITATION: Yes

Articulation: None

For Further Information Contact:

Dr Virginia Pennington, Director
Louisiana Tech University
PO Box 3152 TS
Ruston, LA 71270
(318) 257-2572

McNeese State University
—Lake Charles—

Full-Time Enrollments:	—	Evening Classes:	—
Part-Time Enrollments:	24	Weekend Classes:	—
Affiliation:	Private	Distance Learning:	—

NLN ACCREDITATION: No

Articulation: None

For Further Information Contact:

Dr Jeannine Babineaux, Acting Coordinator
McNeese State University
College of nursing
Lake Charles, LA 70601
(318) 475-8863

Nicholls State University Department of Nursing
—Thibodaux—

Full-Time Enrollments:	49	Evening Classes:	No
Part-Time Enrollments:	44	Weekend Classes:	No
Affiliation:	Public	Distance Learning:	No

NLN ACCREDITATION: Yes

Articulation: Associate to Baccalaureate
LPN to Baccalaureate
LPN to Associate

For Further Information Contact:

Mrs Cheryl Franklin, Director
Nicholls State University Department of Nursing
College Sta, PO Box 2143
Thibodaux, LA 70310
(504) 448-4696

Northwestern State University of Louisiana
—Shreveport—

Full-Time Enrollments:	465	Evening Classes:	No
Part-Time Enrollments:	342	Weekend Classes:	No
Affiliation:	Public	Distance Learning:	Yes

NLN ACCREDITATION: Yes

Articulation: LPN to Associate

For Further Information Contact:

Dr Norann Planchock, Acting Director
Northwestern State University of Louisiana
1800 Line Ave
Shreveport, LA 71103
(318) 677-3100

Our Lady of the Lake College
—Baton Rouge—

Full-Time Enrollments:	211	Evening Classes:	No
Part-Time Enrollments:	—	Weekend Classes:	No
Affiliation:	Religious	Distance Learning:	No

NLN ACCREDITATION: Yes

Articulation: LPN to Associate

For Further Information Contact:

Dr Joe Ann Clark, Dean
Our Lady of the Lake College
7500 Hennessy Blvd
Baton Rouge, LA 70808
(504) 768-7799

Maine

Central Maine Medical Center-School of Nursing
—Lewiston—

Full-Time Enrollments:	76	Evening Classes:	No
Part-Time Enrollments:	12	Weekend Classes:	No
Affiliation:	Private	Distance Learning:	No

NLN ACCREDITATION: Yes

Articulation: Associate to Baccalaureate

For Further Information Contact:

Mrs Fay E Ingersoll, Director
Central Maine Medical Center-School of Nursing
300 Main St
Lewiston, ME 04240
(207) 795-2858

Central Maine Technical College
—Auburn—

Full-Time Enrollments:	18	Evening Classes:	No
Part-Time Enrollments:	32	Weekend Classes:	No
Affiliation:	Public	Distance Learning:	No

NLN ACCREDITATION: Yes

Articulation: Associate to Baccalaureate

For Further Information Contact:

Mrs Patricia Vampatella, Assistant Dean
Central Maine Technical College
1250 Turner St
Auburn, ME 04210
(207) 784-2385

Eastern Maine Technical College
—Bangor—

Full-Time Enrollments:	32	Evening Classes:	Yes
Part-Time Enrollments:	22	Weekend Classes:	—
Affiliation:	Public	Distance Learning:	—

NLN ACCREDITATION: Yes

Articulation: Associate to Baccalaureate

For Further Information Contact:

Ms Marilyn A Lavelle, Chair
Eastern Maine Technical College
354 Hogan Rd
Bangor, ME 04401
(207) 941-4600

Kennebec Valley Technical College
—Fairfield—

Full-Time Enrollments:	4	Evening Classes:	No
Part-Time Enrollments:	70	Weekend Classes:	No
Affiliation:	Public	Distance Learning:	No

NLN ACCREDITATION: Yes

Articulation: Associate to Baccalaureate
LPN to Associate

For Further Information Contact:

Mrs Marcia Parker, Chair
Kennebec Valley Technical College
92 Western Ave
Fairfield, ME 04937
(207) 453-9762

Northern Maine Technical College
—Presque Isle—

Full-Time Enrollments:	56	Evening Classes:	No
Part-Time Enrollments:	—	Weekend Classes:	No
Affiliation:	Public	Distance Learning:	No

NLN ACCREDITATION: Yes

Articulation: Associate to Baccalaureate
LPN to Associate

For Further Information Contact:

Mrs Betty Kent Conant, Chair
Northern Maine Technical College
33 Edgemont Dr
Presque Isle, ME 04769
(207) 768-2700

Southern Maine Technical College
—So Portland—

Full-Time Enrollments:	66	Evening Classes:	No
Part-Time Enrollments:	—	Weekend Classes:	No
Affiliation:	Public	Distance Learning:	No

NLN ACCREDITATION: Yes

Articulation: Associate to Baccalaureate
LPN to Associate
RN to MSN

For Further Information Contact:

Mrs Nancy Smith, Chair
Southern Maine Technical College
Fort Rd
So Portland, ME 04106
(207) 767-9588

University of Maine at Augusta
—Augusta—

Full-Time Enrollments:	86	Evening Classes:	No
Part-Time Enrollments:	40	Weekend Classes:	No
Affiliation:	Public	Distance Learning:	Yes

NLN ACCREDITATION: Yes

Articulation: Associate to Baccalaureate
LPN to Associate

For Further Information Contact:

Ms Marianne Steinhacker, Chair
University of Maine at Augusta
46 University Dr
Augusta, ME 04330
(207) 621-3226

University of New England
—Biddeford—

Full-Time Enrollments:	65	Evening Classes:	No
Part-Time Enrollments:	21	Weekend Classes:	No
Affiliation:	Private	Distance Learning:	No

NLN ACCREDITATION: Yes

Articulation: Associate to Baccalaureate

For Further Information Contact:

Ms Barbara E Teague, Chair
University of New England
Eleven Hills Beach Rd
Biddeford, ME 04005
(207) 283-0171

Maryland

Allegany College of Maryland
—Cumberland—

Full-Time Enrollments:	158	Evening Classes:	—
Part-Time Enrollments:	—	Weekend Classes:	—
Affiliation:	Public	Distance Learning:	—

NLN ACCREDITATION: No

Articulation: None

For Further Information Contact:

Mrs Fran Leibfreid, Director
Allegany College of Maryland
12401 Willowbrook Rd
Cumberland, MD 21502
(301) 724-7700

Anne Arundel Community College
—Arnold—

Full-Time Enrollments:	201	Evening Classes:	Yes
Part-Time Enrollments:	—	Weekend Classes:	No
Affiliation:	Public	Distance Learning:	No

NLN ACCREDITATION: Yes

Articulation: Associate to Baccalaureate
LPN to Associate

For Further Information Contact:

Ms Linda Epstein, Dept Head
Anne Arundel Community College
101 College Pkwy
Arnold, MD 21021
(410) 315-7352

Baltimore City Community College
—Baltimore—

Full-Time Enrollments:	—	Evening Classes:	—
Part-Time Enrollments:	—	Weekend Classes:	—
Affiliation:	Public	Distance Learning:	—

NLN ACCREDITATION: Yes

Articulation: None

For Further Information Contact:

Mrs Gertrude T Hodges, Chair
Baltimore City Community College
2901 Liberty Hts
Baltimore, MD 21215
(410) 333-5969

Catonsville Community College
—Catonsville—

Full-Time Enrollments:	155	Evening Classes:	Yes
Part-Time Enrollments:	—	Weekend Classes:	Yes
Affiliation:	Public	Distance Learning:	Yes

NLN ACCREDITATION: No

Articulation: Associate to Baccalaureate
LPN to Associate

For Further Information Contact:

Mrs Ann E Miller, Chair
Catonsville Community College
800 S Rolling Rd
Catonsville, MD 21228
(410) 455-4570

Cecil Community College
—North East—

Full-Time Enrollments:	15	Evening Classes:	Yes
Part-Time Enrollments:	92	Weekend Classes:	Yes
Affiliation:	Public	Distance Learning:	No

NLN ACCREDITATION: Yes

Articulation: Associate to Baccalaureate

For Further Information Contact:

Mrs Mary Way Bolt, Acting Director
Cecil Community College
1000 North East Rd
North East, MD 21901
(410) 287-6060

ASSOCIATE DEGREE

Charles County Community College
—La Plata—

Full-Time Enrollments: 27 — Evening Classes: Yes
Part-Time Enrollments: 93 — Weekend Classes: No
Affiliation: Public — Distance Learning: Yes

NLN ACCREDITATION: Yes

Articulation: Associate to Baccalaureate
Diploma to Associate
LPN to Associate

For Further Information Contact:

Ms Margaret DeStefanis, Chair
Charles County Community College
Mitchell Rd, Box 910
La Plata, MD 20646
(301) 934-2251

Essex Community College
—Baltimore County—

Full-Time Enrollments: 211 — Evening Classes: —
Part-Time Enrollments: — — Weekend Classes: —
Affiliation: Public — Distance Learning: —

NLN ACCREDITATION: Yes

Articulation: None

For Further Information Contact:

Mrs Teresa M Bianco, Coordinator
Essex Community College
7201 Rossville Blvd
Baltimore County, MD 21237
(410) 780-6433

Frederick Community College
—Frederick—

Full-Time Enrollments: 56 — Evening Classes: —
Part-Time Enrollments: 39 — Weekend Classes: —
Affiliation: Public — Distance Learning: —

NLN ACCREDITATION: No

Articulation: None

For Further Information Contact:

Ms Jane Garvin, Director
Frederick Community College
7932 Opossumtown Pike
Frederick, MD 21701
(301) 846-2525

Hagerstown Jr College
—Hagerstown—

Full-Time Enrollments: 36 — Evening Classes: —
Part-Time Enrollments: 31 — Weekend Classes: —
Affiliation: Public — Distance Learning: —

NLN ACCREDITATION: No

Articulation: None

For Further Information Contact:

Ms Virginia A Gossard, Director
Hagerstown Jr College
11400 Robinwood Dr
Hagerstown, MD 21742
(301) 790-2800

Harford Community College
—Bel Air—

Full-Time Enrollments: 35 — Evening Classes: Yes
Part-Time Enrollments: 116 — Weekend Classes: No
Affiliation: Public — Distance Learning: No

NLN ACCREDITATION: Yes

Articulation: Associate to Baccalaureate
LPN to Associate

For Further Information Contact:

Mrs Tina Zimmerman, Chair
Harford Community College
401 Thomas Run Rd
Bel Air, MD 21015
(410) 836-4000

Howard Community College
—Columbia—

Full-Time Enrollments: 60 — Evening Classes: Yes
Part-Time Enrollments: 124 — Weekend Classes: Yes
Affiliation: Public — Distance Learning: Yes

NLN ACCREDITATION: Yes

Articulation: Associate to Baccalaureate
LPN to Associate

For Further Information Contact:

Dr Emily Slunt, Chair
Howard Community College
Little Patuxent Pkwy
Columbia, MD 21044
(410) 992-4888

Montgomery Community College
—Takoma Park—

Full-Time Enrollments: 84
Part-Time Enrollments: 131
Affiliation: Public

Evening Classes: Yes
Weekend Classes: Yes
Distance Learning: No

NLN ACCREDITATION: Yes

Articulation: Associate to Baccalaureate

For Further Information Contact:

Dr Sharon Bernier, Director
Montgomery Community College
7600 New York Ave
Takoma Park, MD 20012
(301) 650-1355

Prince George's Community College
—Largo—

Full-Time Enrollments: 9
Part-Time Enrollments: 184
Affiliation: Public

Evening Classes: Yes
Weekend Classes: Yes
Distance Learning: No

NLN ACCREDITATION: Yes

Articulation: Associate to Baccalaureate
LPN to Associate

For Further Information Contact:

Dr Lois Neuman, Chair
Prince George's Community College
301 Largo Rd
Largo, MD 20772-2199
(301) 322-0734

Wor-Wic Community College-Nursing Department
—Cambridge—

Full-Time Enrollments: 43
Part-Time Enrollments: 16
Affiliation: Public

Evening Classes: Yes
Weekend Classes: Yes
Distance Learning: No

NLN ACCREDITATION: No

Articulation: Associate to Baccalaureate
LPN to Associate

For Further Information Contact:

Ms Denise Marshall, Head
Wor-Wic Community College-Nursing Department
PO Box 800
Cambridge, MD 21613
(410) 221-2555

Massachusetts

Atlantic Union College
—South Lancaster—

Full-Time Enrollments: —
Part-Time Enrollments: —
Affiliation: Religious

Evening Classes: —
Weekend Classes: —
Distance Learning: —

NLN ACCREDITATION: Yes

Articulation: —

For Further Information Contact:

Mrs Vera B Davis, Chair
Atlantic Union College
South Lancaster, MA 01561
(508) 368-2400

Becker College
—Worcester—

Full-Time Enrollments: 44
Part-Time Enrollments: 59
Affiliation: Private

Evening Classes: No
Weekend Classes: No
Distance Learning: No

NLN ACCREDITATION: Yes

Articulation: Associate to Baccalaureate

For Further Information Contact:

Mrs Madge McNair, Director
Becker College
Box 15071 61 Sever St
Worcester, MA 01615-0071
(508) 791-9221

Berkshire Community College
—Pittsfield—

Full-Time Enrollments: 22
Part-Time Enrollments: 74
Affiliation: Public

Evening Classes: Yes
Weekend Classes: Yes
Distance Learning: No

NLN ACCREDITATION: Yes

Articulation: Associate to Baccalaureate
LPN to Associate

For Further Information Contact:

Mrs Patricia Brien, Chair
Berkshire Community College
1350 West St
Pittsfield, MA 01201
(413) 499-4660

Bristol Community College
—Fall River—

Full-Time Enrollments:	19	Evening Classes:	—
Part-Time Enrollments:	100	Weekend Classes:	—
Affiliation:	Public	Distance Learning:	—

NLN ACCREDITATION: Yes

Articulation: None

For Further Information Contact:

Dr Marie G Marshall, Chair
Bristol Community College
777 Elsbree St
Fall River, MA 02720
(508) 678-2811

Bunker Hill Community College
—Charlestown—

Full-Time Enrollments:	140	Evening Classes:	Yes
Part-Time Enrollments:	—	Weekend Classes:	No
Affiliation:	Public	Distance Learning:	No

NLN ACCREDITATION: Yes

Articulation: Associate to Baccalaureate

For Further Information Contact:

Ms Marjorie J Langway, Chair
Bunker Hill Community College
New Rutherford Ave
Charlestown, MA 02129
(617) 228-2443

Cape Cod Community College
—W Barnstable—

Full-Time Enrollments:	119	Evening Classes:	Yes
Part-Time Enrollments:	25	Weekend Classes:	Yes
Affiliation:	Public	Distance Learning:	Yes

NLN ACCREDITATION: Yes

Articulation: Associate to Baccalaureate
LPN to Associate

For Further Information Contact:

Ms Luise Speakman, Chair
Cape Cod Community College
2240 Iyanouth Rd
W Barnstable, MA 02668-1599
(508) 362-2131 Ext 4548

Endicott College
—Beverly—

Full-Time Enrollments:	66	Evening Classes:	No
Part-Time Enrollments:	3	Weekend Classes:	No
Affiliation:	Private	Distance Learning:	No

NLN ACCREDITATION: Yes

Articulation: None

For Further Information Contact:

Dr Sherry Merrow, Assoc Dean
Endicott College
376 Hale St
Beverly, MA 01915
(508) 927-0585

Greenfield Community College
—Greenfield—

Full-Time Enrollments:	77	Evening Classes:	No
Part-Time Enrollments:	1	Weekend Classes:	No
Affiliation:	Public	Distance Learning:	No

NLN ACCREDITATION: Yes

Articulation: Associate to Baccalaureate
LPN to Associate

For Further Information Contact:

Mrs Margaret M Craig, Director
Greenfield Community College
270 Main St
Greenfield, MA 01301
(413) 774-3131

Holyoke Community College
—Holyoke—

Full-Time Enrollments:	100	Evening Classes:	—
Part-Time Enrollments:	—	Weekend Classes:	—
Affiliation:	Public	Distance Learning:	—

NLN ACCREDITATION: Yes

Articulation: None

For Further Information Contact:

Ms Patricia Triggs, Chair
Holyoke Community College
303 Homestead Ave
Holyoke, MA 01040
(413) 538-7000

Laboure College
—Boston—

Full-Time Enrollments:	179	Evening Classes:	Yes
Part-Time Enrollments:	69	Weekend Classes:	—
Affiliation:	Private	Distance Learning:	—

NLN ACCREDITATION: Yes

Articulation: Associate to Baccalaureate

For Further Information Contact:

Ms Roberta Pazyra, Chair
Laboure College
2120 Dorchester Ave
Boston, MA 02124
(617) 296-8300

Lasell College
—Medford—

Full-Time Enrollments:	33	Evening Classes:	—
Part-Time Enrollments:	—	Weekend Classes:	—
Affiliation:	Private	Distance Learning:	—

NLN ACCREDITATION: No

Articulation: None

For Further Information Contact:

Dr Cathy Livingston, Dean
Lasell College
1844 Commonwealth Ave
Medford, MA 02166
(617) 243-2111

Massachusetts Bay Community College
—Wellesley Hills—

Full-Time Enrollments:	143	Evening Classes:	Yes
Part-Time Enrollments:	233	Weekend Classes:	Yes
Affiliation:	Public	Distance Learning:	No

NLN ACCREDITATION: Yes

Articulation: Associate to Baccalaureate
LPN to Associate

For Further Information Contact:

Dr Patricia Schuldenfrei, Coordinator
Massachusetts Bay Community College
50 Oakland St
Wellesley Hills, MA 02181
(617) 239-2261

Massasoit Community College
—Brockton—

Full-Time Enrollments:	112	Evening Classes:	No
Part-Time Enrollments:	—	Weekend Classes:	No
Affiliation:	Public	Distance Learning:	No

NLN ACCREDITATION: Yes

Articulation: LPN to Associate

For Further Information Contact:

Mrs Barbara Waible, Chair
Massasoit Community College
1 Massasoit Blvd
Brockton, MA 02402
(508) 588-9100

Middlesex Community College
—Lowell—

Full-Time Enrollments:	22	Evening Classes:	No
Part-Time Enrollments:	73	Weekend Classes:	No
Affiliation:	Public	Distance Learning:	No

NLN ACCREDITATION: Yes

Articulation: Associate to Baccalaureate
LPN to Associate

For Further Information Contact:

Miss Mary Foley, Assistant Dean
Middlesex Community College
44 Middle St
Lowell, MA 01852-1901
(508) 656-3046

Mount Wachusett Community College
—Gardner—

Full-Time Enrollments:	5	Evening Classes:	Yes
Part-Time Enrollments:	106	Weekend Classes:	Yes
Affiliation:	Public	Distance Learning:	Yes

NLN ACCREDITATION: Yes

Articulation: Associate to Baccalaureate
LPN to Associate

For Further Information Contact:

Ms Frances S Strother, Chair
Mount Wachusett Community College
444 Green St
Gardner, MA 01440
(508) 632-6600

ASSOCIATE DEGREE

North Shore Community College
—Danvers—

Full-Time Enrollments:	112	Evening Classes:	No
Part-Time Enrollments:	—	Weekend Classes:	No
Affiliation:	Public	Distance Learning:	Yes

NLN ACCREDITATION: Yes

Articulation: Associate to Baccalaureate
LPN to Associate

For Further Information Contact:

Mrs Susan Maciewicz, Chair
North Shore Community College
1 Ferncroft Rd
Danvers, MA 01923
(508) 762-4000

Northern Essex Community College
—Lawrence—

Full-Time Enrollments:	83	Evening Classes:	Yes
Part-Time Enrollments:	124	Weekend Classes:	Yes
Affiliation:	Public	Distance Learning:	No

NLN ACCREDITATION: Yes

Articulation: Associate to Baccalaureate
LPN to Associate

For Further Information Contact:

Dr Sylvia G Hallsworth, Director
Northern Essex Community College
45 Franklin St
Lawrence, MA 01841
(508) 688-3181

Quincy College
—Quincy—

Full-Time Enrollments:	140	Evening Classes:	Yes
Part-Time Enrollments:	133	Weekend Classes:	—
Affiliation:	Private	Distance Learning:	—

NLN ACCREDITATION: Yes

Articulation: Associate to Baccalaureate
LPN to Associate

For Further Information Contact:

Ms Kristin Parks, Chair
Quincy College
34 Coddington St
Quincy, MA 02169
(617) 984-1742

Quinsigamond Community College
—Worcester—

Full-Time Enrollments:	165	Evening Classes:	No
Part-Time Enrollments:	—	Weekend Classes:	No
Affiliation:	Public	Distance Learning:	No

NLN ACCREDITATION: Yes

Articulation: Associate to Baccalaureate
LPN to Associate

For Further Information Contact:

Mrs Ruth Pelkey, Coordinator
Quinsigamond Community College
670 W Boylston St
Worcester, MA 01606
(508) 854-4273

Roxbury Community College
—Roxbury Crossing—

Full-Time Enrollments:	68	Evening Classes:	No
Part-Time Enrollments:	—	Weekend Classes:	No
Affiliation:	Public	Distance Learning:	No

NLN ACCREDITATION: No

Articulation: Associate to Baccalaureate

For Further Information Contact:

Ms Shellie Simons, Chair
Roxbury Community College
1234 Columbus Ave
Roxbury Crossing, MA 02120
(617) 541-5313

Springfield Tech Community College
—Springfield—

Full-Time Enrollments:	30	Evening Classes:	No
Part-Time Enrollments:	99	Weekend Classes:	No
Affiliation:	Public	Distance Learning:	No

NLN ACCREDITATION: Yes

Articulation: Associate to Baccalaureate

For Further Information Contact:

Dr Eileen Neville, Dean
Springfield Tech Community College
One Armory Sq
Springfield, MA 01105
(413) 781-7822

Michigan

Alpena Community College
—Alpena—

Full-Time Enrollments:	26	Evening Classes:	No
Part-Time Enrollments:	—	Weekend Classes:	No
Affiliation:	Public	Distance Learning:	No

NLN ACCREDITATION: No

Articulation: Associate to Baccalaureate
LPN to Associate

For Further Information Contact:

Mrs Kathleen McGillis, Assistant Dean
Alpena Community College
666 Johnson St
Alpena, MI 49707
(517) 356-9021

Bay de Noc Community College
—Escanaba—

Full-Time Enrollments:	23	Evening Classes:	Yes
Part-Time Enrollments:	91	Weekend Classes:	No
Affiliation:	Public	Distance Learning:	Yes

NLN ACCREDITATION: No

Articulation: Associate to Baccalaureate

For Further Information Contact:

Mrs Patricia Valensky, Dean
Bay de Noc Community College
2001 North Lincoln Rd
Escanaba, MI 49829
(906) 786-5802

Charles Stewart Mott Community College
—Flint—

Full-Time Enrollments:	—	Evening Classes:	—
Part-Time Enrollments:	—	Weekend Classes:	—
Affiliation:	Public	Distance Learning:	—

NLN ACCREDITATION: Yes

Articulation: —

For Further Information Contact:

Ms Patricia Markowicz, Associate Dean
Charles Stewart Mott Community College
1401 E Court St
Flint, MI 48503
(810) 232-6592

Delta College
—University Center—

Full-Time Enrollments:	—	Evening Classes:	—
Part-Time Enrollments:	—	Weekend Classes:	—
Affiliation:	Public	Distance Learning:	—

NLN ACCREDITATION: Yes

Articulation: —

For Further Information Contact:

Mrs Louise Brentin, Chair
Delta College
University Center, MI 48710
(517) 686-9274

Ferris State University
—Big Rapids—

Full-Time Enrollments:	98	Evening Classes:	Yes
Part-Time Enrollments:	20	Weekend Classes:	Yes
Affiliation:	Public	Distance Learning:	No

NLN ACCREDITATION: No

Articulation: Associate to Baccalaureate
Diploma to Baccalaureate

For Further Information Contact:

Dr Sally K Johnson, Dept Head
Ferris State University
Birkam Hlth Ctr Rm 210
Big Rapids, MI 49307-2295
(616) 592-2267

Glen Oaks Community College
—Centreville—

Full-Time Enrollments:	43	Evening Classes:	Yes
Part-Time Enrollments:	—	Weekend Classes:	Yes
Affiliation:	Public	Distance Learning:	No

NLN ACCREDITATION: No

Articulation: None

For Further Information Contact:

Mrs Gail Brown, Director
Glen Oaks Community College
Centreville, MI 49032
(616) 467-9945

Gogebic Community College
—Ironwood—

Full-Time Enrollments: 32 Evening Classes: No
Part-Time Enrollments: — Weekend Classes: No
Affiliation: Public Distance Learning: No

NLN ACCREDITATION: No

Articulation: Associate to Baccalaureate
LPN to Associate

For Further Information Contact:

Ms Kathryn Encalada, Director
Gogebic Community College
E 4946 Jackson Rd
Ironwood, MI 49938
(906) 932-4231

Grand Rapids Community College
—Grand Rapids—

Full-Time Enrollments: 93 Evening Classes: No
Part-Time Enrollments: 88 Weekend Classes: No
Affiliation: Public Distance Learning: No

NLN ACCREDITATION: Yes

Articulation: Associate to Baccalaureate
LPN to Associate

For Further Information Contact:

Mrs Marilyn Smidt, Director
Grand Rapids Community College
143 Bostwick Ave, NE
Grand Rapids, MI 49502
(616) 771-4231

Great Lakes Jr College
—Midland—

Full-Time Enrollments: 51 Evening Classes: Yes
Part-Time Enrollments: 29 Weekend Classes: Yes
Affiliation: Private Distance Learning: —

NLN ACCREDITATION: No

Articulation: LPN to Associate

For Further Information Contact:

Mrs Barbara Carter, Director
Great Lakes Jr College
3555 East Patrick Rd
Midland, MI 48642-5837
(517) 835-4501

Henry Ford Community College
—Dearborn—

Full-Time Enrollments: — Evening Classes: —
Part-Time Enrollments: — Weekend Classes: —
Affiliation: Public Distance Learning: —

NLN ACCREDITATION: Yes

Articulation: None

For Further Information Contact:

Ms Genevieve Czarnecki, Director
Henry Ford Community College
5101 Evergreen Rd
Dearborn, MI 48128
(313) 845-9661

Jackson Community College
—Jackson—

Full-Time Enrollments: 61 Evening Classes: —
Part-Time Enrollments: 39 Weekend Classes: —
Affiliation: Public Distance Learning: —

NLN ACCREDITATION: No

Articulation: None

For Further Information Contact:

Mrs Linda Williams, Chair
Jackson Community College
2111 Emmons Rd
Jackson, MI 49201
(517) 787-3881

Kalamazoo Valley Community College
—Kalamazoo—

Full-Time Enrollments: 123 Evening Classes: No
Part-Time Enrollments: 22 Weekend Classes: No
Affiliation: Public Distance Learning: No

NLN ACCREDITATION: No

Articulation: Associate to Baccalaureate

For Further Information Contact:

Mrs Carol Roe, Director
Kalamazoo Valley Community College
6767 West O Ave
Kalamazoo, MI 49009
(616) 372-5389

Kellogg Community College (2 Programs)
—Battle Creek—

Full-Time Enrollments:	95	Evening Classes:	Yes
Part-Time Enrollments:	114	Weekend Classes:	—
Affiliation:	Public	Distance Learning:	—

NLN ACCREDITATION: No

Articulation: Associate to Baccalaureate
LPN to Associate

For Further Information Contact:

Mrs Cynthia Sublett, Director
Kellogg Community College (2 Programs)
450 North Ave
Battle Creek, MI 49016
(616) 965-3931

Kirtland Community College
—Roscommon—

Full-Time Enrollments:	37	Evening Classes:	No
Part-Time Enrollments:	—	Weekend Classes:	No
Affiliation:	Public	Distance Learning:	No

NLN ACCREDITATION: No

Articulation: Associate to Baccalaureate
LPN to Associate

For Further Information Contact:

Ms Michelle Marineau, Director
Kirtland Community College
Rte 4 Box 59A
Roscommon, MI 48653
(517) 275-5121

Lake Michigan College
—Benton Harbor—

Full-Time Enrollments:	72	Evening Classes:	Yes
Part-Time Enrollments:	47	Weekend Classes:	Yes
Affiliation:	Public	Distance Learning:	Yes

NLN ACCREDITATION: Yes

Articulation: None

For Further Information Contact:

Mrs Alice Rasmussen, Coordinator
Lake Michigan College
2755 E Napier Ave
Benton Harbor, MI 49022
(616) 927-3571

Lansing Community College
—Lansing—

Full-Time Enrollments:	195	Evening Classes:	Yes
Part-Time Enrollments:	—	Weekend Classes:	Yes
Affiliation:	Public	Distance Learning:	No

NLN ACCREDITATION: Yes

Articulation: Associate to Baccalaureate

For Further Information Contact:

Ms Dorothy Linau Mirkil, Coordinator
Lansing Community College
PO Box 40010
Lansing, MI 48901-7210
(517) 483-1410

Macomb Community College
—Clinton Township—

Full-Time Enrollments:	220	Evening Classes:	No
Part-Time Enrollments:	—	Weekend Classes:	No
Affiliation:	Public	Distance Learning:	No

NLN ACCREDITATION: Yes

Articulation: Associate to Baccalaureate

For Further Information Contact:

Ms Maureen T Neal, Director
Macomb Community College
44575 Garfield Rd
Clinton Township, MI 48038
(810) 286-2097

Mid-Michigan Community College
—Harrison—

Full-Time Enrollments:	111	Evening Classes:	Yes
Part-Time Enrollments:	—	Weekend Classes:	No
Affiliation:	Public	Distance Learning:	No

NLN ACCREDITATION: No

Articulation: LPN to Associate

For Further Information Contact:

Ms Beth Sendre, Director
Mid-Michigan Community College
1375 S Clare Ave
Harrison, MI 48625
(517) 386-7792

Monroe County Community College
—Monroe—

Full-Time Enrollments:	18	Evening Classes:	Yes
Part-Time Enrollments:	53	Weekend Classes:	No
Affiliation:	Public	Distance Learning:	No

NLN ACCREDITATION: Yes

Articulation: Associate to Baccalaureate

For Further Information Contact:

Ms Gail Odneal, Chair
Monroe County Community College
1555 S Raisinville Rd
Monroe, MI 48161
(313) 242-7300

Montcalm Community College
—Sidney—

Full-Time Enrollments:	6	Evening Classes:	Yes
Part-Time Enrollments:	31	Weekend Classes:	Yes
Affiliation:	Public	Distance Learning:	Yes

NLN ACCREDITATION: No

Articulation: LPN to Associate

For Further Information Contact:

Ms Catherine Earl, Director
Montcalm Community College
1464 Sidney Rd
Sidney, MI 48885
(517) 328-2111

Muskegon Community College
—Muskegon—

Full-Time Enrollments:	—	Evening Classes:	—
Part-Time Enrollments:	—	Weekend Classes:	—
Affiliation:	Public	Distance Learning:	—

NLN ACCREDITATION: No

Articulation: None

For Further Information Contact:

Mrs Darlene Collet, Director
Muskegon Community College
221 S Quarterline Rd
Muskegon, MI 49442
(616) 777-0332

North Central Michigan College
—Petoskey—

Full-Time Enrollments:	84	Evening Classes:	No
Part-Time Enrollments:	8	Weekend Classes:	No
Affiliation:	Public	Distance Learning:	No

NLN ACCREDITATION: No

Articulation: Associate to Baccalaureate

For Further Information Contact:

Mrs Peggy Comstock, Director
North Central Michigan College
1515 Howard St
Petoskey, MI 49770
(616) 348-6604

Northwestern Michigan College
—Traverse City—

Full-Time Enrollments:	28	Evening Classes:	Yes
Part-Time Enrollments:	72	Weekend Classes:	No
Affiliation:	Public	Distance Learning:	No

NLN ACCREDITATION: No

Articulation: Associate to Baccalaureate
LPN to Associate

For Further Information Contact:

Ms Mary Vanderkolk, Dept Head
Northwestern Michigan College
1701 E Front St
Traverse City, MI 49684
(616) 922-1239

Oakland Community College
—Waterford—

Full-Time Enrollments:	435	Evening Classes:	Yes
Part-Time Enrollments:	—	Weekend Classes:	No
Affiliation:	Public	Distance Learning:	No

NLN ACCREDITATION: Yes

Articulation: Associate to Baccalaureate
LPN to Associate

For Further Information Contact:

Ms Jane Ditri, Interim Dean
Oakland Community College
7350 Cooley Lake Rd
Waterford, MI 48327
(810) 360-3111

Schoolcraft College
—Livonia—

Full-Time Enrollments:	3	Evening Classes:	Yes
Part-Time Enrollments:	163	Weekend Classes:	Yes
Affiliation:	Public	Distance Learning:	Yes

NLN ACCREDITATION: No

Articulation: LPN to Associate

For Further Information Contact:

Mrs Midge Carleton, Assistant Dean
Schoolcraft College
18600 Haggerty Rd
Livonia, MI 48152
(313) 462-4400

Southwestern Michigan College
—Dowagiac—

Full-Time Enrollments:	98	Evening Classes:	Yes
Part-Time Enrollments:	50	Weekend Classes:	Yes
Affiliation:	Public	Distance Learning:	Yes

NLN ACCREDITATION: No

Articulation: Associate to Baccalaureate

For Further Information Contact:

Miss Marilouise Hagenberg, Dean
Southwestern Michigan College
Cherry Grove Rd
Dowagiac, MI 49047
(616) 782-5113

St Clair County Community College
—Port Huron—

Full-Time Enrollments:	3	Evening Classes:	No
Part-Time Enrollments:	182	Weekend Classes:	No
Affiliation:	Public	Distance Learning:	Yes

NLN ACCREDITATION: No

Articulation: LPN to Associate

For Further Information Contact:

Mrs Susan J Meeker, Director
St Clair County Community College
323 Erie St Po Box 5015
Port Huron, MI 48061-5015
(810) 989-5675

Suomi College
—Hancock—

Full-Time Enrollments:	42	Evening Classes:	No
Part-Time Enrollments:	9	Weekend Classes:	No
Affiliation:	Religious	Distance Learning:	No

NLN ACCREDITATION: No

Articulation: Associate to Baccalaureate
LPN to Associate

For Further Information Contact:

Mrs Barbara Whitman, Chair
Suomi College
Hancock, MI 49930
(906) 482-5300

Washtenaw Community College
—Ann Arbor—

Full-Time Enrollments:	18	Evening Classes:	Yes
Part-Time Enrollments:	207	Weekend Classes:	Yes
Affiliation:	Public	Distance Learning:	No

NLN ACCREDITATION: Yes

Articulation: None

For Further Information Contact:

Dr Phyllis Grzegorczyk, Dean
Washtenaw Community College
PO Box D-1
Ann Arbor, MI 48106
(313) 973-3358

Wayne County Community College
—Detroit—

Full-Time Enrollments:	190	Evening Classes:	Yes
Part-Time Enrollments:	190	Weekend Classes:	Yes
Affiliation:	Public	Distance Learning:	No

NLN ACCREDITATION: Yes

Articulation: Associate to Baccalaureate

For Further Information Contact:

Ms Katherine Bradley, Director
Wayne County Community College
8551 Greenfield Rm 305A
Detroit, MI 48228
(313) 496-2566

West Shore Community College
—Scottville—

Full-Time Enrollments:	63	Evening Classes:	No
Part-Time Enrollments:	1	Weekend Classes:	No
Affiliation:	Public	Distance Learning:	No

NLN ACCREDITATION: No

Articulation: Associate to Baccalaureate
LPN to Associate

For Further Information Contact:

Mrs Patricia Collins, Director
West Shore Community College
PO Box 277 3000 N Stiles Rd
Scottville, MI 49454
(616) 845-6211

Minnesota

Anoka-Ramsey Community College
—Coon Rapids—

Full-Time Enrollments:	116	Evening Classes:	No
Part-Time Enrollments:	72	Weekend Classes:	No
Affiliation:	Public	Distance Learning:	No

NLN ACCREDITATION: Yes

Articulation: Associate to Baccalaureate
LPN to Associate

For Further Information Contact:

Mrs Charlyne Foss, Director
Anoka-Ramsey Community College
11200 Mississippi Blvd, NW
Coon Rapids, MN 55433-3470
(612) 422-3321

Central Lakes College
—Brainerd—

Full-Time Enrollments:	37	Evening Classes:	Yes
Part-Time Enrollments:	—	Weekend Classes:	—
Affiliation:	Public	Distance Learning:	Yes

NLN ACCREDITATION: No

Articulation: LPN to Associate

For Further Information Contact:

Mrs Lois Fielding, Director
Central Lakes College
501 West College Dr
Brainerd, MN 56401
(218) 828-2515

College of St Catherine-Minneapolis
—Minneapolis—

Full-Time Enrollments:	115	Evening Classes:	Yes
Part-Time Enrollments:	264	Weekend Classes:	Yes
Affiliation:	Religious	Distance Learning:	No

NLN ACCREDITATION: Yes

Articulation: None

For Further Information Contact:

Ms Kathleen A Hartmann, Director
College of St Catherine-Minneapolis
601 25th Ave So
Minneapolis, MN 55454
(612) 690-7712

Fergus Falls Community College
—Fergus Falls—

Full-Time Enrollments:	24	Evening Classes:	Yes
Part-Time Enrollments:	14	Weekend Classes:	Yes
Affiliation:	Public	Distance Learning:	Yes

NLN ACCREDITATION: No

Articulation: Associate to Baccalaureate
LPN to Associate

For Further Information Contact:

Mrs Shirley Seyfried, Coordinator
Fergus Falls Community College
1414 College Way
Fergus Falls, MN 56537
(218) 739-7548

Hibbing Community College
—Hibbing—

Full-Time Enrollments:	81	Evening Classes:	Yes
Part-Time Enrollments:	—	Weekend Classes:	No
Affiliation:	Public	Distance Learning:	Yes

NLN ACCREDITATION: No

Articulation: Associate to Baccalaureate
LPN to Associate

For Further Information Contact:

Mrs Susan Hyndman, Director
Hibbing Community College
1515 East 25th St
Hibbing, MN 55746
(218) 262-6700

Inver Hills-Century Community College
—White Bear Lake—

Full-Time Enrollments:	185	Evening Classes:	—
Part-Time Enrollments:	119	Weekend Classes:	—
Affiliation:	Public	Distance Learning:	—

NLN ACCREDITATION: Yes

Articulation: None

For Further Information Contact:

Ms Ellie Slette, Dean
Inver Hills-Century Community College
3401 Century Ave North
White Bear Lake, MN 55110
(612) 779-3438

Lake Superior College
—Duluth—

Full-Time Enrollments:	32	Evening Classes:	—
Part-Time Enrollments:	2	Weekend Classes:	—
Affiliation:	Public	Distance Learning:	—

NLN ACCREDITATION: No

Articulation: None

For Further Information Contact:

Mrs Mary Vnuk, Director
Lake Superior College
2101 Trinity Rd
Duluth, MN 55811
(218) 725-7713

Minneapolis Community Technical College
—Minneapolis—

Full-Time Enrollments:	—	Evening Classes:	—
Part-Time Enrollments:	—	Weekend Classes:	—
Affiliation:	Public	Distance Learning:	—

NLN ACCREDITATION: Yes

Articulation: —

For Further Information Contact:

Ms Nancy Miller, Coordinator
Minneapolis Community Technical College
1501 Hennepin Ave
Minneapolis, MN 55403
(612) 373-2783

Normandale Community College
—Bloomington—

Full-Time Enrollments:	70	Evening Classes:	No
Part-Time Enrollments:	112	Weekend Classes:	No
Affiliation:	Public	Distance Learning:	No

NLN ACCREDITATION: Yes

Articulation: Associate to Baccalaureate

For Further Information Contact:

Dr Kathleen F Manahan, Associate Dean
Normandale Community College
9700 France Ave S
Bloomington, MN 55431
(612) 832-6348

North Hennepin Community College
—Brooklyn Park—

Full-Time Enrollments:	177	Evening Classes:	Yes
Part-Time Enrollments:	—	Weekend Classes:	Yes
Affiliation:	Public	Distance Learning:	Yes

NLN ACCREDITATION: Yes

Articulation: None

For Further Information Contact:

Ms Miriam Hazzard, Associate Dean
North Hennepin Community College
7411 85th Ave N
Brooklyn Park, MN 55445
(612) 424-0761

Northland Community and Technical College
—Thief River Falls—

Full-Time Enrollments:	35	Evening Classes:	Yes
Part-Time Enrollments:	22	Weekend Classes:	No
Affiliation:	Public	Distance Learning:	Yes

NLN ACCREDITATION: No

Articulation: LPN to Associate

For Further Information Contact:

Ms Debra Filer, Director
Northland Community and Technical College
1101 Highway One East
Thief River Falls, MN 56701
(218) 681-2101

Ridgewater College
—Willmar—

Full-Time Enrollments:	12	Evening Classes:	Yes
Part-Time Enrollments:	16	Weekend Classes:	Yes
Affiliation:	Public	Distance Learning:	Yes

NLN ACCREDITATION: No

Articulation: None

For Further Information Contact:

Ms C Lynn Johnson, Director
Ridgewater College
PO Box 797
Willmar, MN 56201
(612) 231-5102

Riverland Community College
—Austin—

Full-Time Enrollments:	54	Evening Classes:	No
Part-Time Enrollments:	13	Weekend Classes:	No
Affiliation:	Public	Distance Learning:	No

NLN ACCREDITATION: Yes

Articulation: LPN to Associate

For Further Information Contact:

Ms Patricia Parsons, Director
Riverland Community College
1900 8th Ave NW
Austin, MN 55912-1470
(507) 433-0826

Rochester Community Technical College
—Rochester—

Full-Time Enrollments:	81	Evening Classes:	Yes
Part-Time Enrollments:	138	Weekend Classes:	—
Affiliation:	Public	Distance Learning:	—

NLN ACCREDITATION: Yes

Articulation: LPN to Associate

For Further Information Contact:

Dr Julie Goodman, Dean
Rochester Community Technical College
851 30th Ave SE
Rochester, MN 55904-4999
(507) 285-7143

Worthington Community College
—Worthington—

Full-Time Enrollments:	4	Evening Classes:	No
Part-Time Enrollments:	20	Weekend Classes:	No
Affiliation:	Public	Distance Learning:	No

NLN ACCREDITATION: No

Articulation: LPN to Associate

For Further Information Contact:

Ms Kathi Haberman, Director
Worthington Community College
1450 Collegeway
Worthington, MN 56187
(507) 372-3443

Mississippi

Alcorn State University
—Natchez—

Full-Time Enrollments:	23	Evening Classes:	—
Part-Time Enrollments:	52	Weekend Classes:	—
Affiliation:	Public	Distance Learning:	—

NLN ACCREDITATION: Yes

Articulation: None

For Further Information Contact:

Mrs Linda Godley, Chair
Alcorn State University
PO Box 18399
Natchez, MS 39122
(601) 442-3901

Copiah Lincoln Community College
—Wesson—

Full-Time Enrollments:	90	Evening Classes:	—
Part-Time Enrollments:	—	Weekend Classes:	—
Affiliation:	Public	Distance Learning:	—

NLN ACCREDITATION: No

Articulation: None

For Further Information Contact:

Dr Susan Hart, Director
Copiah Lincoln Community College
PO Box 649
Wesson, MS 39191
(601) 643-8413

East Central Community College
—Decatur—

Full-Time Enrollments:	70	Evening Classes:	No
Part-Time Enrollments:	—	Weekend Classes:	No
Affiliation:	Public	Distance Learning:	No

NLN ACCREDITATION:

Articulation: None

For Further Information Contact:

Mrs Nancy Harris, Director
East Central Community College
PO Box 129
Decatur, MS 39327
(601) 635-2111

Hinds Community College
—Jackson—

Full-Time Enrollments:	336	Evening Classes:	No
Part-Time Enrollments:	—	Weekend Classes:	No
Affiliation:	Public	Distance Learning:	No

NLN ACCREDITATION: Yes

Articulation: LPN to Associate

For Further Information Contact:

Mrs Gloria Coxwell, Assistant Dean
Hinds Community College
1750 Chadwick Dr
Jackson, MS 39204
(601) 371-3503

Holmes Community College
—Grenada—

Full-Time Enrollments:	108	Evening Classes:	No
Part-Time Enrollments:	1	Weekend Classes:	No
Affiliation:	Public	Distance Learning:	No

NLN ACCREDITATION: Yes

Articulation: Associate to Baccalaureate
LPN to Associate

For Further Information Contact:

Ms Joyce Vaughn, Director
Holmes Community College
1060 Avent Dr
Grenada, MS 38901
(601) 226-0830

Itawamba Community College
—Fulton—

Full-Time Enrollments:	189	Evening Classes:	No
Part-Time Enrollments:	1	Weekend Classes:	No
Affiliation:	Public	Distance Learning:	No

NLN ACCREDITATION: Yes

Articulation: Associate to Baccalaureate
LPN to Associate

For Further Information Contact:

Ms Carolyn Prestage, Chair
Itawamba Community College
Fulton, MS 38843
(601) 862-3101

Jones County Jr College
—Ellisville—

Full-Time Enrollments:	114	Evening Classes:	No
Part-Time Enrollments:	—	Weekend Classes:	No
Affiliation:	Public	Distance Learning:	No

NLN ACCREDITATION: Yes

Articulation: LPN to Associate

For Further Information Contact:

Mrs Linda Suttle, Director
Jones County Jr College
900 South Court St
Ellisville, MS 39437
(601) 477-9311

Meridian Community College
—Meridian—

Full-Time Enrollments:	269	Evening Classes:	Yes
Part-Time Enrollments:	—	Weekend Classes:	Yes
Affiliation:	Public	Distance Learning:	—

NLN ACCREDITATION: Yes

Articulation: LPN to Associate

For Further Information Contact:

Mrs Shirley Griffin, Assistant Dean
Meridian Community College
910 Highway 19 North
Meridian, MS 39307
(601) 483-8241

Mississippi Delta Community College
—Moorhead—

Full-Time Enrollments:	120	Evening Classes:	No
Part-Time Enrollments:	—	Weekend Classes:	No
Affiliation:	Public	Distance Learning:	No

NLN ACCREDITATION: Yes

Articulation: Associate to Baccalaureate
LPN to Associate

For Further Information Contact:

Ms Martha Catlette, Director
Mississippi Delta Community College
PO Box 668
Moorhead, MS 38761
(601) 246-5631

Mississippi Gulf Coast Community College
Jackson County Campus
—Gautier—

Full-Time Enrollments:	156	Evening Classes:	Yes
Part-Time Enrollments:	—	Weekend Classes:	No
Affiliation:	Public	Distance Learning:	No

NLN ACCREDITATION: Yes

Articulation: LPN to Associate

For Further Information Contact:

Ms Nica Cason, Chair
Mississippi Gulf Coast Community College Jackson
County Campus
PO Box 100
Gautier, MS 39553
(601) 497-7662

Mississippi Gulf Coast Community College-
District Davis Campus
—Gulfport—

Full-Time Enrollments:	160	Evening Classes:	No
Part-Time Enrollments:	3	Weekend Classes:	No
Affiliation:	Public	Distance Learning:	No

NLN ACCREDITATION: Yes

Articulation: LPN to Associate

For Further Information Contact:

Mrs Wanda Brignac, Director
Mississippi Gulf Coast Community College-District
Davis Campus
2226 Switzer Rd
Gulfport, MS 39507
(601) 896-2501

Mississippi University for Women
—Columbus—

Full-Time Enrollments:	93	Evening Classes:	No
Part-Time Enrollments:	—	Weekend Classes:	No
Affiliation:	Public	Distance Learning:	No

NLN ACCREDITATION: Yes

Articulation: Associate to Baccalaureate

For Further Information Contact:

Mrs Mary Jo Kirkpatrick, Director
Mississippi University for Women
W Box 910
Columbus, MS 39701
(601) 329-7299

Northeast Mississippi Community College
—Booneville—

Full-Time Enrollments:	209	Evening Classes:	No
Part-Time Enrollments:	—	Weekend Classes:	No
Affiliation:	Public	Distance Learning:	No

NLN ACCREDITATION: Yes

Articulation: LPN to Associate

For Further Information Contact:

Mrs Debbie Ricks, Head
Northeast Mississippi Community College
Cunningham Blvd
Booneville, MS 38829
(601) 728-7751

Northwest Mississippi Community College
—Senatobia—

Full-Time Enrollments:	184	Evening Classes:	No
Part-Time Enrollments:	2	Weekend Classes:	No
Affiliation:	Public	Distance Learning:	No

NLN ACCREDITATION: Yes

Articulation: Associate to Baccalaureate
LPN to Associate

For Further Information Contact:

Mrs Victoria P Hale, Director
Northwest Mississippi Community College
Highway 51 North
Senatobia, MS 38668
(601) 562-3284

Pearl River Community College
—Poplarville—

Full-Time Enrollments:	154	Evening Classes:	No
Part-Time Enrollments:	—	Weekend Classes:	No
Affiliation:	Public	Distance Learning:	No

NLN ACCREDITATION: Yes

Articulation: None

For Further Information Contact:

Mrs Peggy Dease, Director
Pearl River Community College
Box 5760 101 Highway 11 N
Poplarville, MS 39470
(601) 795-6801

Southwest Mississippi Community College
—Summit—

Full-Time Enrollments:	189	Evening Classes:	Yes
Part-Time Enrollments:	—	Weekend Classes:	No
Affiliation:	Public	Distance Learning:	Yes

NLN ACCREDITATION: Yes

Articulation: LPN to Associate

For Further Information Contact:

Mrs Truda J McGrew, Director
Southwest Mississippi Community College
College Dr
Summit, MS 39666
(601) 276-2008

Missouri

Central Methodist College
—Fayette—

Full-Time Enrollments:	6	Evening Classes:	No
Part-Time Enrollments:	—	Weekend Classes:	No
Affiliation:	Religious	Distance Learning:	No

NLN ACCREDITATION: No

Articulation: Associate to Baccalaureate
Diploma to Baccalaureate

For Further Information Contact:

Dr Shirley J Peterson, Chair
Central Methodist College
411 Central Methodist Sq
Fayette, MO 65248
(816) 248-3391

Columbia College
—Columbia—

Full-Time Enrollments:	—	Evening Classes:	Yes
Part-Time Enrollments:	25	Weekend Classes:	No
Affiliation:	Private	Distance Learning:	No

NLN ACCREDITATION: Yes

Articulation: LPN to Associate

For Further Information Contact:

Mrs Sharon K Taylor, Director
Columbia College
500 Strawn Rd
Columbia, MO 65203-6100
(573) 886-2276

Crowder College
—Neosho—

Full-Time Enrollments:	53	Evening Classes:	Yes
Part-Time Enrollments:	—	Weekend Classes:	No
Affiliation:	Public	Distance Learning:	No

NLN ACCREDITATION: No

Articulation: Associate to Baccalaureate

For Further Information Contact:

Mrs D'ann Dennis, Director
Crowder College
601 Laclede
Neosho, MO 64850
(417) 451-4700

Deaconess College of Nursing
—St Louis—

Full-Time Enrollments:	4	Evening Classes:	Yes
Part-Time Enrollments:	41	Weekend Classes:	Yes
Affiliation:	Private	Distance Learning:	No

NLN ACCREDITATION: Yes

Articulation: Associate to Baccalaureate
LPN to Associate

For Further Information Contact:

Mrs Carmel T White, Director
Deaconess College of Nursing
6150 Oakland Ave
St Louis, MO 63139-3297
(314) 768-3044

East Central College
—Union—

Full-Time Enrollments:	26	Evening Classes:	No
Part-Time Enrollments:	16	Weekend Classes:	No
Affiliation:	Public	Distance Learning:	No

NLN ACCREDITATION: No

Articulation: LPN to Associate

For Further Information Contact:

Ms Patrice O'Connor, Director
East Central College
PO Box 529
Union, MO 63084-3720
(314) 583-5195

Hannibal-La Grange College
—Hannibal—

Full-Time Enrollments:	16	Evening Classes:	Yes
Part-Time Enrollments:	7	Weekend Classes:	No
Affiliation:	Religious	Distance Learning:	No

NLN ACCREDITATION: Yes

Articulation: Associate to Baccalaureate

For Further Information Contact:

Mrs Senda Guertzgen, Interim Director
Hannibal-La Grange College
2800 Palmyra Rd
Hannibal, MO 63401-1999
(573) 221-3675

Jefferson College
—Hillsboro—

Full-Time Enrollments:	41	Evening Classes:	No
Part-Time Enrollments:	—	Weekend Classes:	No
Affiliation:	Public	Distance Learning:	No

NLN ACCREDITATION: No

Articulation: Associate to Baccalaureate
RN to MSN

For Further Information Contact:

Ms Michele Soest, Director
Jefferson College
1000 Viking Dr
Hillsboro, MO 63050
(314) 789-3951

Jewish Hospital College of Nursing
—St Louis—

Full-Time Enrollments:	133	Evening Classes:	Yes
Part-Time Enrollments:	64	Weekend Classes:	Yes
Affiliation:	Private	Distance Learning:	No

NLN ACCREDITATION: Yes

Articulation: Diploma to Baccalaureate
LPN to Associate

For Further Information Contact:

Dr Sharon Pontious, President
Jewish Hospital College of Nursing
306 S Kinsgshighway
St Louis, MO 63110
(314) 454-8686

Lester L Cox College of Nursing and Health Sciences
—Springfield—

Full-Time Enrollments:	40	Evening Classes:	Yes
Part-Time Enrollments:	86	Weekend Classes:	No
Affiliation:	Private	Distance Learning:	No

NLN ACCREDITATION:

Articulation: None

For Further Information Contact:

Mrs Vickie L Donnell, Director
Lester L Cox College of Nursing and Health Sciences
1423 North Jefferson
Springfield, MO 65802
(417) 269-3067

Lincoln University
—Jefferson City—

Full-Time Enrollments:	31	Evening Classes:	Yes
Part-Time Enrollments:	74	Weekend Classes:	No
Affiliation:	Public	Distance Learning:	No

NLN ACCREDITATION: Yes

Articulation: None

For Further Information Contact:

Mrs Linda S Bickel, Dept Head
Lincoln University
100 Elliff Hall
Jefferson City, MO 65102-0029
(573) 681-5421

Lincoln University-Ft Leonard Wood
—Ft Leonard Wood—

Full-Time Enrollments:	—	Evening Classes:	Yes
Part-Time Enrollments:	37	Weekend Classes:	No
Affiliation:	Public	Distance Learning:	No

NLN ACCREDITATION: Yes

Articulation: None

For Further Information Contact:

Mrs Linda S Bickel, Dept Head
Lincoln University-Ft Leonard Wood
Truman Educ Center Blg 499
Ft Leonard Wood, MO 65473
(573) 681-5421

Mineral Area College
—Park Hills—

Full-Time Enrollments:	65	Evening Classes:	No
Part-Time Enrollments:	—	Weekend Classes:	No
Affiliation:	Public	Distance Learning:	No

NLN ACCREDITATION: No

Articulation: LPN to Associate

For Further Information Contact:

Mrs Teri Douglas, Chair
Mineral Area College
PO Box 1000
Park Hills, MO 63601
(573) 431-4593

Moberly Area Community College
—Moberly—

Full-Time Enrollments:	90	Evening Classes:	—
Part-Time Enrollments:	20	Weekend Classes:	—
Affiliation:	Public	Distance Learning:	—

NLN ACCREDITATION: No

Articulation: None

For Further Information Contact:

Ruth Jones, Director
Moberly Area Community College
College & Rollin St
Moberly, MO 65270
(816) 263-4110

North Central Missouri College
—Trenton—

Full-Time Enrollments:	—	Evening Classes:	—
Part-Time Enrollments:	—	Weekend Classes:	—
Affiliation:	Public	Distance Learning:	—

NLN ACCREDITATION: No

Articulation: None

For Further Information Contact:

Mrs Carol Elliott, Associate Dean
North Central Missouri College
1301 Main Street
Trenton, MO 64683
(816) 359-3948

Park College
—Parkville—

Full-Time Enrollments:	81	Evening Classes:	No
Part-Time Enrollments:	—	Weekend Classes:	No
Affiliation:	Private	Distance Learning:	No

NLN ACCREDITATION: Yes

Articulation: Associate to Baccalaureate
LPN to Associate

For Further Information Contact:

Dr Marvel Williamson, Director
Park College
8700 River Park Dr
Parkville, MO 64152
(816) 741-2000

Park College
—Rolla—

Full-Time Enrollments:	—	Evening Classes:	—
Part-Time Enrollments:	—	Weekend Classes:	—
Affiliation:	Private	Distance Learning:	—

NLN ACCREDITATION: Yes

Articulation: None

For Further Information Contact:

Dr Marvel Williamson, Director
Park College
600 Elm St
Rolla, MO 64501
(573) 341-2750

No longer there (handwritten)

Park College
—Sikeston—

Full-Time Enrollments:	—	Evening Classes:	—
Part-Time Enrollments:	—	Weekend Classes:	—
Affiliation:	Private	Distance Learning:	—

NLN ACCREDITATION: Yes

Articulation: None

No longer there

For Further Information Contact:

Dr Marvel Williamson, Director
Park College
312 E Center St
Sikeston, MO
(573) 472-3182

Penn Valley Community College
—Kansas City—

Full-Time Enrollments:	157	Evening Classes:	Yes
Part-Time Enrollments:	102	Weekend Classes:	Yes
Affiliation:	Public	Distance Learning:	Yes

NLN ACCREDITATION: Yes

Articulation: LPN to Associate

For Further Information Contact:

Ms Karen Komoroski, Chair
Penn Valley Community College
3201 SW Trafficway
Kansas City, MO 64111
(816) 759-4175

Sanford Brown College
—Kansas City—

Full-Time Enrollments:	—	Evening Classes:	—
Part-Time Enrollments:	—	Weekend Classes:	—
Affiliation:	Private	Distance Learning:	—

NLN ACCREDITATION: No

Articulation: None

For Further Information Contact:

To be named
Sanford Brown College
2702 Rockcreek Pkwy Suite 300
Kansas City, MO 64117
(816) 472-7400

Sanford Brown College
—St Charles—

Full-Time Enrollments:	—	Evening Classes:	—
Part-Time Enrollments:	—	Weekend Classes:	—
Affiliation:	Private	Distance Learning:	—

NLN ACCREDITATION: No

Articulation: None

For Further Information Contact:

Ms Maria Rapert, Director
Sanford Brown College
3555 Franks Dr
St Charles, MO 63301
(314) 949-2620

Sanford Brown College
—St Louis—

Full-Time Enrollments:	—	Evening Classes:	—
Part-Time Enrollments:	—	Weekend Classes:	—
Affiliation:	Private	Distance Learning:	—

NLN ACCREDITATION: No

Articulation: None

For Further Information Contact:

Ms Maryann Shrader, Director
Sanford Brown College
12006 Manchester Rd
St Louis, MO
(314) 822-7100

Southeast Missouri Hospital College
—Cape Girardeau—

Full-Time Enrollments:	23	Evening Classes:	Yes
Part-Time Enrollments:	12	Weekend Classes:	—
Affiliation:	Private	Distance Learning:	—

NLN ACCREDITATION: No

Articulation: Associate to Baccalaureate
LPN to Associate

For Further Information Contact:

Ms Tonya Buttry, Chair
Southeast Missouri Hospital College
1819 Brodway
Cape Girardeau, MO 63701
(573) 334-6825

Southeast Missouri State University
—Cape Girardeau—

Full-Time Enrollments:	—	Evening Classes:	Yes
Part-Time Enrollments:	106	Weekend Classes:	Yes
Affiliation:	Public	Distance Learning:	No

NLN ACCREDITATION: Yes

Articulation: Associate to Baccalaureate

For Further Information Contact:

Dr A Louise Hart, Chair
Southeast Missouri State University
One University Plaza
Cape Girardeau, MO 63701
(573) 651-2585

Southwest Missouri State University
—West Plains—

Full-Time Enrollments:	61	Evening Classes:	No
Part-Time Enrollments:	—	Weekend Classes:	No
Affiliation:	Public	Distance Learning:	Yes

NLN ACCREDITATION: Yes

Articulation: Associate to Baccalaureate
LPN to Associate

For Further Information Contact:

Mrs Juanita Roth, Director
Southwest Missouri State University
128 Garfield Ave
West Plains, MO 65775
(417) 256-1118

St Charles County Community College
—St Peter—

Full-Time Enrollments:	3	Evening Classes:	Yes
Part-Time Enrollments:	100	Weekend Classes:	No
Affiliation:	Public	Distance Learning:	No

NLN ACCREDITATION: Yes

Articulation: LPN to Associate

For Further Information Contact:

Mrs Patricia Porterfield, Chair
St Charles County Community College
4601 Mid River Mall Dr
St Peter, MO 63376
(314) 922-8000

St Louis Community College at Florissant Valley
—St Louis—

Full-Time Enrollments:	116	Evening Classes:	Yes
Part-Time Enrollments:	—	Weekend Classes:	—
Affiliation:	Public	Distance Learning:	—

NLN ACCREDITATION: Yes

Articulation: Associate to Baccalaureate
LPN to Associate

For Further Information Contact:

Mrs Frances Robbins Dennis, Chair
St Louis Community College at Florissant Valley
3400 Pershall Rd
St Louis, MO 63135-1499
(314) 595-4316

St Louis Community College at Forest Park
—St Louis—

Full-Time Enrollments:	90	Evening Classes:	—
Part-Time Enrollments:	59	Weekend Classes:	—
Affiliation:	Public	Distance Learning:	—

NLN ACCREDITATION: Yes

Articulation: None

For Further Information Contact:

Ms Marybelle Barnes, Chair
St Louis Community College at Forest Park
5600 Oakland Ave
St Louis, MO 63110-1393
(314) 644-9315

St Louis Community College at Meramec
—St Louis—

Full-Time Enrollments:	189	Evening Classes:	No
Part-Time Enrollments:	—	Weekend Classes:	No
Affiliation:	Public	Distance Learning:	No

NLN ACCREDITATION: Yes

Articulation: Associate to Baccalaureate

For Further Information Contact:

Mrs Sharon S Godwin, Chair
St Louis Community College at Meramec
11333 Big Bend Blvd
St Louis, MO 63122
(314) 984-7759

State Fair Community College
—Sedalia—

Full-Time Enrollments:	43	Evening Classes:	No
Part-Time Enrollments:	—	Weekend Classes:	No
Affiliation:	Public	Distance Learning:	No

NLN ACCREDITATION: No

Articulation: Associate to Baccalaureate
LPN to Associate

For Further Information Contact:

Ms Beverly Wilkerson, Director
State Fair Community College
3201 W 16th St
Sedalia, MO 65301
(816) 530-7100

Three Rivers Community College
—Poplar Bluff—

Full-Time Enrollments:	27	Evening Classes:	No
Part-Time Enrollments:	29	Weekend Classes:	No
Affiliation:	Public	Distance Learning:	No

NLN ACCREDITATION: Yes

Articulation: Associate to Baccalaureate
LPN to Associate

For Further Information Contact:

Ms Catherine F Wampler, Director
Three Rivers Community College
2080 Three Rivers Blvd
Poplar Bluff, MO 63901
(573) 840-9681

Montana

Miles Community College
—Miles City—

Full-Time Enrollments:	48	Evening Classes:	—
Part-Time Enrollments:	16	Weekend Classes:	—
Affiliation:	Public	Distance Learning:	—

NLN ACCREDITATION: Yes

Articulation: None

For Further Information Contact:

Ms Laura Lenau, Chair
Miles Community College
Miles City, MT 59301
(406) 232-3031

Montana State University Northern
—Havre—

Full-Time Enrollments:	106	Evening Classes:	No
Part-Time Enrollments:	—	Weekend Classes:	No
Affiliation:	Public	Distance Learning:	No

NLN ACCREDITATION: Yes

Articulation: Associate to Baccalaureate
LPN to Associate

For Further Information Contact:

Dr Jackie Swanson, Chair
Montana State University Northern
PO Box 7751
Havre, MT 59501-7751
(406) 265-4196

Salish Kootenai College
—Pablo—

Full-Time Enrollments:	48	Evening Classes:	No
Part-Time Enrollments:	—	Weekend Classes:	No
Affiliation:	Private	Distance Learning:	No

NLN ACCREDITATION: Yes

Articulation: Associate to Baccalaureate

For Further Information Contact:

Ms Jacque Dolberry, Director
Salish Kootenai College
PO Box 117 Hwy 93
Pablo, MT 59855-0117
(406) 675-4800

Nebraska

Central Community College
—Grand Island—

Full-Time Enrollments:	66	Evening Classes:	No
Part-Time Enrollments:	14	Weekend Classes:	No
Affiliation:	Public	Distance Learning:	No

NLN ACCREDITATION: Yes

Articulation: LPN to Associate

For Further Information Contact:

Mrs Linda Walline, Associate Dean
Central Community College
3134 West Hwy 34 PO Box 4903
Grand Island, NE 68802-0240
(308) 389-5220

ASSOCIATE DEGREE

College of St Mary
—Omaha—

Full-Time Enrollments:	88	Evening Classes:	Yes
Part-Time Enrollments:	20	Weekend Classes:	Yes
Affiliation:	Private	Distance Learning:	No

NLN ACCREDITATION: Yes

Articulation: Associate to Baccalaureate
LPN to Associate

For Further Information Contact:

Dr Mary A Hoefler, Chair
College of St Mary
72nd and Mercy Rd
Omaha, NE 68124
(402) 399-2636

Metropolitan Community College
—Omaha—

Full-Time Enrollments:	39	Evening Classes:	No
Part-Time Enrollments:	26	Weekend Classes:	No
Affiliation:	Public	Distance Learning:	No

NLN ACCREDITATION: Yes

Articulation: LPN to Associate

For Further Information Contact:

Ms Nina Wardell, Director
Metropolitan Community College
PO Box 3777
Omaha, NE 68103
(402) 449-8367

Mid Plains Community College
—North Platte—

Full-Time Enrollments:	47	Evening Classes:	No
Part-Time Enrollments:	—	Weekend Classes:	No
Affiliation:	Public	Distance Learning:	Yes

NLN ACCREDITATION: Yes

Articulation: Associate to Baccalaureate
LPN to Baccalaureate
LPN to Associate
RN to MSN

For Further Information Contact:

Mrs Diane Hoffmann, Head
Mid Plains Community College
1101 Halligan Dr
North Platte, NE 69101
(308) 532-8740

Nebraska Methodist College
—Coucil Bluff-IA—

Full-Time Enrollments:	50	Evening Classes:	—
Part-Time Enrollments:	—	Weekend Classes:	—
Affiliation:	Private	Distance Learning:	—

NLN ACCREDITATION: No

Articulation: None

For Further Information Contact:

Ms Carol Maxwell, Coordinator
Nebraska Methodist College
933 E Pierce St
Coucil Bluff-IA, NE 31503
(712) 328-6100

Northeast Community College
—Norfolk—

Full-Time Enrollments:	30	Evening Classes:	No
Part-Time Enrollments:	12	Weekend Classes:	No
Affiliation:	Public	Distance Learning:	Yes

NLN ACCREDITATION: Yes

Articulation: Associate to Baccalaureate
LPN to Associate

For Further Information Contact:

Ms Elaine Gardner, Director
Northeast Community College
801 E Benjamin Ave Box 469
Norfolk, NE 68702
(402) 644-0612

Southeast Community College
—Lincoln—

Full-Time Enrollments:	26	Evening Classes:	Yes
Part-Time Enrollments:	61	Weekend Classes:	No
Affiliation:	Public	Distance Learning:	No

NLN ACCREDITATION: Yes

Articulation: LPN to Associate

For Further Information Contact:

Ms Virginia Hess, Chair
Southeast Community College
8800 "O" St
Lincoln, NE 68520
(402) 471-3333

Nevada

Community College of Southern Nevada
—Las Vegas—

Full-Time Enrollments:	105	Evening Classes:	—
Part-Time Enrollments:	68	Weekend Classes:	—
Affiliation:	Public	Distance Learning:	—

NLN ACCREDITATION: Yes

Articulation: None

For Further Information Contact:

Frances Brown, Director
Community College of Southern Nevada
6375 W Charleston Blvd
Las Vegas, NV 89102-1124
(702) 877-1133

Great Basin College
—Elko—

Full-Time Enrollments:	12	Evening Classes:	No
Part-Time Enrollments:	16	Weekend Classes:	No
Affiliation:	Public	Distance Learning:	No

NLN ACCREDITATION: Yes

Articulation: Associate to Baccalaureate

For Further Information Contact:

Mrs Georgeanna Smith, Director
Great Basin College
1500 College Parkway
Elko, NV 89801
(702) 753-2216

Truckee Meadows Community College
—Reno—

Full-Time Enrollments:	75	Evening Classes:	No
Part-Time Enrollments:	—	Weekend Classes:	No
Affiliation:	Public	Distance Learning:	No

NLN ACCREDITATION: Yes

Articulation: Associate to Baccalaureate

For Further Information Contact:

Mrs Sandi Emerson, Director
Truckee Meadows Community College
7000 Dandini Blvd
Reno, NV 89512
(702) 673-7115

Western Nevada Community College
—Carson City—

Full-Time Enrollments:	38	Evening Classes:	No
Part-Time Enrollments:	30	Weekend Classes:	No
Affiliation:	Public	Distance Learning:	Yes

NLN ACCREDITATION: Yes

Articulation: Associate to Baccalaureate

For Further Information Contact:

Ms Mildred Wade, Director
Western Nevada Community College
2201 W College Parkway
Carson City, NV 89701
(702) 887-3176

New Hampshire

New Hampshire Community Technical College
—Claremont—

Full-Time Enrollments:	51	Evening Classes:	No
Part-Time Enrollments:	33	Weekend Classes:	No
Affiliation:	Public	Distance Learning:	No

NLN ACCREDITATION: Yes

Articulation: None

For Further Information Contact:

Mrs Susan Henderson, Chair
New Hampshire Community Technical College
1 College Dr RR#3 Box 550
Claremont, NH 03743-9707
(603) 542-7744

New Hampshire Community Technical College
—Manchester—

Full-Time Enrollments:	40	Evening Classes:	Yes
Part-Time Enrollments:	54	Weekend Classes:	No
Affiliation:	Public	Distance Learning:	No

NLN ACCREDITATION: Yes

Articulation: None

For Further Information Contact:

Mrs Mary Wheeler, Chair
New Hampshire Community Technical College
1066 Front St
Manchester, NH 03102
(603) 668-6706

New Hampshire Community Technical College-Berlin
—Berlin—

Full-Time Enrollments:	40	Evening Classes:	No
Part-Time Enrollments:	14	Weekend Classes:	No
Affiliation:	Public	Distance Learning:	No

NLN ACCREDITATION: No

Articulation: LPN to Associate

For Further Information Contact:

Ms Terrie Judge, Director
New Hampshire Community Technical College-Berlin
2020 Riverside Dr
Berlin, NH 03570
(603) 752-1113x

New Hampshire Community Technical College
—Stratham—

Full-Time Enrollments:	20	Evening Classes:	No
Part-Time Enrollments:	48	Weekend Classes:	No
Affiliation:	Public	Distance Learning:	No

NLN ACCREDITATION: No

Articulation: None

For Further Information Contact:

Mrs Mary Wheeler, Chair
New Hamsphire Community Technical College
277 Portsmouth Ave
Stratham, NH 03885
(603) 772-1194

New Hampshire Technical Institute
—Concord—

Full-Time Enrollments:	73	Evening Classes:	Yes
Part-Time Enrollments:	128	Weekend Classes:	—
Affiliation:	Public	Distance Learning:	—

NLN ACCREDITATION: Yes

Articulation: Associate to Baccalaureate

For Further Information Contact:

Mrs Joyce Myles, Dept Head
New Hampshire Technical Institute
11 Institute Dr
Concord, NH 03301-7412
(603) 225-1800

Rivier College/St Joseph Nursing
—Nashua—

Full-Time Enrollments:	149	Evening Classes:	Yes
Part-Time Enrollments:	96	Weekend Classes:	Yes
Affiliation:	Religious	Distance Learning:	Yes

NLN ACCREDITATION: Yes

Articulation: Associate to Baccalaureate
LPN to Associate

For Further Information Contact:

Dr Judith Haywood, Dean
Rivier College/St Joseph Nursing
South Main St
Nashua, NH 03060
(603) 888-1311

New Jersey

Atlantic Community College
—Mays Landing—

Full-Time Enrollments:	28	Evening Classes:	No
Part-Time Enrollments:	60	Weekend Classes:	No
Affiliation:	Public	Distance Learning:	Yes

NLN ACCREDITATION: Yes

Articulation: None

For Further Information Contact:

Ms Muriel Jacoby, Chair
Atlantic Community College
5100 Black Horse Pike
Mays Landing, NJ 08330-2699
(609) 343-5035

Bergen Community College
—Paramus—

Full-Time Enrollments:	—	Evening Classes:	—
Part-Time Enrollments:	—	Weekend Classes:	—
Affiliation:	Public	Distance Learning:	—

NLN ACCREDITATION: Yes

Articulation: —

For Further Information Contact:

Ms Joan Murko, Director
Bergen Community College
400 Paramus Rd
Paramus, NJ 07652
(201) 447-7181

ASSOCIATE DEGREE

Brookdale Community College
—Lincroft—

Full-Time Enrollments:	50	**Evening Classes:**	Yes
Part-Time Enrollments:	223	**Weekend Classes:**	No
Affiliation:	Public	**Distance Learning:**	No

NLN ACCREDITATION: Yes

Articulation: Associate to Baccalaureate
Diploma to Associate
LPN to Associate

For Further Information Contact:

Mrs Maris A Lown, Director
Brookdale Community College
765 Newman Springs Rd
Lincroft, NJ 07738
(908) 842-1900

Burlington County College
—Pemberton—

Full-Time Enrollments:	82	**Evening Classes:**	Yes
Part-Time Enrollments:	40	**Weekend Classes:**	—
Affiliation:	Public	**Distance Learning:**	—

NLN ACCREDITATION: Yes

Articulation: Associate to Baccalaureate
Diploma to Associate
LPN to Associate

For Further Information Contact:

Ms Charlotte McCarraher, Director
Burlington County College
Pemberton-Browns Mills Rd
Pemberton, NJ 08068
(609) 894-9311

County College of Morris
—Randolph—

Full-Time Enrollments:	29	**Evening Classes:**	—
Part-Time Enrollments:	265	**Weekend Classes:**	—
Affiliation:	Public	**Distance Learning:**	—

NLN ACCREDITATION: Yes

Articulation: None

For Further Information Contact:

Ms Margaret Kinsella Warshaw, Chair
County College of Morris
Route 10 & Center Grove Rd
Randolph, NJ 07869
(201) 328-5000

Cumberland County College
—Vineland—

Full-Time Enrollments:	33	**Evening Classes:**	Yes
Part-Time Enrollments:	85	**Weekend Classes:**	Yes
Affiliation:	Public	**Distance Learning:**	Yes

NLN ACCREDITATION: Yes

Articulation: Associate to Baccalaureate
LPN to Associate

For Further Information Contact:

Dr Noreen Sisko, Chair
Cumberland County College
PO Box 517
Vineland, NJ 08360
(609) 691-8600

Essex County College
—Newark—

Full-Time Enrollments:	27	**Evening Classes:**	No
Part-Time Enrollments:	89	**Weekend Classes:**	No
Affiliation:	Public	**Distance Learning:**	No

NLN ACCREDITATION: Yes

Articulation: Associate to Baccalaureate
RN to MSN

For Further Information Contact:

Ms Vickie A Grosso, Chair
Essex County College
303 Univ Ave
Newark, NJ 07102
(201) 877-1868

Felician College
—Lodi—

Full-Time Enrollments:	—	**Evening Classes:**	—
Part-Time Enrollments:	—	**Weekend Classes:**	—
Affiliation:	Religious	**Distance Learning:**	—

NLN ACCREDITATION: Yes

Articulation: —

For Further Information Contact:

Dr Rona Levin, Director
Felician College
262 South Main St
Lodi, NJ 07644
(201) 778-1190

Gloucester County College
—Sewell—

Full-Time Enrollments: 147
Part-Time Enrollments: 95
Affiliation: Public
Evening Classes: Yes
Weekend Classes: Yes
Distance Learning: No

NLN ACCREDITATION: Yes

Articulation: Associate to Baccalaureate

For Further Information Contact:

Mr Earl Goldberg, Chair
Gloucester County College
1400 Tanyard Rd
Sewell, NJ 08080
(609) 468-5000

Mercer County College
—Trenton—

Full-Time Enrollments: 8
Part-Time Enrollments: 128
Affiliation: Public
Evening Classes: Yes
Weekend Classes: Yes
Distance Learning: No

NLN ACCREDITATION: Yes

Articulation: Associate to Baccalaureate
LPN to Associate

For Further Information Contact:

Ms Clara Lidz, Director
Mercer County College
1200 Old Trenton Rd, Box B
Trenton, NJ 08690
(609) 586-4800

Ocean County College
—Toms River—

Full-Time Enrollments: 92
Part-Time Enrollments: 112
Affiliation: Public
Evening Classes: Yes
Weekend Classes: No
Distance Learning: No

NLN ACCREDITATION: Yes

Articulation: LPN to Associate

For Further Information Contact:

Dr Nancy Sweeney, Dean
Ocean County College
College Dr, Box 2001
Toms River, NJ 08754-2001
(908) 255-0395

Passaic County Community College
—Paterson—

Full-Time Enrollments: 26
Part-Time Enrollments: 96
Affiliation: Public
Evening Classes: Yes
Weekend Classes: No
Distance Learning: No

NLN ACCREDITATION: Yes

Articulation: Associate to Baccalaureate
LPN to Associate

For Further Information Contact:

Ms Sylvia Edge, Director
Passaic County Community College
College Boulevard
Paterson, NJ 07509
(201) 684-5221

Raritan Valley Community College
—Somerville—

Full-Time Enrollments: 112
Part-Time Enrollments: 31
Affiliation: Public
Evening Classes: No
Weekend Classes: No
Distance Learning: Yes

NLN ACCREDITATION: Yes

Articulation: Associate to Baccalaureate

For Further Information Contact:

Mrs Rosalia Hamilton, Chair
Raritan Valley Community College
PO Box 3300
Somerville, NJ 08876
(908) 218-8877

University of Medicine & Dentistry of New Jersey
—Edison—

Full-Time Enrollments: 48
Part-Time Enrollments: 82
Affiliation: Public
Evening Classes: —
Weekend Classes: —
Distance Learning: —

NLN ACCREDITATION: Yes

Articulation: None

For Further Information Contact:

Dr Minerva Guttman, Assistant Dean
University of Medicine & Dentistry of New Jersey
155 Mill Rd PO Box 3050
Edison, NJ 08818
(908) 906-4660

ASSOCIATE DEGREE

New Mexico

Albuquerque Technical Vocational Institute
—Albuquerque—

Full-Time Enrollments:	5	Evening Classes:	Yes
Part-Time Enrollments:	100	Weekend Classes:	Yes
Affiliation:	Public	Distance Learning:	—

NLN ACCREDITATION: Yes

Articulation: Associate to Baccalaureate
LPN to Associate

For Further Information Contact:

Mrs Patricia Stephens, Director
Albuquerque Technical Vocational Institute
2000 Coal SE
Albuquerque, NM 87106
(505) 224-4141

Clovis Community College
—Clovis—

Full-Time Enrollments:	27	Evening Classes:	Yes
Part-Time Enrollments:	—	Weekend Classes:	No
Affiliation:	Public	Distance Learning:	Yes

NLN ACCREDITATION: Yes

Articulation: LPN to Associate

For Further Information Contact:

Mrs Ione Wood, Director
Clovis Community College
417 Schepps Blvd
Clovis, NM 88101
(505) 769-4100

Dona Ana Branch Community College
—Las Cruces—

Full-Time Enrollments:	34	Evening Classes:	Yes
Part-Time Enrollments:	5	Weekend Classes:	Yes
Affiliation:	Public	Distance Learning:	No

NLN ACCREDITATION:

Articulation: Associate to Baccalaureate

For Further Information Contact:

Dr Sarah Stark, Head
Dona Ana Branch Community College
Box 30001-3 DA
Las Cruces, NM 88003
(505) 527-7639

Eastern New Mexico University-Roswell
—Roswell—

Full-Time Enrollments:	63	Evening Classes:	No
Part-Time Enrollments:	29	Weekend Classes:	No
Affiliation:	Public	Distance Learning:	No

NLN ACCREDITATION: Yes

Articulation: Associate to Baccalaureate

For Further Information Contact:

Mrs Eloise A Blake, Chair
Eastern New Mexico University-Roswell
PO Box 6000
Roswell, NM 88201
(505) 624-7235

Luna Technical Vocational Institute
—Las Vegas—

Full-Time Enrollments:	48	Evening Classes:	—
Part-Time Enrollments:	—	Weekend Classes:	—
Affiliation:	Public	Distance Learning:	—

NLN ACCREDITATION: No

Articulation: None

For Further Information Contact:

Mrs Faith T Edwards, Director
Luna Technical Vocational Institute
PO Drawer K
Las Vegas, NM 87701
(505) 454-2527

New Mexico Jr College
—Hobbs—

Full-Time Enrollments:	90	Evening Classes:	Yes
Part-Time Enrollments:	39	Weekend Classes:	Yes
Affiliation:	Public	Distance Learning:	—

NLN ACCREDITATION: Yes

Articulation: None

For Further Information Contact:

Mr Steven Davis, Director
New Mexico Jr College
5317 Lovington Hwy
Hobbs, NM 88240
(505) 392-5714

New Mexico State University
—Alamogordo—

Full-Time Enrollments: 52
Part-Time Enrollments: 23
Affiliation: Public

Evening Classes: —
Weekend Classes: —
Distance Learning: —

NLN ACCREDITATION: Yes

Articulation: Associate to Baccalaureate

For Further Information Contact:

Mrs Joanna Giglio, Coordinator
New Mexico State University
Box 477
Alamogordo, NM 88310
(505) 439-0593

New Mexico State University at Carlsbad
—Carlsbad—

Full-Time Enrollments: 62
Part-Time Enrollments: —
Affiliation: Public

Evening Classes: Yes
Weekend Classes: Yes
Distance Learning: No

NLN ACCREDITATION: Yes

Articulation: Associate to Baccalaureate
LPN to Associate

For Further Information Contact:

Ms Sharon Souter, Director
New Mexico State University at Carlsbad
1500 Univ Dr
Carlsbad, NM 88220
(505) 885-8831

Northern New Mexico Community College
—Espanola—

Full-Time Enrollments: —
Part-Time Enrollments: —
Affiliation: Public

Evening Classes: —
Weekend Classes: —
Distance Learning: —

NLN ACCREDITATION: No

Articulation: —

For Further Information Contact:

Mrs Ramona Gonzales, Director
Northern New Mexico Community College
1002 N Onate
Espanola, NM 87532
(505) 747-2209

San Juan College
—Farmington—

Full-Time Enrollments: 67
Part-Time Enrollments: —
Affiliation: Public

Evening Classes: No
Weekend Classes: No
Distance Learning: No

NLN ACCREDITATION: Yes

Articulation: Associate to Baccalaureate
LPN to Associate

For Further Information Contact:

Mrs Judy Lund-Green, Director
San Juan College
4601 College Blvd
Farmington, NM 87402
(505) 599-0224

Santa Fe Community College
—Santa Fe—

Full-Time Enrollments: 26
Part-Time Enrollments: 20
Affiliation: Public

Evening Classes: No
Weekend Classes: No
Distance Learning: No

NLN ACCREDITATION: Yes

Articulation: Associate to Baccalaureate
LPN to Associate

For Further Information Contact:

Ms Sue MacMillan, Director
Santa Fe Community College
PO Box 4187
Santa Fe, NM 87502-4187
(505) 438-1324

University of New Mexico-Gallup
—Gallup—

Full-Time Enrollments: 65
Part-Time Enrollments: 5
Affiliation: Public

Evening Classes: Yes
Weekend Classes: No
Distance Learning: No

NLN ACCREDITATION: Yes

Articulation: Associate to Baccalaureate

For Further Information Contact:

Ms Jane Bruker, Chair
University of New Mexico-Gallup
200 College Rd
Gallup, NM 87301
(505) 863-7514

Western New Mexico University
—Silver City—

Full-Time Enrollments: 36
Part-Time Enrollments: —
Affiliation: Public
Evening Classes: Yes
Weekend Classes: No
Distance Learning: —

NLN ACCREDITATION: Yes

Articulation: LPN to Associate

For Further Information Contact:

Mrs Patricia McIntire, Chair
Western New Mexico University
PO Box 680
Silver City, NM 88062
(505) 538-6348

New York

Adirondack Community College
—Queensbury—

Full-Time Enrollments: 61
Part-Time Enrollments: 106
Affiliation: Public
Evening Classes: Yes
Weekend Classes: No
Distance Learning: Yes

NLN ACCREDITATION: No

Articulation: LPN to Associate

For Further Information Contact:

Dr Susan Letvak, Chair
Adirondack Community College
Queensbury, NY 12804
(518) 793-2262

Borough of Manhattan Community College of CUNY
—New York—

Full-Time Enrollments: 236
Part-Time Enrollments: 157
Affiliation: Public
Evening Classes: Yes
Weekend Classes: Yes
Distance Learning: —

NLN ACCREDITATION: Yes

Articulation: Associate to Baccalaureate

For Further Information Contact:

Prof Veronica Coleman, Chair
Borough of Manhattan Community College of CUNY
199 Chambers St-Rm S786
New York, NY 10007
(212) 346-8700

Bronx Community College of CUNY
—Bronx—

Full-Time Enrollments: 61
Part-Time Enrollments: 120
Affiliation: Public
Evening Classes: —
Weekend Classes: —
Distance Learning: —

NLN ACCREDITATION: Yes

Articulation: None

For Further Information Contact:

Prof Ann Smith, Chair
Bronx Community College of CUNY
181th St & Univ Ave
Bronx, NY 10453
(718) 289-5100

Broome Community College
—Binghamton—

Full-Time Enrollments: 131
Part-Time Enrollments: 49
Affiliation: Public
Evening Classes: No
Weekend Classes: No
Distance Learning: No

NLN ACCREDITATION: Yes

Articulation: LPN to Associate

For Further Information Contact:

Ms C Ligeikis Clayton, Chair
Broome Community College
901 Front St
Binghamton, NY 13902
(607) 778-5059

Catholic Medical Center of Brooklyn & Queens
—Fresh Meadows—

Full-Time Enrollments: 27
Part-Time Enrollments: 42
Affiliation: Religious
Evening Classes: No
Weekend Classes: No
Distance Learning: No

NLN ACCREDITATION: No

Articulation: None

For Further Information Contact:

Mrs Elisa Dalman Hess, Director
Catholic Medical Center of Brooklyn & Queens
175-05 H Harding Expressway
Fresh Meadows, NY 11365
(718) 357-0500 Ext 127

Cayuga County Community College
—Auburn—

Full-Time Enrollments:	36	Evening Classes:	Yes
Part-Time Enrollments:	61	Weekend Classes:	No
Affiliation:	Public	Distance Learning:	Yes

NLN ACCREDITATION: Yes

Articulation: Associate to Baccalaureate
LPN to Associate

For Further Information Contact:

Mrs Vicki C Condie, Director
Cayuga County Community College
Auburn, NY 13021
(315) 255-1743

Clinton Community College
—Plattsburgh—

Full-Time Enrollments:	53	Evening Classes:	Yes
Part-Time Enrollments:	40	Weekend Classes:	No
Affiliation:	Public	Distance Learning:	No

NLN ACCREDITATION: Yes

Articulation: Associate to Baccalaureate

For Further Information Contact:

Dr Agnes Pearl, Associate Dean
Clinton Community College
136 Clinton Point Dr
Plattsburgh, NY 12901
(518) 562-4162

Cochran School of Nursing-St John's Riverside
—Yonkers—

Full-Time Enrollments:	80	Evening Classes:	Yes
Part-Time Enrollments:	34	Weekend Classes:	—
Affiliation:	Private	Distance Learning:	—

NLN ACCREDITATION: No

Articulation: Associate to Baccalaureate
LPN to Associate

For Further Information Contact:

Mrs Lucetta M Ganley, Vice President
Cochran School of Nursing-St John's Riverside
967 N Broadway
Yonkers, NY 10701
(914) 964-4283

College of Staten Island
—Staten Island—

Full-Time Enrollments:	200	Evening Classes:	No
Part-Time Enrollments:	82	Weekend Classes:	No
Affiliation:	Public	Distance Learning:	No

NLN ACCREDITATION: Yes

Articulation: Associate to Baccalaureate

For Further Information Contact:

Dr Louise M Malarkey, Chair
College of Staten Island
2800 Victoria Blvd
Staten Island, NY 10314
(718) 982-3810

Columbia-Greene Community College
—Hudson—

Full-Time Enrollments:	29	Evening Classes:	No
Part-Time Enrollments:	96	Weekend Classes:	No
Affiliation:	Public	Distance Learning:	No

NLN ACCREDITATION: Yes

Articulation: None

For Further Information Contact:

Mrs Joan Tompkins, Chair
Columbia-Greene Community College
4400 Route 23
Hudson, NY 12534
(518) 828-4181

Corning Community College
—Corning—

Full-Time Enrollments:	103	Evening Classes:	No
Part-Time Enrollments:	43	Weekend Classes:	No
Affiliation:	Public	Distance Learning:	No

NLN ACCREDITATION: Yes

Articulation: Associate to Baccalaureate
LPN to Associate

For Further Information Contact:

Mrs Bonnie Page, Chair
Corning Community College
1 Academic Dr
Corning, NY 14830-3297
(607) 962-9241

Crouse Hospital School of Nursing
—Syracuse—

Full-Time Enrollments:	—	**Evening Classes:**	—
Part-Time Enrollments:	—	**Weekend Classes:**	—
Affiliation:	Private	**Distance Learning:**	—

NLN ACCREDITATION: No

Articulation: None

For Further Information Contact:

Ms Sherry Pearsall, Director
Crouse Hospital School of Nursing
736 Irving Ave
Syracuse, NY 13210
(315) 470-7483

Dutchess Community College
—Poughkeepsie—

Full-Time Enrollments:	75	**Evening Classes:**	Yes
Part-Time Enrollments:	133	**Weekend Classes:**	No
Affiliation:	Public	**Distance Learning:**	No

NLN ACCREDITATION: Yes

Articulation: Associate to Baccalaureate
LPN to Associate

For Further Information Contact:

Dr Edna Gardenier, Dept Head
Dutchess Community College
Pendell Rd
Poughkeepsie, NY 12601
(914) 471-4500

Ellis Hospital School of Nursing
—Schenectady—

Full-Time Enrollments:	39	**Evening Classes:**	No
Part-Time Enrollments:	30	**Weekend Classes:**	No
Affiliation:	Private	**Distance Learning:**	No

NLN ACCREDITATION: No

Articulation: Associate to Baccalaureate

For Further Information Contact:

Mrs Rose Petrak, Director
Ellis Hospital School of Nursing
1101 Nott St
Schenectady, NY 12308
(518) 382-4471

Erie Community College
—Buffalo—

Full-Time Enrollments:	40	**Evening Classes:**	No
Part-Time Enrollments:	63	**Weekend Classes:**	No
Affiliation:	Public	**Distance Learning:**	No

NLN ACCREDITATION: Yes

Articulation: Associate to Baccalaureate

For Further Information Contact:

Dr Marcia Gellin, Dept Head
Erie Community College
121 Elliott St
Buffalo, NY 14203
(716) 851-1098

Erie Community College-North
—Williamsville—

Full-Time Enrollments:	70	**Evening Classes:**	Yes
Part-Time Enrollments:	222	**Weekend Classes:**	No
Affiliation:	Public	**Distance Learning:**	No

NLN ACCREDITATION: Yes

Articulation: Associate to Baccalaureate

For Further Information Contact:

Dr Theresa Ranne, Dept Head
Erie Community College-North
6205 Main St
Williamsville, NY 14221
(716) 851-1357

Finger Lake Community College
—Canandaigua—

Full-Time Enrollments:	55	**Evening Classes:**	No
Part-Time Enrollments:	93	**Weekend Classes:**	No
Affiliation:	Public	**Distance Learning:**	No

NLN ACCREDITATION: Yes

Articulation: Associate to Baccalaureate
LPN to Associate

For Further Information Contact:

Mrs Mary Capozzi, Chair
Finger Lake Community College
4355 Lake Shore Dr
Canandaigua, NY 14424-8395
(716) 394-3500

Fulton Montgomery Community College
—Johnstown—

Full-Time Enrollments:	53	Evening Classes:	—
Part-Time Enrollments:	22	Weekend Classes:	—
Affiliation:	Public	Distance Learning:	—

NLN ACCREDITATION: No

Articulation: None

For Further Information Contact:

Mrs Teresa Becker, Director
Fulton Montgomery Community College
Johnstown, NY 12095
(518) 762-4651

Genesee Community College
—Batavia—

Full-Time Enrollments:	86	Evening Classes:	Yes
Part-Time Enrollments:	24	Weekend Classes:	Yes
Affiliation:	Public	Distance Learning:	Yes

NLN ACCREDITATION: Yes

Articulation: Associate to Baccalaureate

For Further Information Contact:

Mrs Betty Lapp, Director
Genesee Community College
College Rd
Batavia, NY 14020
(716) 343-0055

Helene Fuld School of Nursing-North General Hospital
—New York—

Full-Time Enrollments:	130	Evening Classes:	No
Part-Time Enrollments:	73	Weekend Classes:	No
Affiliation:	Private	Distance Learning:	No

NLN ACCREDITATION: Yes

Articulation: Associate to Baccalaureate
LPN to Associate

For Further Information Contact:

Dr Margaret Wines, President
Helene Fuld School of Nursing-North General Hospital
1879 Madison Ave
New York, NY 10035
(212) 423-1000

Hostos Community College
—Bronx—

Full-Time Enrollments:	45	Evening Classes:	No
Part-Time Enrollments:	5	Weekend Classes:	No
Affiliation:	Public	Distance Learning:	No

NLN ACCREDITATION: No

Articulation: Associate to Baccalaureate

For Further Information Contact:

Dr Elizabeth L Errico, Coordinator
Hostos Community College
475 Grand Concourse
Bronx, NY 10451
(718) 960-1161

Hudson Valley Community College
—Troy—

Full-Time Enrollments:	153	Evening Classes:	Yes
Part-Time Enrollments:	57	Weekend Classes:	—
Affiliation:	Public	Distance Learning:	—

NLN ACCREDITATION: Yes

Articulation: Associate to Baccalaureate

For Further Information Contact:

Dr Dicey O'Malley, Chair
Hudson Valley Community College
80 Vandenburgh Ave
Troy, NY 12180
(518) 283-7409

Interfaith Medical Center
—Brooklyn—

Full-Time Enrollments:	54	Evening Classes:	—
Part-Time Enrollments:	—	Weekend Classes:	—
Affiliation:	Private	Distance Learning:	—

NLN ACCREDITATION: No

Articulation: None

For Further Information Contact:

Ms Meta S Haven, Dean
Interfaith Medical Center
567 Prospect Pl
Brooklyn, NY 11238
(718) 935-7902

Iona College-Yonkers (2 Campuses)
—New Rochelle—

Full-Time Enrollments:	71	Evening Classes:	Yes
Part-Time Enrollments:	—	Weekend Classes:	Yes
Affiliation:	Religious	Distance Learning:	Yes

NLN ACCREDITATION: Yes

Articulation: Associate to Baccalaureate
LPN to Associate

For Further Information Contact:

Mrs Catherine D'Amico, Director
Iona College-Yonkers (2 Campuses)
715 North Ave
New Rochelle, NY 10801
(914) 633-2000

Jamestown Community College
—Jamestown—

Full-Time Enrollments:	107	Evening Classes:	—
Part-Time Enrollments:	57	Weekend Classes:	—
Affiliation:	Public	Distance Learning:	—

NLN ACCREDITATION: Yes

Articulation: None

For Further Information Contact:

Mrs Judith B Cordia, Director
Jamestown Community College
Jamestown, NY 14701
(716) 665-5220

Jefferson Community College
—Watertown—

Full-Time Enrollments:	57	Evening Classes:	Yes
Part-Time Enrollments:	43	Weekend Classes:	Yes
Affiliation:	Public	Distance Learning:	No

NLN ACCREDITATION: Yes

Articulation: Associate to Baccalaureate

For Further Information Contact:

Mrs L M Carlisle, Chair
Jefferson Community College
Watertown, NY 13601
(315) 786-2321

Kingsborough Community College of CUNY
—Brooklyn—

Full-Time Enrollments:	189	Evening Classes:	No
Part-Time Enrollments:	—	Weekend Classes:	No
Affiliation:	Public	Distance Learning:	No

NLN ACCREDITATION: Yes

Articulation: Associate to Baccalaureate

For Further Information Contact:

Prof Dolores Shrimpton, Chair
Kingsborough Community College of CUNY
2001 Oriental Blvd
Brooklyn, NY 11235
(718) 368-5522

LaGuardia Community College
—Long Island City—

Full-Time Enrollments:	168	Evening Classes:	No
Part-Time Enrollments:	—	Weekend Classes:	No
Affiliation:	Public	Distance Learning:	No

NLN ACCREDITATION: Yes

Articulation: Associate to Baccalaureate

For Further Information Contact:

Assoc Prof Marcia Caton, Director
LaGuardia Community College
31-10 Thomsom Ave
Long Island City, NY 11101
(718) 482-5774

Long Island College Hospital School of Nursing
—Brooklyn—

Full-Time Enrollments:	30	Evening Classes:	Yes
Part-Time Enrollments:	130	Weekend Classes:	No
Affiliation:	Private	Distance Learning:	No

NLN ACCREDITATION: Yes

Articulation: Associate to Baccalaureate

For Further Information Contact:

Dr Stephen Holzemer, Dean
Long Island College Hospital School of Nursing
397 Hicks St
Brooklyn, NY 11201
(718) 780-1952

Maria College
—Albany—

Full-Time Enrollments:	100	Evening Classes:	Yes
Part-Time Enrollments:	126	Weekend Classes:	Yes
Affiliation:	Religious	Distance Learning:	No

NLN ACCREDITATION: Yes

Articulation: Associate to Baccalaureate

For Further Information Contact:

Mrs Esther K McEvoy, Chair
Maria College
700 New Scotland Ave
Albany, NY 12208
(518) 489-7436

Medgar Evers College of CUNY
—Brooklyn—

Full-Time Enrollments:	—	Evening Classes:	—
Part-Time Enrollments:	59	Weekend Classes:	—
Affiliation:	Public	Distance Learning:	—

NLN ACCREDITATION: Yes

Articulation: None

For Further Information Contact:

Dr Bertie M Gilmore, Director
Medgar Evers College of CUNY
1650 Bedford Ave
Brooklyn, NY 11222
(718) 270-6441

Millard Fillmore Hospital School of Nursing
—Buffalo—

Full-Time Enrollments:	56	Evening Classes:	No
Part-Time Enrollments:	17	Weekend Classes:	No
Affiliation:	Private	Distance Learning:	No

NLN ACCREDITATION: No

Articulation: Associate to Baccalaureate

For Further Information Contact:

Mrs Cheryl Hausner, Director
Millard Fillmore Hospital School of Nursing
3 Gates Circle
Buffalo, NY 14209
(716) 887-4860

Mohawk Valley Community College
—Utica—

Full-Time Enrollments:	75	Evening Classes:	Yes
Part-Time Enrollments:	131	Weekend Classes:	No
Affiliation:	Public	Distance Learning:	Yes

NLN ACCREDITATION: Yes

Articulation: Associate to Baccalaureate
LPN to Associate

For Further Information Contact:

Mrs Nancy Caputo, Head
Mohawk Valley Community College
1101 Sherman Dr
Utica, NY 13501
(315) 792-5499

Monroe Community College
—Rochester—

Full-Time Enrollments:	55	Evening Classes:	No
Part-Time Enrollments:	233	Weekend Classes:	No
Affiliation:	Public	Distance Learning:	No

NLN ACCREDITATION: Yes

Articulation: Associate to Baccalaureate
LPN to Associate

For Further Information Contact:

Mrs Barbara Connolly Lauder, Chair
Monroe Community College
1000 E Henrietta Rd
Rochester, NY 14623
(716) 424-5200

Nassau Community College
—Garden City—

Full-Time Enrollments:	72	Evening Classes:	Yes
Part-Time Enrollments:	300	Weekend Classes:	Yes
Affiliation:	Public	Distance Learning:	Yes

NLN ACCREDITATION: Yes

Articulation: Associate to Baccalaureate
LPN to Associate

For Further Information Contact:

Dr Roseanna Mills, Chair
Nassau Community College
Stewart Ave
Garden City, NY 11530
(516) 572-7234

New York City Technical College of CUNY
—Brooklyn—

Full-Time Enrollments:	275	Evening Classes:	No
Part-Time Enrollments:	159	Weekend Classes:	No
Affiliation:	Public	Distance Learning:	No

NLN ACCREDITATION: Yes

Articulation: Associate to Baccalaureate

For Further Information Contact:

Prof Kathryn Richardson, Chair
New York City Technical College of CUNY
300 Jay St
Brooklyn, NY 11201
(718) 260-5660

Niagara County Community College
—Sanborn—

Full-Time Enrollments:	—	Evening Classes:	—
Part-Time Enrollments:	—	Weekend Classes:	—
Affiliation:	Public	Distance Learning:	—

NLN ACCREDITATION: Yes

Articulation: —

For Further Information Contact:

Mrs Catherine Peuquet, Director
Niagara County Community College
3111 Saunders Settlement Rd
Sanborn, NY 14132
(716) 731-3271

North County Community College
—Saranac Lake—

Full-Time Enrollments:	29	Evening Classes:	No
Part-Time Enrollments:	10	Weekend Classes:	No
Affiliation:	Public	Distance Learning:	Yes

NLN ACCREDITATION: No

Articulation: Associate to Baccalaureate

For Further Information Contact:

Mrs Barbara Rexilius, Director
North County Community College
20 Winona Ave Box 89
Saranac Lake, NY 12983-0089
(518) 891-2915

Onondaga Community College
—Syracuse—

Full-Time Enrollments:	92	Evening Classes:	Yes
Part-Time Enrollments:	128	Weekend Classes:	Yes
Affiliation:	Public	Distance Learning:	No

NLN ACCREDITATION: Yes

Articulation: Associate to Baccalaureate
LPN to Associate
RN to MSN

For Further Information Contact:

Ms Margaret Powers, Chair
Onondaga Community College
Onondaga Hill
Syracuse, NY 13215
(315) 469-7741

Orange County Community College
—Middletown—

Full-Time Enrollments:	45	Evening Classes:	Yes
Part-Time Enrollments:	168	Weekend Classes:	No
Affiliation:	Public	Distance Learning:	No

NLN ACCREDITATION: Yes

Articulation: Associate to Baccalaureate
LPN to Associate

For Further Information Contact:

Mrs Barbara Kellum, Chair
Orange County Community College
115 South St
Middletown, NY 10940
(914) 344-6222

Pace University Westchester
—Pleasantville—

Full-Time Enrollments:	14	Evening Classes:	Yes
Part-Time Enrollments:	34	Weekend Classes:	No
Affiliation:	Private	Distance Learning:	No

NLN ACCREDITATION: Yes

Articulation: None

For Further Information Contact:

Mrs Eileen Karlik, Chair
Pace University Westchester
861 Bedford Rd
Pleasantville, NY 10570
(914) 773-3347

Phillips Beth Israel School of Nursing
—New York—

Full-Time Enrollments:	37	Evening Classes:	No
Part-Time Enrollments:	74	Weekend Classes:	No
Affiliation:	Private	Distance Learning:	No

NLN ACCREDITATION: Yes

Articulation: Associate to Baccalaureate

For Further Information Contact:

Dr Cynthia Chesner, Dean
Phillips Beth Israel School of Nursing
310 East 22nd St
New York, NY 10010
(212) 614-6107

Queensborough Community College of CUNY
—Bayside—

Full-Time Enrollments:	136	Evening Classes:	No
Part-Time Enrollments:	285	Weekend Classes:	No
Affiliation:	Public	Distance Learning:	No

NLN ACCREDITATION: Yes

Articulation: Associate to Baccalaureate

For Further Information Contact:

Prof Patricia D Irons, Chair
Queensborough Community College of CUNY
Bayside, NY 11364
(718) 631-6362

Regents College-University of the State of New York
—Albany—

Full-Time Enrollments:	—	Evening Classes:	No
Part-Time Enrollments:	8163	Weekend Classes:	No
Affiliation:	Private	Distance Learning:	Yes

NLN ACCREDITATION: Yes

Articulation: Associate to Baccalaureate
Diploma to Baccalaureate

For Further Information Contact:

Dr Mary Beth Hanner, Dean
Regents College-University of the State of New York
7 Columbia Circle
Albany, NY 12203-5159
(518) 464-8500

Rockland Community College
—Suffern—

Full-Time Enrollments:	194	Evening Classes:	Yes
Part-Time Enrollments:	211	Weekend Classes:	No
Affiliation:	Public	Distance Learning:	No

NLN ACCREDITATION: Yes

Articulation: Associate to Baccalaureate

For Further Information Contact:

Dr Frances Monahan, Dept Head
Rockland Community College
145 College Rd
Suffern, NY 10901
(914) 356-4650

SUNY College of Agriculture & Technology Morrisville
—Morrisville—

Full-Time Enrollments:	97	Evening Classes:	—
Part-Time Enrollments:	31	Weekend Classes:	—
Affiliation:	Public	Distance Learning:	Yes

NLN ACCREDITATION: Yes

Articulation: Associate to Baccalaureate
LPN to Associate

For Further Information Contact:

Mrs Margaret Golden, Associate Dean
SUNY College of Agriculture & Technology Morrisville
Morrisville, NY 13408
(315) 684-6049

SUNY College of Technology
—Farmingdale—

Full-Time Enrollments:	61	Evening Classes:	Yes
Part-Time Enrollments:	203	Weekend Classes:	—
Affiliation:	Public	Distance Learning:	—

NLN ACCREDITATION: Yes

Articulation: Associate to Baccalaureate
LPN to Associate

For Further Information Contact:

Prof Loretta Falk, Chair
SUNY College of Technology
RT 110
Farmingdale, NY 11735
(516) 420-2229

SUNY at Delhi
—Delhi—

Full-Time Enrollments:	65	Evening Classes:	No
Part-Time Enrollments:	12	Weekend Classes:	No
Affiliation:	Public	Distance Learning:	No

NLN ACCREDITATION: No

Articulation: Associate to Baccalaureate
LPN to Associate

For Further Information Contact:

Mrs Patricia Judd, Chair
SUNY at Delhi
Delhi, NY 13753
(607) 746-4377

SUNY, College of Technology at Canton
—Canton—

Full-Time Enrollments:	112	Evening Classes:	No
Part-Time Enrollments:	31	Weekend Classes:	No
Affiliation:	Public	Distance Learning:	No

NLN ACCREDITATION: Yes

Articulation: Associate to Baccalaureate
LPN to Associate

For Further Information Contact:

Mrs Margaret P Vining, Associate Dean
SUNY, College of Technology at Canton
Canton, NY 13617
(315) 386-7419

SUNY-College of Technology at Alfred
—Alfred—

Full-Time Enrollments:	134	Evening Classes:	Yes
Part-Time Enrollments:	12	Weekend Classes:	No
Affiliation:	Public	Distance Learning:	Yes

NLN ACCREDITATION: Yes

Articulation: Associate to Baccalaureate
LPN to Associate
RN to MSN

For Further Information Contact:

Mrs Marilyn R Lusk, Chair
SUNY-College of Technology at Alfred
Alfred, NY 14802
(607) 587-3695

Saint Elizabeth College of Nursing
—Utica—

Full-Time Enrollments:	75	Evening Classes:	Yes
Part-Time Enrollments:	40	Weekend Classes:	Yes
Affiliation:	Religious	Distance Learning:	No

NLN ACCREDITATION: No

Articulation: Associate to Baccalaureate
LPN to Associate

For Further Information Contact:

Sr Walter Marie, Director
Saint Elizabeth College of Nursing
2215 Genesee St
Utica, NY 13501
(315) 798-8125

Samaritan Hospital-School of Nursing
—Troy—

Full-Time Enrollments:	31	Evening Classes:	—
Part-Time Enrollments:	55	Weekend Classes:	—
Affiliation:	Private	Distance Learning:	—

NLN ACCREDITATION: No

Articulation: None

For Further Information Contact:

Ms Barbara Wood, Director
Samaritan Hospital-School of Nursing
2215 Burdett Ave
Troy, NY 12180
(518) 271-3285

Sisters of Charity Hospital of Buffalo
—Buffalo—

Full-Time Enrollments:	22	Evening Classes:	No
Part-Time Enrollments:	67	Weekend Classes:	No
Affiliation:	Private	Distance Learning:	No

NLN ACCREDITATION: No

Articulation: Associate to Baccalaureate

For Further Information Contact:

Sr Margaret Ahl, Dean
Sisters of Charity Hospital of Buffalo
2157 Main St
Buffalo, NY 14214
(716) 862-2774

St Joseph's Hospital Health Center
—Syracuse—

Full-Time Enrollments:	68	Evening Classes:	No
Part-Time Enrollments:	48	Weekend Classes:	No
Affiliation:	Private	Distance Learning:	No

NLN ACCREDITATION: No

Articulation: Associate to Baccalaureate

For Further Information Contact:

Mrs Marianne Markowitz, Director
St Joseph's Hospital Health Center
Marian Hall-206 Prospect Ave
Syracuse, NY 13203
(315) 448-5046

St Vincent's Medical Center of Richmond
—Staten Island—

Full-Time Enrollments:	58	Evening Classes:	—
Part-Time Enrollments:	—	Weekend Classes:	—
Affiliation:	Public	Distance Learning:	—

NLN ACCREDITATION: No

Articulation: None

For Further Information Contact:

Dr Roberta Marpet, Dean
St Vincent's Medical Center of Richmond
2 Gridley Ave
Staten Island, NY 10303
(718) 876-1300

Suffolk Community College
—Brentwood—

Full-Time Enrollments:	18	Evening Classes:	No
Part-Time Enrollments:	75	Weekend Classes:	No
Affiliation:	Public	Distance Learning:	No

NLN ACCREDITATION: Yes

Articulation: LPN to Associate

For Further Information Contact:

Ms Joan Garnar, Dept Head
Suffolk Community College
Crooked Hill Rd
Brentwood, NY 11717
(516) 851-6752

Suffolk Community College
—Selden—

Full-Time Enrollments:	42	Evening Classes:	Yes
Part-Time Enrollments:	302	Weekend Classes:	No
Affiliation:	Public	Distance Learning:	No

NLN ACCREDITATION: Yes

Articulation: Associate to Baccalaureate

For Further Information Contact:

Ms Marcia Geraghty, Dept Head
Suffolk Community College
533 College Rd
Selden, NY 11784
(516) 451-4265

Sullivan County Community College
—Loch Sheldrake—

Full-Time Enrollments:	30	Evening Classes:	No
Part-Time Enrollments:	48	Weekend Classes:	No
Affiliation:	Public	Distance Learning:	No

NLN ACCREDITATION: Yes

Articulation: Associate to Baccalaureate
LPN to Associate

For Further Information Contact:

Mrs Anne M Lavelle, Chair
Sullivan County Community College
Loch Sheldrake, NY 12759
(914) 434-5750

The Dorothea Hopfer School of Nursing
—Mt Vernon—

Full-Time Enrollments:	18	Evening Classes:	Yes
Part-Time Enrollments:	68	Weekend Classes:	Yes
Affiliation:	Private	Distance Learning:	No

NLN ACCREDITATION: No

Articulation: Associate to Baccalaureate

For Further Information Contact:

Mrs Patricia Horner, Director
The Dorothea Hopfer School of Nursing
53 Valentine St
Mt Vernon, NY 10550
(914) 664-8000

Tompkins-Cortland Community College
—Dryden—

Full-Time Enrollments:	60	Evening Classes:	Yes
Part-Time Enrollments:	34	Weekend Classes:	Yes
Affiliation:	Public	Distance Learning:	—

NLN ACCREDITATION: Yes

Articulation: Associate to Baccalaureate

For Further Information Contact:

Mrs Catherine Milnor, Chair
Tompkins-Cortland Community College
170 North St
Dryden, NY 13053
(607) 844-8211

Trocaire College
—Buffalo—

Full-Time Enrollments:	142	Evening Classes:	Yes
Part-Time Enrollments:	259	Weekend Classes:	Yes
Affiliation:	Private	Distance Learning:	—

NLN ACCREDITATION: Yes

Articulation: Associate to Baccalaureate
LPN to Associate

For Further Information Contact:

Mrs M Patricia Shanks, Director
Trocaire College
110 Red Jacket Pkwy
Buffalo, NY 14220
(716) 826-1200

Ulster County Community College
—Stone Ridge—

Full-Time Enrollments:	43	Evening Classes:	Yes
Part-Time Enrollments:	72	Weekend Classes:	No
Affiliation:	Public	Distance Learning:	No

NLN ACCREDITATION: Yes

Articulation: Associate to Baccalaureate
LPN to Associate

For Further Information Contact:

Mrs Roberta Gavner, Chair
Ulster County Community College
Nursing Dept
Stone Ridge, NY 12484
(914) 687-5236

Westchester Community College
—Valhalla—

Full-Time Enrollments:	28	Evening Classes:	No
Part-Time Enrollments:	48	Weekend Classes:	No
Affiliation:	Public	Distance Learning:	No

NLN ACCREDITATION: No

Articulation: Associate to Baccalaureate
LPN to Associate

For Further Information Contact:

Mrs Marie Cahill, Chair
Westchester Community College
75 Grasslands Rd
Valhalla, NY 10595
(914) 785-6884

North Carolina

Alamance Community College
—Graham—

Full-Time Enrollments:	80	Evening Classes:	No
Part-Time Enrollments:	—	Weekend Classes:	No
Affiliation:	Public	Distance Learning:	No

NLN ACCREDITATION: No

Articulation: Associate to Baccalaureate

For Further Information Contact:

Ms Suella C Klug, Director
Alamance Community College
PO Box 8000
Graham, NC 27253
(910) 578-2002

Asheville-Buncombe Technical Community College
—Asheville—

Full-Time Enrollments:	—	Evening Classes:	—
Part-Time Enrollments:	—	Weekend Classes:	—
Affiliation:	Public	Distance Learning:	—

NLN ACCREDITATION: No

Articulation: None

For Further Information Contact:

Ms Marti Koch, Chair
Asheville-Buncombe Technical Community College
340 Victoria Rd
Asheville, NC 28801
(704) 254-1921

Beaufort Community College
—Washington—

Full-Time Enrollments: 59   Evening Classes: No
Part-Time Enrollments: —   Weekend Classes: No
Affiliation: Public   Distance Learning: No
NLN ACCREDITATION: No
Articulation: Associate to Baccalaureate

For Further Information Contact:

Mrs Sandra S Edwards, Chair
Beaufort Community College
PO Box 1069
Washington, NC 27889
(919) 946-6194

Blue Ridge Community College
—Flat Rock—

Full-Time Enrollments: 33   Evening Classes: No
Part-Time Enrollments: 18   Weekend Classes: No
Affiliation: Public   Distance Learning: No
NLN ACCREDITATION: No
Articulation: Associate to Baccalaureate

For Further Information Contact:

Miss Rita D Conner, Director
Blue Ridge Community College
Rt 2 Box 133A
Flat Rock, NC 28731
(704) 692-3572

Cabarrus College of Health Sciences
—Concord—

Full-Time Enrollments: 93   Evening Classes: Yes
Part-Time Enrollments: 30   Weekend Classes: No
Affiliation: Private   Distance Learning: No
NLN ACCREDITATION: No
Articulation: Associate to Baccalaureate

For Further Information Contact:

Mrs Anita Brown, Dean
Cabarrus College of Health Sciences
431 Copperfield Blvd NE
Concord, NC 28025-2405
(704) 783-1558

Caldwell Community College
—Hudson—

Full-Time Enrollments: 116   Evening Classes: No
Part-Time Enrollments: —   Weekend Classes: No
Affiliation: Public   Distance Learning: No
NLN ACCREDITATION: No
Articulation: None

For Further Information Contact:

Ms Fredel T Reighard, Director
Caldwell Community College
1000 Hickory Blvd
Hudson, NC 28638
(704) 726-2354

Cape Fear Community College
—Wilmington—

Full-Time Enrollments: 58   Evening Classes: Yes
Part-Time Enrollments: —   Weekend Classes: Yes
Affiliation: Public   Distance Learning: —
NLN ACCREDITATION: Yes
Articulation: LPN to Associate

For Further Information Contact:

Ms Susan Vinson-Greene, Director
Cape Fear Community College
411 N Front
Wilmington, NC 28401
(910) 251-5182

Carolinas College of Health Sciences
—Charlotte—

Full-Time Enrollments: 27   Evening Classes: No
Part-Time Enrollments: 126   Weekend Classes: No
Affiliation: Public   Distance Learning: No
NLN ACCREDITATION: No
Articulation: Associate to Baccalaureate

For Further Information Contact:

Ms Clara Smith, Director
Carolinas College of Health Sciences
PO Box 32861
Charlotte, NC 28232
(704) 355-5043

Catawba Valley Community College
—Hickory—

Full-Time Enrollments:	37	Evening Classes:	No
Part-Time Enrollments:	67	Weekend Classes:	No
Affiliation:	Public	Distance Learning:	No

NLN ACCREDITATION: Yes

Articulation: Associate to Baccalaureate

For Further Information Contact:

Mrs Naomi East, Dept Head
Catawba Valley Community College
2550 Hwy 70 SE
Hickory, NC 28602
(704) 327-7000

Central Carolina Community College
—Sanford—

Full-Time Enrollments:	50	Evening Classes:	Yes
Part-Time Enrollments:	27	Weekend Classes:	—
Affiliation:	Public	Distance Learning:	No

NLN ACCREDITATION: No

Articulation: LPN to Associate

For Further Information Contact:

Mrs Rhonda Evans, Chair
Central Carolina Community College
1105 Kelly Dr
Sanford, NC 27330
(919) 775-5401

Central Piedmont Community College
—Charlotte—

Full-Time Enrollments:	114	Evening Classes:	No
Part-Time Enrollments:	—	Weekend Classes:	No
Affiliation:	Public	Distance Learning:	No

NLN ACCREDITATION: No

Articulation: None

For Further Information Contact:

Ms Eileen Forrester, Director
Central Piedmont Community College
PO Box 35009
Charlotte, NC 28235
(704) 330-6958

Coastal Carolina Community College
—Jacksonville—

Full-Time Enrollments:	26	Evening Classes:	No
Part-Time Enrollments:	22	Weekend Classes:	No
Affiliation:	Public	Distance Learning:	No

NLN ACCREDITATION: No

Articulation: Associate to Baccalaureate
LPN to Associate

For Further Information Contact:

Mrs Paula V Gribble, Chair
Coastal Carolina Community College
444 Western Blvd
Jacksonville, NC 28540
(919) 455-1221

College of the Albemarle
—Elizabeth City—

Full-Time Enrollments:	66	Evening Classes:	No
Part-Time Enrollments:	10	Weekend Classes:	No
Affiliation:	Public	Distance Learning:	No

NLN ACCREDITATION: Yes

Articulation: Associate to Baccalaureate
LPN to Associate

For Further Information Contact:

Mrs Wilma Harris, Chair
College of the Albemarle
PO Box 2327
Elizabeth City, NC 27906
(919) 335-0821

Craven Community College
—New Bern—

Full-Time Enrollments:	40	Evening Classes:	Yes
Part-Time Enrollments:	51	Weekend Classes:	—
Affiliation:	Public	Distance Learning:	—

NLN ACCREDITATION: No

Articulation: Associate to Baccalaureate

For Further Information Contact:

Mrs Carolyn S Jones, Director
Craven Community College
800 College Court
New Bern, NC 28560
(919) 638-4131

Davidson County Community College
—Lexington—

Full-Time Enrollments: 64 Evening Classes: No
Part-Time Enrollments: 17 Weekend Classes: No
Affiliation: Public Distance Learning: No

NLN ACCREDITATION: Yes

Articulation: Associate to Baccalaureate

For Further Information Contact:

Ms Patricia P Shoemaker, Chair
Davidson County Community College
PO Box 1287
Lexington, NC 27293
(910) 249-8186

Durham Technical Community College
—Durham—

Full-Time Enrollments: 62 Evening Classes: —
Part-Time Enrollments: 41 Weekend Classes: —
Affiliation: Public Distance Learning: —

NLN ACCREDITATION: No

Articulation: None

For Further Information Contact:

Ms Margaret Skulnik, Director
Durham Technical Community College
1637 Lawson St
Durham, NC 27703
(919) 598-9289

Fayetteville Technical Community College
—Fayetteville—

Full-Time Enrollments: 57 Evening Classes: No
Part-Time Enrollments: 88 Weekend Classes: No
Affiliation: Public Distance Learning: No

NLN ACCREDITATION: Yes

Articulation: Associate to Baccalaureate
LPN to Associate

For Further Information Contact:

Mrs Kathy Weeks, Chair
Fayetteville Technical Community College
PO Box 35236
Fayetteville, NC 28303
(910) 678-8482

Foothills Nursing Consortium
—Spindale—

Full-Time Enrollments: 70 Evening Classes: No
Part-Time Enrollments: — Weekend Classes: No
Affiliation: Public Distance Learning: No

NLN ACCREDITATION: No

Articulation: Associate to Baccalaureate
LPN to Associate

For Further Information Contact:

Mrs Martha Ledbetter-Baskin, Director
Foothills Nursing Consortium
PO Box 804
Spindale, NC 28160
(704) 286-3636

Forsyth Technical Community College
—Winston-Salem—

Full-Time Enrollments: 195 Evening Classes: No
Part-Time Enrollments: — Weekend Classes: No
Affiliation: Public Distance Learning: No

NLN ACCREDITATION: No

Articulation: LPN to Associate

For Further Information Contact:

Ms Phyllis Sample, Assistant Dean
Forsyth Technical Community College
2100 Silas Creek Pkwy
Winston-Salem, NC 27103
(919) 723-0371

Gardner-Webb University
—Boiling Springs—

Full-Time Enrollments: 75 Evening Classes: No
Part-Time Enrollments: 45 Weekend Classes: No
Affiliation: Religious Distance Learning: No

NLN ACCREDITATION: Yes

Articulation: Associate to Baccalaureate
LPN to Associate

For Further Information Contact:

Dr Shirley Toney, Dean
Gardner-Webb University
Box 997
Boiling Springs, NC 28017-0997
(704) 434-2361

Gaston College
—Dallas—

Full-Time Enrollments:	113	Evening Classes:	No
Part-Time Enrollments:	—	Weekend Classes:	No
Affiliation:	Public	Distance Learning:	No

NLN ACCREDITATION: No

Articulation: Associate to Baccalaureate
LPN to Associate

For Further Information Contact:

Ms Lois Bradley, Chair
Gaston College
201 Hwy 321 South
Dallas, NC 28034-1499
(704) 922-6367

Guilford Technical Community College
—Jamestown—

Full-Time Enrollments:	—	Evening Classes:	—
Part-Time Enrollments:	148	Weekend Classes:	—
Affiliation:	Public	Distance Learning:	—

NLN ACCREDITATION: No

Articulation: None

For Further Information Contact:

Mrs Cecelia G Ray, Dept Chair
Guilford Technical Community College
PO Box 309
Jamestown, NC 27282
(910) 454-1126

James Sprunt Community College
—Kenansville—

Full-Time Enrollments:	40	Evening Classes:	Yes
Part-Time Enrollments:	37	Weekend Classes:	No
Affiliation:	Public	Distance Learning:	Yes

NLN ACCREDITATION: No

Articulation: Associate to Baccalaureate
LPN to Associate

For Further Information Contact:

Mrs Rhonda B Ferrell, Chair
James Sprunt Community College
PO Box 398
Kenansville, NC 28349
(910) 296-1341

Johnston Community College
—Smithfield—

Full-Time Enrollments:	36	Evening Classes:	—
Part-Time Enrollments:	29	Weekend Classes:	—
Affiliation:	Public	Distance Learning:	—

NLN ACCREDITATION: No

Articulation: None

For Further Information Contact:

Mrs Donnye B Rooks, Director
Johnston Community College
PO Box 2350
Smithfield, NC 27577
(919) 934-3051

Lenoir Community College
—Kinston—

Full-Time Enrollments:	56	Evening Classes:	Yes
Part-Time Enrollments:	—	Weekend Classes:	Yes
Affiliation:	Public	Distance Learning:	Yes

NLN ACCREDITATION: No

Articulation: Associate to Baccalaureate
LPN to Associate

For Further Information Contact:

Mrs Alexis Welch, Associate Dean
Lenoir Community College
PO Box 188
Kinston, NC 28502-0188
(919) 527-6223

Mayland Community College
—Spruce Pine—

Full-Time Enrollments:	45	Evening Classes:	No
Part-Time Enrollments:	—	Weekend Classes:	No
Affiliation:	Public	Distance Learning:	No

NLN ACCREDITATION: No

Articulation: Associate to Baccalaureate

For Further Information Contact:

Mrs Carol Ingram, Coordinator
Mayland Community College
PO Box 547
Spruce Pine, NC 28777
(704) 765-0814

Mitchell Community College
—Statesville—

Full-Time Enrollments: 84   Evening Classes: No
Part-Time Enrollments: —   Weekend Classes: No
Affiliation: Public   Distance Learning: No

NLN ACCREDITATION: No

Articulation: Associate to Baccalaureate

For Further Information Contact:

Ms Kaye Miller, Director
Mitchell Community College
500 W Broad St
Statesville, NC 28677
(704) 878-3300

NEWH Nursing Education Options Program
—Rocky Mount—

Full-Time Enrollments: —   Evening Classes: —
Part-Time Enrollments: —   Weekend Classes: —
Affiliation: Public   Distance Learning: —

NLN ACCREDITATION: No

Articulation: None

For Further Information Contact:

Ms V Diane Gibb, Dean
NEWH Nursing Education Options Program
225 Tarboro St
Rocky Mount, NC 27801
(919) 446-0436

Piedmont Community College
—Roxboro—

Full-Time Enrollments: 45   Evening Classes: Yes
Part-Time Enrollments: —   Weekend Classes: No
Affiliation: Public   Distance Learning: Yes

NLN ACCREDITATION: No

Articulation: Associate to Baccalaureate

For Further Information Contact:

Mrs Reba N Walters, Chair
Piedmont Community College
PO Box 1197
Roxboro, NC 27573
(910) 599-1181

Pitt Community College
—Greenville—

Full-Time Enrollments: 117   Evening Classes: Yes
Part-Time Enrollments: —   Weekend Classes: —
Affiliation: Public   Distance Learning: —

NLN ACCREDITATION: No

Articulation: Associate to Baccalaureate
LPN to Associate

For Further Information Contact:

Mrs Carla Lewis, Chair
Pitt Community College
PO Drawer 7007
Greenville, NC 27835-7007
(919) 321-4337

Randolph Community College
—Asheboro—

Full-Time Enrollments: 25   Evening Classes: No
Part-Time Enrollments: 51   Weekend Classes: No
Affiliation: Public   Distance Learning: No

NLN ACCREDITATION: Yes

Articulation: Associate to Baccalaureate

For Further Information Contact:

Mrs Lynn Tesh, Chair
Randolph Community College
PO Box 1009
Asheboro, NC 27204
(910) 629-1471

Region A Nursing Consortium
—Clyde—

Full-Time Enrollments: —   Evening Classes: —
Part-Time Enrollments: —   Weekend Classes: —
Affiliation: Public   Distance Learning: —

NLN ACCREDITATION: No

Articulation: None

For Further Information Contact:

Ms Sue A Morgan, Director
Region A Nursing Consortium
Freedlander Dr
Clyde, NC 28721
(704) 627-2821

Richmond Community College
—Hamlet—

Full-Time Enrollments:	76	Evening Classes:	No
Part-Time Enrollments:	—	Weekend Classes:	No
Affiliation:	Public	Distance Learning:	No

NLN ACCREDITATION: No

Articulation: Associate to Baccalaureate

For Further Information Contact:

Mrs Nancy C Sumner, Chair
Richmond Community College
PO Box 1189
Hamlet, NC 28345
(910) 582-7061

Roanoke-Chowan Community College
—Ahoskie—

Full-Time Enrollments:	27	Evening Classes:	No
Part-Time Enrollments:	13	Weekend Classes:	No
Affiliation:	Public	Distance Learning:	No

NLN ACCREDITATION: No

Articulation: Associate to Baccalaureate

For Further Information Contact:

Ms Claudia Hall Morris, Director
Roanoke-Chowan Community College
Rt 2, Box 46-A
Ahoskie, NC 27910
(919) 332-5921

Robeson Community College
—Lumberton—

Full-Time Enrollments:	79	Evening Classes:	Yes
Part-Time Enrollments:	—	Weekend Classes:	—
Affiliation:	Public	Distance Learning:	Yes

NLN ACCREDITATION: No

Articulation: LPN to Associate

For Further Information Contact:

Mrs Elizabeth T Nye, Chair
Robeson Community College
PO Box 1420
Lumberton, NC 28359
(910) 738-7101

Rockingham Community College
—Wentworth—

Full-Time Enrollments:	59	Evening Classes:	No
Part-Time Enrollments:	—	Weekend Classes:	No
Affiliation:	Public	Distance Learning:	No

NLN ACCREDITATION: No

Articulation: Associate to Baccalaureate

For Further Information Contact:

Mrs Cathy Franklin-Griffin, Dean
Rockingham Community College
PO Box 38
Wentworth, NC 27375
(910) 342-4261

Rowan Cabarrus Community College
—Salisbury—

Full-Time Enrollments:	67	Evening Classes:	No
Part-Time Enrollments:	34	Weekend Classes:	No
Affiliation:	Public	Distance Learning:	No

NLN ACCREDITATION: Yes

Articulation: LPN to Associate

For Further Information Contact:

Mrs Laura C Norris, Director
Rowan Cabarrus Community College
PO Box 1595
Salisbury, NC 28145
(704) 637-0760

Sampson Community College
—Clinton—

Full-Time Enrollments:	71	Evening Classes:	No
Part-Time Enrollments:	—	Weekend Classes:	No
Affiliation:	Public	Distance Learning:	No

NLN ACCREDITATION: No

Articulation: LPN to Associate

For Further Information Contact:

Mrs Mary B Brown, Chair
Sampson Community College
PO Drawer 318
Clinton, NC 28329
(910) 592-8081

Sandhills Community College
—Pinehurst—

Full-Time Enrollments:	—	Evening Classes:	—
Part-Time Enrollments:	—	Weekend Classes:	—
Affiliation:	Public	Distance Learning:	—

NLN ACCREDITATION: No

Articulation: None

For Further Information Contact:

Ms Star Mitchell, Chair
Sandhills Community College
2200 Airport Rd
Pinehurst, NC 28374
(910) 692-6185

Southeastern Community College
—Whiteville—

Full-Time Enrollments:	109	Evening Classes:	No
Part-Time Enrollments:	—	Weekend Classes:	No
Affiliation:	Public	Distance Learning:	No

NLN ACCREDITATION: No

Articulation: Associate to Baccalaureate
LPN to Associate

For Further Information Contact:

Mrs Peggy Blackmon, Dean
Southeastern Community College
PO Box 151
Whiteville, NC 28472
(910) 642-7141

Stanly Community College
—Albemarle—

Full-Time Enrollments:	30	Evening Classes:	No
Part-Time Enrollments:	37	Weekend Classes:	No
Affiliation:	Public	Distance Learning:	No

NLN ACCREDITATION: No

Articulation: Associate to Baccalaureate

For Further Information Contact:

Mrs Mary Anne Laney, Chair
Stanly Community College
141 College Dr
Albemarle, NC 28001
(704) 982-0121

Surry Community College
—Dobson—

Full-Time Enrollments:	52	Evening Classes:	Yes
Part-Time Enrollments:	63	Weekend Classes:	Yes
Affiliation:	Public	Distance Learning:	No

NLN ACCREDITATION: No

Articulation: Associate to Baccalaureate

For Further Information Contact:

Ms Sharon Shook Kallam, Chair
Surry Community College
PO Box 304
Dobson, NC 27017
(910) 386-8121

Vance-Granville Community College
—Henderson—

Full-Time Enrollments:	80	Evening Classes:	No
Part-Time Enrollments:	—	Weekend Classes:	No
Affiliation:	Public	Distance Learning:	No

NLN ACCREDITATION: No

Articulation: Associate to Baccalaureate

For Further Information Contact:

Mrs JoAnne Alston, Director
Vance-Granville Community College
PO Box 917
Henderson, NC 27536
(919) 492-2061

Wake Technical Community College
—Raleigh—

Full-Time Enrollments:	188	Evening Classes:	—
Part-Time Enrollments:	—	Weekend Classes:	—
Affiliation:	Public	Distance Learning:	—

NLN ACCREDITATION: No

Articulation: None

For Further Information Contact:

Ms Patsy L Hawkins, Director
Wake Technical Community College
9101 Fayetteville Rd
Raleigh, NC 27603
(919) 772-0551

Wayne Community College
—Goldsboro—

Full-Time Enrollments:	71	Evening Classes:	Yes
Part-Time Enrollments:	—	Weekend Classes:	No
Affiliation:	Public	Distance Learning:	No

NLN ACCREDITATION: No

Articulation: Associate to Baccalaureate
LPN to Associate

For Further Information Contact:

Mrs Cynthia B Archie, Head
Wayne Community College
Box 8002
Goldsboro, NC 27533
(919) 735-5151

Western Piedmont Community College
—Morganton—

Full-Time Enrollments:	93	Evening Classes:	No
Part-Time Enrollments:	—	Weekend Classes:	No
Affiliation:	Public	Distance Learning:	No

NLN ACCREDITATION: Yes

Articulation: Associate to Baccalaureate

For Further Information Contact:

Mrs Patricia Crumpler, Coordinator
Western Piedmont Community College
1001 Burkemont Ave
Morganton, NC 28655
(704) 438-6122

Wilkes Community College
—Wilkesboro—

Full-Time Enrollments:	69	Evening Classes:	Yes
Part-Time Enrollments:	—	Weekend Classes:	No
Affiliation:	Public	Distance Learning:	No

NLN ACCREDITATION: No

Articulation: Associate to Baccalaureate

For Further Information Contact:

Mrs Kathryn H Tisdale, Chair
Wilkes Community College
PO Drawer 120
Wilkesboro, NC 28697
(910) 651-8674

Ohio

Belmont Technical College
—St Clairsville—

Full-Time Enrollments:	20	Evening Classes:	No
Part-Time Enrollments:	80	Weekend Classes:	No
Affiliation:	Public	Distance Learning:	Yes

NLN ACCREDITATION: No

Articulation: Associate to Baccalaureate
LPN to Associate

For Further Information Contact:

Ms Rebecca Kurtz, Assistant Dean
Belmont Technical College
120 Fox-Shannon Pl
St Clairsville, OH 43950-9735
(614) 695-9500

Central Ohio Technical College
—Newark—

Full-Time Enrollments:	38	Evening Classes:	Yes
Part-Time Enrollments:	101	Weekend Classes:	No
Affiliation:	Public	Distance Learning:	No

NLN ACCREDITATION: Yes

Articulation: LPN to Associate

For Further Information Contact:

Mrs Mona Myers, Interim Chair
Central Ohio Technical College
1179 University Dr
Newark, OH 43055-1767
(614) 366-9285

Cincinnati State Technical Community College
—Cincinnati—

Full-Time Enrollments:	—	Evening Classes:	—
Part-Time Enrollments:	—	Weekend Classes:	—
Affiliation:	Public	Distance Learning:	—

NLN ACCREDITATION: Yes

Articulation: None

For Further Information Contact:

Ms Brenda Heck, Asst Dean
Cincinnati State Technical Community College
3520 Central Parkway
Cincinnati, OH 45223-2690
(513) 569-6331

Clark State Community College
—Springfield—

Full-Time Enrollments:	149	Evening Classes:	Yes
Part-Time Enrollments:	38	Weekend Classes:	—
Affiliation:	Public	Distance Learning:	—

NLN ACCREDITATION: Yes

Articulation: LPN to Associate

For Further Information Contact:

Mrs Carolyn Swanger, Assistant Dean
Clark State Community College
570 E Leffel Lane Box 570
Springfield, OH 45505-0570
(513) 328-6058

Columbus State Community College
—Columbus—

Full-Time Enrollments:	174	Evening Classes:	No
Part-Time Enrollments:	155	Weekend Classes:	No
Affiliation:	Public	Distance Learning:	No

NLN ACCREDITATION: Yes

Articulation: Associate to Baccalaureate

For Further Information Contact:

Ms Polly Owen, Chair
Columbus State Community College
550 E Spring St PO Box 1609
Columbus, OH 43216
(614) 227-2606

Cuyahoga Community College/Eastern Campus
—Cleveland—

Full-Time Enrollments:	350	Evening Classes:	Yes
Part-Time Enrollments:	—	Weekend Classes:	Yes
Affiliation:	Public	Distance Learning:	No

NLN ACCREDITATION: Yes

Articulation: Associate to Baccalaureate
LPN to Associate

For Further Information Contact:

Dr Barbara Pennell, Assistant Dean
Cuyahoga Community College/Eastern Campus
2900 Community College Ave
Cleveland, OH 44115
(216) 987-4106

Edison State Community College
—Piqua—

Full-Time Enrollments:	35	Evening Classes:	Yes
Part-Time Enrollments:	71	Weekend Classes:	—
Affiliation:	Public	Distance Learning:	—

NLN ACCREDITATION: Yes

Articulation: Associate to Baccalaureate
LPN to Associate

For Further Information Contact:

Ms Sharon Brown, Associate Dean
Edison State Community College
1973 Edison Dr
Piqua, OH 45356-9253
(937) 778-8600

Hocking College
—Nelsonville—

Full-Time Enrollments:	147	Evening Classes:	Yes
Part-Time Enrollments:	—	Weekend Classes:	Yes
Affiliation:	Public	Distance Learning:	Yes

NLN ACCREDITATION: Yes

Articulation: Associate to Baccalaureate
LPN to Associate

For Further Information Contact:

Mrs Nadine Goebel, Dean
Hocking College
3301 Hocking Parkway
Nelsonville, OH 45764-9704
(614) 753-3591

Kent State University-Ashtabula Campus
—Ashtabula—

Full-Time Enrollments:	—	Evening Classes:	—
Part-Time Enrollments:	—	Weekend Classes:	—
Affiliation:	Public	Distance Learning:	—

NLN ACCREDITATION: Yes

Articulation: —

For Further Information Contact:

Mrs Frances Briggs, Director
Kent State University-Ashtabula Campus
3325 W 13th St
Ashtabula, OH 44004-2299
(216) 964-4234

Kent State University-East Liverpool Campus
—East Liverpool—

Full-Time Enrollments:	—	Evening Classes:	—
Part-Time Enrollments:	—	Weekend Classes:	—
Affiliation:	Public	Distance Learning:	—

NLN ACCREDITATION: Yes

Articulation: None

For Further Information Contact:

Ms Joyce Heise, Director
Kent State University-East Liverpool Campus
400 E 4th St
East Liverpool, OH 43920
(230) 385-3805

Kent State University-Tuscarawas Campus
—New Philadelphia—

Full-Time Enrollments:	75	Evening Classes:	No
Part-Time Enrollments:	65	Weekend Classes:	No
Affiliation:	Public	Distance Learning:	Yes

NLN ACCREDITATION: Yes

Articulation: Associate to Baccalaureate
LPN to Associate

For Further Information Contact:

Mrs Dorothy Ervin, Director
Kent State University-Tuscarawas Campus
330 University Dr, NE
New Philadelphia, OH 44663-9422
(330) 339-3391

Kettering College of Medical Arts
—Kettering—

Full-Time Enrollments:	44	Evening Classes:	Yes
Part-Time Enrollments:	51	Weekend Classes:	No
Affiliation:	Religious	Distance Learning:	No

NLN ACCREDITATION: Yes

Articulation: Associate to Baccalaureate

For Further Information Contact:

Ms Lavonne Beck, Director
Kettering College of Medical Arts
3737 Southern Blvd
Kettering, OH 45429-1299
(513) 296-7219

Lakeland Community College
—Kirtland—

Full-Time Enrollments:	76	Evening Classes:	No
Part-Time Enrollments:	161	Weekend Classes:	No
Affiliation:	Public	Distance Learning:	No

NLN ACCREDITATION: Yes

Articulation: Associate to Baccalaureate
LPN to Associate
RN to MSN

For Further Information Contact:

Mrs Judith Greig, Director
Lakeland Community College
7700 Clocktower Dr
Kirtland, OH 44094-5198
(216) 953-7172

Lima Technical College
—Lima—

Full-Time Enrollments:	142	Evening Classes:	Yes
Part-Time Enrollments:	130	Weekend Classes:	Yes
Affiliation:	Public	Distance Learning:	No

NLN ACCREDITATION: Yes

Articulation: Associate to Baccalaureate

For Further Information Contact:

Dr Lois Deleruyelle, Chair
Lima Technical College
4240 Campus Dr
Lima, OH 45804-3597
(419) 221-1112

Lorain County Community College
—Elyria—

Full-Time Enrollments:	264	Evening Classes:	Yes
Part-Time Enrollments:	162	Weekend Classes:	Yes
Affiliation:	Public	Distance Learning:	—

NLN ACCREDITATION: Yes

Articulation: Associate to Baccalaureate
LPN to Associate
RN to MSN

For Further Information Contact:

Mr Robert A Schloss, Director
Lorain County Community College
1005 N Abbe Rd
Elyria, OH 44035-1691
(216) 366-4191

Marion Technical College
—Marion—

Full-Time Enrollments:	69	Evening Classes:	Yes
Part-Time Enrollments:	51	Weekend Classes:	Yes
Affiliation:	Public	Distance Learning:	No

NLN ACCREDITATION: Yes

Articulation: Associate to Baccalaureate
LPN to Associate

For Further Information Contact:

Mrs Janice E Hinkle, Dean
Marion Technical College
1467 Mt Vernon Ave
Marion, OH 43302-5694
(614) 389-4636

Mercy College of Northwest Ohio
—Toledo—

Full-Time Enrollments:	54	Evening Classes:	Yes
Part-Time Enrollments:	119	Weekend Classes:	No
Affiliation:	Religious	Distance Learning:	No

NLN ACCREDITATION: Yes

Articulation: None

For Further Information Contact:

Dr Maria Nowicki, Director
Mercy College of Northwest Ohio
2238 Jefferson Ave
Toledo, OH 43624-1197
(419) 259-1279

Miami University-Hamilton Campus
—Hamilton—

Full-Time Enrollments:	68	Evening Classes:	No
Part-Time Enrollments:	11	Weekend Classes:	No
Affiliation:	Public	Distance Learning:	Yes

NLN ACCREDITATION: Yes

Articulation: None

For Further Information Contact:

Dr Eugenia Mills, Chair
Miami University-Hamilton Campus
1601 Peck Blvd
Hamilton, OH 45011-3399
(513) 863-8833

Miami University-Middletown Campus
—Middletown—

Full-Time Enrollments:	56	Evening Classes:	No
Part-Time Enrollments:	24	Weekend Classes:	No
Affiliation:	Public	Distance Learning:	Yes

NLN ACCREDITATION: Yes

Articulation: None

For Further Information Contact:

Dr Eugenia Mills, Chair
Miami University-Middletown Campus
4200 E Univ Blvd
Middletown, OH 45042-3497
(513) 727-3359

North Central Technical College
—Mansfield—

Full-Time Enrollments:	147	Evening Classes:	No
Part-Time Enrollments:	—	Weekend Classes:	No
Affiliation:	Public	Distance Learning:	No

NLN ACCREDITATION: Yes

Articulation: LPN to Associate

For Further Information Contact:

Ms Carol Lepley, Director
North Central Technical College
2441 Kenwood Cir Box 698
Mansfield, OH 44901-0698
(419) 755-4800

Northwest State Community College
—Archbold—

Full-Time Enrollments:	29	Evening Classes:	No
Part-Time Enrollments:	57	Weekend Classes:	No
Affiliation:	Public	Distance Learning:	No

NLN ACCREDITATION: Yes

Articulation: Associate to Baccalaureate

For Further Information Contact:

Mrs Debora J Barcy, Dean
Northwest State Community College
22-600 State Rt 34
Archbold, OH 43502-9502
(419) 267-5511

ASSOCIATE DEGREE

Ohio University-Chillicothe
—Chillicothe—

Full-Time Enrollments:	68	Evening Classes:	No
Part-Time Enrollments:	—	Weekend Classes:	No
Affiliation:	Public	Distance Learning:	No

NLN ACCREDITATION: Yes

Articulation: LPN to Associate

For Further Information Contact:

Ms Barbara Montgomery, Associate Director
Ohio University-Chillicothe
571 W 5th St
Chillicothe, OH 45601-0621
(614) 774-7282

Ohio University-Zanesville Campus
—Zanesville—

Full-Time Enrollments:	95	Evening Classes:	No
Part-Time Enrollments:	61	Weekend Classes:	No
Affiliation:	Public	Distance Learning:	No

NLN ACCREDITATION: Yes

Articulation: LPN to Associate

For Further Information Contact:

Dr Linda L Hunt, Director
Ohio University-Zanesville Campus
1425 Newark Rd
Zanesville, OH 43701
(614) 453-0762

Owens Community College
—Toledo—

Full-Time Enrollments:	298	Evening Classes:	Yes
Part-Time Enrollments:	165	Weekend Classes:	Yes
Affiliation:	Public	Distance Learning:	—

NLN ACCREDITATION: Yes

Articulation: Associate to Baccalaureate
LPN to Associate

For Further Information Contact:

Mrs Elizabeth Ream, Chair
Owens Community College
10000 Oregon Rd
Toledo, OH 43619-1947
(419) 666-0580

Shawnee State University
—Portsmouth—

Full-Time Enrollments:	60	Evening Classes:	—
Part-Time Enrollments:	39	Weekend Classes:	—
Affiliation:	Public	Distance Learning:	—

NLN ACCREDITATION: No

Articulation: None

For Further Information Contact:

Dr Mary Lubno, Chair
Shawnee State University
940 Second St
Portsmouth, OH 45662-4344
(614) 355-2252

Sinclair Community College
—Dayton—

Full-Time Enrollments:	140	Evening Classes:	Yes
Part-Time Enrollments:	299	Weekend Classes:	No
Affiliation:	Public	Distance Learning:	Yes

NLN ACCREDITATION: Yes

Articulation: Associate to Baccalaureate
LPN to Associate

For Further Information Contact:

Ms Gloria Goldman, Chair
Sinclair Community College
444 W 3rd St
Dayton, OH 45402-1454
(513) 226-2848

Southern State Community College
—Hillsboro—

Full-Time Enrollments:	38	Evening Classes:	No
Part-Time Enrollments:	46	Weekend Classes:	No
Affiliation:	Public	Distance Learning:	No

NLN ACCREDITATION: Yes

Articulation: Associate to Baccalaureate
LPN to Associate

For Further Information Contact:

Mrs Jo Carol Laymon, Director
Southern State Community College
200 Hobart Dr
Hillsboro, OH 45133-9488
(513) 393-3431

Stark Technical College
—Canton—

Full-Time Enrollments:	14	Evening Classes:	—
Part-Time Enrollments:	75	Weekend Classes:	—
Affiliation:	Public	Distance Learning:	—

NLN ACCREDITATION: Yes

Articulation: None

For Further Information Contact:

Ms Gloria Kline, Dept Head
Stark Technical College
6200 Frank Ave NW
Canton, OH 44720
(330) 494-6170

University of Cincinnati-R Walters College
—Cincinnati—

Full-Time Enrollments:	29	Evening Classes:	Yes
Part-Time Enrollments:	117	Weekend Classes:	Yes
Affiliation:	Public	Distance Learning:	Yes

NLN ACCREDITATION: Yes

Articulation: Associate to Baccalaureate

For Further Information Contact:

Prof Joan Purdon, Chair
University of Cincinnati-R Walters College
9555 Plainfield Rd
Cincinnati, OH 45236-1096
(513) 745-5665

University of Rio Grande - Holzer School of Nursing
—Rio Grande—

Full-Time Enrollments:	78	Evening Classes:	—
Part-Time Enrollments:	50	Weekend Classes:	—
Affiliation:	Public	Distance Learning:	—

NLN ACCREDITATION: Yes

Articulation: None

For Further Information Contact:

Dr Janet M Byers, Dean
University of Rio Grande - Holzer School of Nursing
PO Box F-36
Rio Grande, OH 45674
(614) 245-5353

University of Toledo Community Technical College
—Toledo—

Full-Time Enrollments:	98	Evening Classes:	—
Part-Time Enrollments:	50	Weekend Classes:	—
Affiliation:	Public	Distance Learning:	—

NLN ACCREDITATION: Yes

Articulation: None

For Further Information Contact:

Ms Mirella Pardee, Director
University of Toledo Community Technical College
2801 W Bancroft St
Toledo, OH 43606-3391
(419) 537-3374

Walsh University
—North Canton—

Full-Time Enrollments:	57	Evening Classes:	Yes
Part-Time Enrollments:	50	Weekend Classes:	No
Affiliation:	Religious	Distance Learning:	No

NLN ACCREDITATION: Yes

Articulation: Associate to Baccalaureate
LPN to Associate

For Further Information Contact:

Dr Joyce K Soehnlen, Interim Chair
Walsh University
2020 Easton St NW
North Canton, OH 44720-3396
(330) 490-7250

Washington State Community College
—Marietta—

Full-Time Enrollments:	—	Evening Classes:	—
Part-Time Enrollments:	—	Weekend Classes:	—
Affiliation:	Public	Distance Learning:	—

NLN ACCREDITATION: No

Articulation: None

For Further Information Contact:

Dr Betty Miller, Director
Washington State Community College
710 Colegate Dr
Marietta, OH 45750-9614
(614) 374-8716

Xavier University-Deaconess Hospital
—Cincinnati—

Full-Time Enrollments:	—	**Evening Classes:**	—
Part-Time Enrollments:	—	**Weekend Classes:**	—
Affiliation:	Religious	**Distance Learning:**	—

NLN ACCREDITATION: Yes

Articulation: None

For Further Information Contact:

Dr Evelyn Lutz, Interim Chair
Xavier University-Deaconess Hospital
3800 Victory Parkway
Cincinnati, OH 45207-7351
(513) 745-3814

Oklahoma

Bacone College
—Muskogee—

Full-Time Enrollments:	28	**Evening Classes:**	Yes
Part-Time Enrollments:	55	**Weekend Classes:**	No
Affiliation:	Religious	**Distance Learning:**	No

NLN ACCREDITATION: Yes

Articulation: LPN to Associate

For Further Information Contact:

Mrs Nancy Diede, Director
Bacone College
2299 Old Bacone Rd
Muskogee, OK 74403
(918) 683-4581

Bartlesville Wesleyan College
—Bartlesville—

Full-Time Enrollments:	35	**Evening Classes:**	Yes
Part-Time Enrollments:	16	**Weekend Classes:**	No
Affiliation:	Religious	**Distance Learning:**	No

NLN ACCREDITATION: Yes

Articulation: LPN to Associate

For Further Information Contact:

Mrs Carol Coose, Chair
Bartlesville Wesleyan College
2201 Silver Lake Rd
Bartlesville, OK 74006-6299
(918) 335-6200

Cameron University
—Lawton—

Full-Time Enrollments:	73	**Evening Classes:**	No
Part-Time Enrollments:	—	**Weekend Classes:**	No
Affiliation:	Public	**Distance Learning:**	No

NLN ACCREDITATION: Yes

Articulation: LPN to Associate

For Further Information Contact:

Ms Lynn Barnhart, Chair
Cameron University
2800 Gore Blvd
Lawton, OK 73505
(405) 581-2310

Carl Albert State College
—Poteau—

Full-Time Enrollments:	44	**Evening Classes:**	No
Part-Time Enrollments:	47	**Weekend Classes:**	No
Affiliation:	Public	**Distance Learning:**	No

NLN ACCREDITATION: Yes

Articulation: LPN to Associate

For Further Information Contact:

Ms Norma F Divine, Chair
Carl Albert State College
1507 S McKenna
Poteau, OK 74953
(918) 647-8660

Connors State College
—Warner—

Full-Time Enrollments:	—	**Evening Classes:**	No
Part-Time Enrollments:	118	**Weekend Classes:**	No
Affiliation:	Public	**Distance Learning:**	No

NLN ACCREDITATION: Yes

Articulation: LPN to Associate

For Further Information Contact:

Ms Sallie Carney, Director
Connors State College
Post Office Box 389
Warner, OK 74469
(918) 463-6257

Eastern Oklahoma State College
—Wilburton—

Full-Time Enrollments:	32	Evening Classes:	Yes
Part-Time Enrollments:	31	Weekend Classes:	No
Affiliation:	Public	Distance Learning:	Yes

NLN ACCREDITATION: Yes

Articulation: LPN to Associate

For Further Information Contact:

Mrs Marsha A Green, Director
Eastern Oklahoma State College
1301 West Main
Wilburton, OK 74578
(918) 465-2361

Murray State College
—Tishomingo—

Full-Time Enrollments:	1	Evening Classes:	No
Part-Time Enrollments:	82	Weekend Classes:	No
Affiliation:	Public	Distance Learning:	No

NLN ACCREDITATION: Yes

Articulation: LPN to Associate

For Further Information Contact:

Ms Joni R Jeter, Dean
Murray State College
Tishomingo, OK 73460
(405) 371-2371

Northeastern Oklahoma A & M College
—Miami—

Full-Time Enrollments:	100	Evening Classes:	—
Part-Time Enrollments:	—	Weekend Classes:	—
Affiliation:	Public	Distance Learning:	—

NLN ACCREDITATION: Yes

Articulation: LPN to Associate

For Further Information Contact:

Ms Bethene Fahnestock, Chair
Northeastern Oklahoma A & M College
2nd and I St, NE
Miami, OK 74354
(918) 542-8441

Northern Oklahoma College
—Tonkawa—

Full-Time Enrollments:	46	Evening Classes:	Yes
Part-Time Enrollments:	52	Weekend Classes:	No
Affiliation:	Public	Distance Learning:	Yes

NLN ACCREDITATION: Yes

Articulation: Associate to Baccalaureate
LPN to Associate

For Further Information Contact:

Mrs Kim Sherer, Chair
Northern Oklahoma College
1220 E Grand PO Box 310
Tonkawa, OK 74653
(405) 628-6679

Oklahoma City Community College
—Oklahoma City—

Full-Time Enrollments:	—	Evening Classes:	Yes
Part-Time Enrollments:	208	Weekend Classes:	No
Affiliation:	Public	Distance Learning:	No

NLN ACCREDITATION: Yes

Articulation: LPN to Associate

For Further Information Contact:

Ms Anita Jones, Dean
Oklahoma City Community College
7777 S May Ave
Oklahoma City, OK 73159
(405) 682-7573

Oklahoma State University-Oklahoma City
—Oklahoma City—

Full-Time Enrollments:	203	Evening Classes:	No
Part-Time Enrollments:	—	Weekend Classes:	No
Affiliation:	Public	Distance Learning:	No

NLN ACCREDITATION: Yes

Articulation: Associate to Baccalaureate
LPN to Associate

For Further Information Contact:

Dr Lois Salmeron, Div Head
Oklahoma State University-Oklahoma City
900 N Portland
Oklahoma City, OK 73107
(405) 945-3295

Redlands Community College
—El Reno—

Full-Time Enrollments:	54	Evening Classes:	No
Part-Time Enrollments:	36	Weekend Classes:	No
Affiliation:	Public	Distance Learning:	No

NLN ACCREDITATION: Yes

Articulation: LPN to Associate

For Further Information Contact:

Ms Rose Marie Bolton, Director
Redlands Community College
Box 370 1300 Country Club Rd
El Reno, OK 73036
(405) 262-2552

Seminole Jr College
—Seminole—

Full-Time Enrollments:	60	Evening Classes:	No
Part-Time Enrollments:	—	Weekend Classes:	No
Affiliation:	Public	Distance Learning:	No

NLN ACCREDITATION: Yes

Articulation: LPN to Associate

For Further Information Contact:

Dr Jorge Neuhaus, Div Chair
Seminole Jr College
PO Box 351 2701 State St
Seminole, OK 74868
(405) 382-9950

Rogers University at Claremore
—Claremore—

Full-Time Enrollments:	60	Evening Classes:	Yes
Part-Time Enrollments:	70	Weekend Classes:	No
Affiliation:	Public	Distance Learning:	Yes

NLN ACCREDITATION: Yes

Articulation: LPN to Associate

For Further Information Contact:

Ms Linda Dennis Andrews, Director
Rogers University at Claremore
College Hill
Claremore, OK 74017
(918) 343-7510

Tulsa Community College
—Tulsa—

Full-Time Enrollments:	19	Evening Classes:	No
Part-Time Enrollments:	230	Weekend Classes:	No
Affiliation:	Public	Distance Learning:	No

NLN ACCREDITATION: Yes

Articulation: LPN to Associate

For Further Information Contact:

Ms Carole Thompson, Chair
Tulsa Community College
909 S Boston
Tulsa, OK 74119
(918) 595-7188

Rose State College
—Midwest City—

Full-Time Enrollments:	74	Evening Classes:	Yes
Part-Time Enrollments:	48	Weekend Classes:	No
Affiliation:	Public	Distance Learning:	No

NLN ACCREDITATION: Yes

Articulation: LPN to Associate

For Further Information Contact:

Ms Gayle McNish, Director
Rose State College
6420 SE 15th St
Midwest City, OK 73110
(405) 733-7546

Western Oklahoma State College
—Altus—

Full-Time Enrollments:	7	Evening Classes:	No
Part-Time Enrollments:	40	Weekend Classes:	No
Affiliation:	Public	Distance Learning:	No

NLN ACCREDITATION: Yes

Articulation: LPN to Associate

For Further Information Contact:

Ms Margaret Thomas, Director
Western Oklahoma State College
2801 North Main
Altus, OK 73521
(405) 477-2000

Oregon

Blue Mountain Community College
—Pendleton—

Full-Time Enrollments:	55	Evening Classes:	No
Part-Time Enrollments:	—	Weekend Classes:	No
Affiliation:	Public	Distance Learning:	No

NLN ACCREDITATION: No

Articulation: LPN to Associate

For Further Information Contact:

Mrs Elizabeth Sullivan, Chair
Blue Mountain Community College
PO Box 100
Pendleton, OR 97801
(541) 276-1260

Central Oregon Community College
—Bend—

Full-Time Enrollments:	—	Evening Classes:	—
Part-Time Enrollments:	—	Weekend Classes:	—
Affiliation:	Public	Distance Learning:	—

NLN ACCREDITATION: No

Articulation: None

For Further Information Contact:

Ms Ellen Howe, Chair
Central Oregon Community College
2600 NW College Way
Bend, OR 97701
(541) 383-6112

Chemeketa Community College
—Salem—

Full-Time Enrollments:	118	Evening Classes:	Yes
Part-Time Enrollments:	—	Weekend Classes:	Yes
Affiliation:	Public	Distance Learning:	Yes

NLN ACCREDITATION: Yes

Articulation: Associate to Baccalaureate
LPN to Associate

For Further Information Contact:

Dr Doris M Williams, Director
Chemeketa Community College
4000 Lancaster Dr NE
Salem, OR 97309
(503) 399-5058

Clackmas Community College
—Oregon City—

Full-Time Enrollments:	65	Evening Classes:	No
Part-Time Enrollments:	—	Weekend Classes:	No
Affiliation:	Public	Distance Learning:	No

NLN ACCREDITATION: Yes

Articulation: None

For Further Information Contact:

Ms Arlene Jurgens, Chair
Clackmas Community College
19600 S Molalla Ave
Oregon City, OR 97045
(503) 657-6900

Clatsop Community College
—Astoria—

Full-Time Enrollments:	27	Evening Classes:	No
Part-Time Enrollments:	7	Weekend Classes:	No
Affiliation:	Public	Distance Learning:	No

NLN ACCREDITATION: No

Articulation: None

For Further Information Contact:

Ms Karen M Burke, Director
Clatsop Community College
16th and Jerome
Astoria, OR 97103
(503) 325-0910

Lane Community College
—Eugene—

Full-Time Enrollments:	100	Evening Classes:	Yes
Part-Time Enrollments:	41	Weekend Classes:	No
Affiliation:	Public	Distance Learning:	No

NLN ACCREDITATION: Yes

Articulation: LPN to Associate

For Further Information Contact:

Mrs Joyce Godels, Director
Lane Community College
4000 E 30th Ave
Eugene, OR 97405
(541) 747-4501

Linn-Benton Community College
—Albany—

Full-Time Enrollments:	60	Evening Classes:	Yes
Part-Time Enrollments:	—	Weekend Classes:	No
Affiliation:	Public	Distance Learning:	No

NLN ACCREDITATION: Yes

Articulation: Associate to Baccalaureate

For Further Information Contact:

Ms Jacqueline Paulson, Chair
Linn-Benton Community College
6500 S Pacific Blvd
Albany, OR 97321
(541) 917-4512

Mt Hood Community College
—Gresham—

Full-Time Enrollments:	88	Evening Classes:	Yes
Part-Time Enrollments:	—	Weekend Classes:	Yes
Affiliation:	Public	Distance Learning:	No

NLN ACCREDITATION: Yes

Articulation: Associate to Baccalaureate
LPN to Associate

For Further Information Contact:

Dr Joan Carley Oliver, Director
Mt Hood Community College
26000 SE Stark
Gresham, OR 97030
(503) 667-7406

Portland Community College
—Portland—

Full-Time Enrollments:	156	Evening Classes:	No
Part-Time Enrollments:	—	Weekend Classes:	No
Affiliation:	Public	Distance Learning:	No

NLN ACCREDITATION: Yes

Articulation: LPN to Associate

For Further Information Contact:

Dr Priscilla Loanzon, Chair
Portland Community College
12000 SW 49th Box 19000
Portland, OR 97219-0990
(503) 244-6111

Rogue Community College
—Grants Pass—

Full-Time Enrollments:	40	Evening Classes:	No
Part-Time Enrollments:	—	Weekend Classes:	No
Affiliation:	Public	Distance Learning:	No

NLN ACCREDITATION: Yes

Articulation: Associate to Baccalaureate
LPN to Associate

For Further Information Contact:

Mrs Linda Wagner, Director
Rogue Community College
3345 Redwood Highway
Grants Pass, OR 97527
(541) 471-3500

Southwestern Oregon Community College
—Coos Bay—

Full-Time Enrollments:	16	Evening Classes:	—
Part-Time Enrollments:	19	Weekend Classes:	No
Affiliation:	Public	Distance Learning:	No

NLN ACCREDITATION: No

Articulation: Associate to Baccalaureate

For Further Information Contact:

Ms Kristen Crusoe, Director
Southwestern Oregon Community College
1988 Newmark
Coos Bay, OR 97420
(503) 888-2525

Treasure Valley Community College
—Ontario—

Full-Time Enrollments:	—	Evening Classes:	—
Part-Time Enrollments:	—	Weekend Classes:	—
Affiliation:	Public	Distance Learning:	—

NLN ACCREDITATION: No

Articulation: None

For Further Information Contact:

Mrs Maureen McDonough, Director
Treasure Valley Community College
650 College Blvd, Box 840
Ontario, OR 97914
(541) 889-6493

Umpqua Community College
—Roseburg—

Full-Time Enrollments:	50	Evening Classes:	No
Part-Time Enrollments:	28	Weekend Classes:	No
Affiliation:	Public	Distance Learning:	No

NLN ACCREDITATION: Yes

Articulation: Associate to Baccalaureate
LPN to Associate

For Further Information Contact:

Mr Duane D Alexenko, Director
Umpqua Community College
PO Box 967
Roseburg, OR 97470
(541) 440-4600

Pennsylvania

Allegheny University of the Health Sciences
—Philadelphia—

Full-Time Enrollments:	88	Evening Classes:	Yes
Part-Time Enrollments:	77	Weekend Classes:	Yes
Affiliation:	Private	Distance Learning:	—

NLN ACCREDITATION: Yes

Articulation: Associate to Baccalaureate
RN to MSN

For Further Information Contact:

Ms Mary E Smith, Director
Allegheny University of the Health Sciences
1505 Rare St Ms501
Philadelphia, PA 19102-1192
(215) 448-7989

Alvernia College
—Reading—

Full-Time Enrollments:	20	Evening Classes:	No
Part-Time Enrollments:	50	Weekend Classes:	No
Affiliation:	Religious	Distance Learning:	No

NLN ACCREDITATION: Yes

Articulation: None

For Further Information Contact:

Dr Deborah Castellucci, Director
Alvernia College
400 St Bernardine St
Reading, PA 19607
(610) 796-8256

Bucks County Community College
—Newtown—

Full-Time Enrollments:	27	Evening Classes:	No
Part-Time Enrollments:	152	Weekend Classes:	No
Affiliation:	Public	Distance Learning:	No

NLN ACCREDITATION: Yes

Articulation: Associate to Baccalaureate

For Further Information Contact:

Mrs Patricia Noone, Director
Bucks County Community College
Swamp Rd
Newtown, PA 18940
(215) 968-8319

Butler County Community College
—Butler—

Full-Time Enrollments:	56	Evening Classes:	No
Part-Time Enrollments:	76	Weekend Classes:	No
Affiliation:	Public	Distance Learning:	No

NLN ACCREDITATION: Yes

Articulation: Associate to Baccalaureate

For Further Information Contact:

Mrs Sharon Brewer, Assistant Dean
Butler County Community College
PO Box 1203 Coll Dr Oak Hills
Butler, PA 16003-1203
(412) 287-8711

Clarion University of Pennsylvania-Venango Campus
—Oil City—

Full-Time Enrollments:	39	Evening Classes:	Yes
Part-Time Enrollments:	22	Weekend Classes:	No
Affiliation:	Public	Distance Learning:	Yes

NLN ACCREDITATION: Yes

Articulation: Associate to Baccalaureate
Diploma to Baccalaureate

For Further Information Contact:

Dr T Audean Duespohl, Dean
Clarion University of Pennsylvania-Venango Campus
1801 W First St
Oil City, PA 16301
(814) 677-6107

Community College of Allegheny County-So Campus
—West Miffin—

Full-Time Enrollments:	397	Evening Classes:	Yes
Part-Time Enrollments:	254	Weekend Classes:	Yes
Affiliation:	Public	Distance Learning:	No

NLN ACCREDITATION: Yes

Articulation: Associate to Baccalaureate
LPN to Associate
RN to MSN

For Further Information Contact:

Dr Kathleen Malloy, Dean
Community College of Allegheny County-So Campus
1750 Clairton Rd
West Miffin, PA 15122
(412) 469-6310

Community College of Beaver County
—Monaca—

Full-Time Enrollments:	13	Evening Classes:	No
Part-Time Enrollments:	87	Weekend Classes:	No
Affiliation:	Public	Distance Learning:	No

NLN ACCREDITATION: Yes

Articulation: Associate to Baccalaureate
LPN to Associate

For Further Information Contact:

Mrs Linda Gallagher, Director
Community College of Beaver County
1 Campus Dr
Monaca, PA 15061
(412) 775-8561

Community College of Philadelphia
—Philadelphia—

Full-Time Enrollments:	48	Evening Classes:	Yes
Part-Time Enrollments:	150	Weekend Classes:	Yes
Affiliation:	Public	Distance Learning:	—

NLN ACCREDITATION: Yes

Articulation: Associate to Baccalaureate
LPN to Associate

For Further Information Contact:

Dr Andrea Mengel, Dept Head
Community College of Philadelphia
1700 Spring Garden St
Philadelphia, PA 19130
(215) 751-8422

Delaware County Community College
—Media—

Full-Time Enrollments:	80	Evening Classes:	Yes
Part-Time Enrollments:	97	Weekend Classes:	Yes
Affiliation:	Public	Distance Learning:	—

NLN ACCREDITATION: Yes

Articulation: Associate to Baccalaureate

For Further Information Contact:

Dr Mary J Boyer, Associate Dean
Delaware County Community College
901 So Media Line Rd
Media, PA 19063
(215) 359-5285

Gannon University-Department of Nursing
—Erie—

Full-Time Enrollments:	90	Evening Classes:	Yes
Part-Time Enrollments:	40	Weekend Classes:	Yes
Affiliation:	Religious	Distance Learning:	No

NLN ACCREDITATION: Yes

Articulation: Associate to Baccalaureate
Diploma to Baccalaureate
RN to MSN

For Further Information Contact:

Dr Beverly Bartlett, Interim Chair
Gannon University-Department of Nursing
University Square
Erie, PA 16541
(814) 871-5463

Gwynedd-Mercy College
—Gwynedd Valley—

Full-Time Enrollments:	160	Evening Classes:	Yes
Part-Time Enrollments:	35	Weekend Classes:	Yes
Affiliation:	Religious	Distance Learning:	No

NLN ACCREDITATION: Yes

Articulation: Associate to Baccalaureate
Diploma to Baccalaureate
LPN to Associate

For Further Information Contact:

Dr Mary Dressler, Dean
Gwynedd-Mercy College
Sunneytown Pike Box 901
Gwynedd Valley, PA 19437
(215) 641-5501

Harrisburg Area Community College
—Harrisburg—

Full-Time Enrollments: 41   Evening Classes: Yes
Part-Time Enrollments: 162   Weekend Classes: No
Affiliation: Public   Distance Learning: Yes

NLN ACCREDITATION: Yes

Articulation: Associate to Baccalaureate
LPN to Associate

For Further Information Contact:

Mrs Diana Wells, Director
Harrisburg Area Community College
One HACC Drive
Harrisburg, PA 17110
(717) 780-2316

Lehigh Carbon Community College
—Schnecksville—

Full-Time Enrollments: —   Evening Classes: —
Part-Time Enrollments: —   Weekend Classes: —
Affiliation: Public   Distance Learning: —

NLN ACCREDITATION: Yes

Articulation: —

For Further Information Contact:

Ms Nancy Becker, Director
Lehigh Carbon Community College
4525 Education Park Dr
Schnecksville, PA 18078-2598
(610) 799-1550

Lock Haven University Nursing Department
—Clearfield—

Full-Time Enrollments: —   Evening Classes: —
Part-Time Enrollments: —   Weekend Classes: —
Affiliation: Public   Distance Learning: —

NLN ACCREDITATION: Yes

Articulation: —

For Further Information Contact:

Mrs Helen J Hummel, Director
Lock Haven University Nursing Department
119 Byers St
Clearfield, PA 16830
(814) 765-0616

Luzerne County Community College
—Nanticoke—

Full-Time Enrollments: 223   Evening Classes: No
Part-Time Enrollments: —   Weekend Classes: No
Affiliation: Public   Distance Learning: No

NLN ACCREDITATION: Yes

Articulation: Associate to Baccalaureate

For Further Information Contact:

Dr Jane Brown, Director
Luzerne County Community College
1333 South Prospect St
Nanticoke, PA 18634-3899
(717) 829-7463

Montgomery County Community College
—Blue Bell—

Full-Time Enrollments: 148   Evening Classes: —
Part-Time Enrollments: 100   Weekend Classes: —
Affiliation: Public   Distance Learning: —

NLN ACCREDITATION: Yes

Articulation: None

For Further Information Contact:

Mrs Dorothy N Campbell, Director
Montgomery County Community College
340 DeKalb Pike Box 400
Blue Bell, PA 19422-0796
(215) 641-6471

Mount Aloysius College
—Cresson—

Full-Time Enrollments: 224   Evening Classes: No
Part-Time Enrollments: —   Weekend Classes: No
Affiliation: Religious   Distance Learning: No

NLN ACCREDITATION: Yes

Articulation: LPN to Associate

For Further Information Contact:

Mrs Nedra Farcus, Chair
Mount Aloysius College
7373 Admiral Peary Hwy
Cresson, PA 16630
(814) 886-4131

Northampton County Area Community College
—Bethlehem—

Full-Time Enrollments:	57	Evening Classes:	No
Part-Time Enrollments:	109	Weekend Classes:	No
Affiliation:	Public	Distance Learning:	No

NLN ACCREDITATION: Yes

Articulation: Associate to Baccalaureate
LPN to Associate

For Further Information Contact:

Ms Aurora Weaver, Director
Northampton County Area Community College
3835 Green Pond Rd
Bethlehem, PA 18017
(215) 861-5376

Pennsylvania College of Technology
—Williamsport—

Full-Time Enrollments:	48	Evening Classes:	Yes
Part-Time Enrollments:	52	Weekend Classes:	Yes
Affiliation:	Public	Distance Learning:	No

NLN ACCREDITATION: Yes

Articulation: LPN to Associate

For Further Information Contact:

Mrs Linda Moran, Director
Pennsylvania College of Technology
1 College Ave
Williamsport, PA 17701-5799
(717) 327-4525

Pennsylvania State University
—Univerity Park—

Full-Time Enrollments:	152	Evening Classes:	No
Part-Time Enrollments:	152	Weekend Classes:	No
Affiliation:	Public	Distance Learning:	No

NLN ACCREDITATION: Yes

Articulation: None

For Further Information Contact:

Dr Sarah Hall Gueldner, Director
Pennsylvania State University
201 Hlth & Human Dev East
Univerity Park, PA 16802
(814) 863-0245

Reading Area Community College
—Reading—

Full-Time Enrollments:	18	Evening Classes:	Yes
Part-Time Enrollments:	91	Weekend Classes:	No
Affiliation:	Public	Distance Learning:	Yes

NLN ACCREDITATION: Yes

Articulation: Associate to Baccalaureate
LPN to Associate

For Further Information Contact:

Mrs Elissa Sauer, Director
Reading Area Community College
10 S Second St Box 1706
Reading, PA 19603
(610) 372-6226

University of Pittsburgh at Bradford
—Bradford—

Full-Time Enrollments:	44	Evening Classes:	No
Part-Time Enrollments:	22	Weekend Classes:	No
Affiliation:	Public	Distance Learning:	No

NLN ACCREDITATION: Yes

Articulation: None

For Further Information Contact:

Ms Lisa Fiorentino, Director
University of Pittsburgh at Bradford
300 Campus Dr
Bradford, PA 16701
(814) 362-7640

Westmoreland County Community College-Ctl Campus
—Youngwood—

Full-Time Enrollments:	96	Evening Classes:	Yes
Part-Time Enrollments:	70	Weekend Classes:	Yes
Affiliation:	Public	Distance Learning:	Yes

NLN ACCREDITATION: No

Articulation: Associate to Baccalaureate

For Further Information Contact:

Dr Patricia Mihalcin, Chair
Westmoreland County Community College-Ctl Campus
Armbrust Rd
Youngwood, PA 15697-1895
(412) 925-4000

Puerto Rico

Antillian Adventist University
—Mayaguez—

Full-Time Enrollments:	135	Evening Classes:	Yes
Part-Time Enrollments:	22	Weekend Classes:	No
Affiliation:	Religious	Distance Learning:	No

NLN ACCREDITATION: No

Articulation: Associate to Baccalaureate
Diploma to Baccalaureate

For Further Information Contact:

Prof Alicia Bruno, Director
Antillian Adventist University
PO Box 118
Mayaguez, PR 00681
(787) 834-9595

Colegio Tecnologico Del Municipio De San Juan
—San Juan—

Full-Time Enrollments:	191	Evening Classes:	Yes
Part-Time Enrollments:	30	Weekend Classes:	No
Affiliation:	Public	Distance Learning:	No

NLN ACCREDITATION: Yes

Articulation: None

For Further Information Contact:

Mrs Ivonne Rodriguez, Chair
College Tecnologico Del Municipio De San Juan
Box 70179
San Juan, PR 00936
(787) 250-7395

Columbia College
—Caguas—

Full-Time Enrollments:	—	Evening Classes:	—
Part-Time Enrollments:	—	Weekend Classes:	—
Affiliation:	Private	Distance Learning:	—

NLN ACCREDITATION: No

Articulation: None

For Further Information Contact:

Mr Hector Colon Del Valle, Coordinator
Columbia College
PO Box 8517
Caguas, PR 00726
(787) 743-4041

Electronic Data Processing College
—San Sebastian—

Full-Time Enrollments:	355	Evening Classes:	—
Part-Time Enrollments:	30	Weekend Classes:	—
Affiliation:	Public	Distance Learning:	—

NLN ACCREDITATION: No

Articulation: None

For Further Information Contact:

Mr Roberto Salas, Coordinator
Electronic Data Processing College
PO Box 1674
San Sebastian, PR 00685
(787) 896-2137

Instituto De Educacion Universal
—San Juan—

Full-Time Enrollments:	34	Evening Classes:	—
Part-Time Enrollments:	—	Weekend Classes:	—
Affiliation:	Private	Distance Learning:	—

NLN ACCREDITATION: No

Articulation: None

For Further Information Contact:

Dr Miguel Ortiz, Director
Instituto De Educacion Universal
Box 195432
San Juan, PR 00919-5432
(787) 758-6410

Instituto Tecnologico-San Juan
—Rio Piedras—

Full-Time Enrollments:	66	Evening Classes:	Yes
Part-Time Enrollments:	—	Weekend Classes:	—
Affiliation:	Public	Distance Learning:	—

NLN ACCREDITATION: No

Articulation: None

For Further Information Contact:

Ms Maria Alonzo Amaro, Director
Instituto Tecnologico-San Juan
9 Calle Alegria Final
Rio Piedras, PR 00924
(787) 764-2559

Interamerican University
—Aguadilla—

Full-Time Enrollments: 105 **Evening Classes:** —
Part-Time Enrollments: — **Weekend Classes:** —
Affiliation: Private **Distance Learning:** —

NLN ACCREDITATION: No

Articulation: None

For Further Information Contact:

Mrs Ana Delgado Hernandez, Coordinator
Interamerican University
Box 925
Aguadilla, PR 00605
(787) 857-2585

Interamerican University
—Arecibo—

Full-Time Enrollments: — **Evening Classes:** —
Part-Time Enrollments: — **Weekend Classes:** —
Affiliation: Private **Distance Learning:** —

NLN ACCREDITATION: No

Articulation: None

For Further Information Contact:

Mrs Delia Brenes, Director
Interamerican University
PO Box 4050
Arecibo, PR 00614-4050
(787) 878-5475

Interamerican University
—Barranquitas—

Full-Time Enrollments: — **Evening Classes:** —
Part-Time Enrollments: — **Weekend Classes:** —
Affiliation: Religious **Distance Learning:** —

NLN ACCREDITATION: No

Articulation: None

For Further Information Contact:

Mrs Hilda Ortiz, Coordinator
Interamerican University
Box 517
Barranquitas, PR 00618
(787) 857-3600

Interamerican University
—Ponce—

Full-Time Enrollments: — **Evening Classes:** —
Part-Time Enrollments: — **Weekend Classes:** —
Affiliation: Private **Distance Learning:** —

NLN ACCREDITATION: No

Articulation: None

For Further Information Contact:

Ms Hilda G Nazario, Director
Interamerican University
Carretera Num 1 Mercedita Sta
Ponce, PR 00731
(787) 840-9090

Interamerican University
—San German—

Full-Time Enrollments: — **Evening Classes:** —
Part-Time Enrollments: — **Weekend Classes:** —
Affiliation: Private **Distance Learning:** —

NLN ACCREDITATION: No

Articulation: None

For Further Information Contact:

Mrs Maritza Ortiz, Director
Interamerican University
PO Box 5106
San German, PR 00683
(787) 264-1912

Interamerican University of Puerto Rico
—Guayama—

Full-Time Enrollments: 198 **Evening Classes:** Yes
Part-Time Enrollments: 8 **Weekend Classes:** —
Affiliation: Private **Distance Learning:** —

NLN ACCREDITATION: No

Articulation: Associate to Baccalaureate

For Further Information Contact:

Dr Angela DeJesus Alicea, Director
Interamerican University of Puerto Rico
Box 1559
Guayama, PR 00785
(787) 864-2222

Interamerican University of Puerto Rico
—San Juan—

Full-Time Enrollments:	—	Evening Classes:	—
Part-Time Enrollments:	—	Weekend Classes:	—
Affiliation:	Private	Distance Learning:	—

NLN ACCREDITATION: No

Articulation: None

For Further Information Contact:

Dr Gloria E Ortiz, Director
Interamerican University of Puerto Rico
PO Box 191293
San Juan, PR 00919
(787) 766-3066

Ponce Jr College
—Ponce—

Full-Time Enrollments:	24	Evening Classes:	No
Part-Time Enrollments:	—	Weekend Classes:	No
Affiliation:	Private	Distance Learning:	No

NLN ACCREDITATION: No

Articulation: None

For Further Information Contact:

Mrs Roxana Lanause, Dean
Ponce Jr College
Salud No 23
Ponce, PR 00731
(787) 259-2969

Universidad Central De Bayamon
—Bayamon—

Full-Time Enrollments:	—	Evening Classes:	—
Part-Time Enrollments:	—	Weekend Classes:	—
Affiliation:	Private	Distance Learning:	—

NLN ACCREDITATION: No

Articulation: None

For Further Information Contact:

Prof Lydia Villamil, Director
Universidad Central De Bayamon
PO Box 1725
Bayamon, PR 00960
(787) 786-3030

Universidad Metropolitana
—Rio Piedras—

Full-Time Enrollments:	128	Evening Classes:	Yes
Part-Time Enrollments:	7	Weekend Classes:	No
Affiliation:	Private	Distance Learning:	Yes

NLN ACCREDITATION: Yes

Articulation: None

For Further Information Contact:

Mrs Carmen Bigas, Director
Universidad Metropolitana
Box 21150
Rio Piedras, PR 00928
(787) 766-1717

University of Puerto Rico-Arecibo Technical College
—Arecibo—

Full-Time Enrollments:	166	Evening Classes:	Yes
Part-Time Enrollments:	53	Weekend Classes:	No
Affiliation:	Public	Distance Learning:	No

NLN ACCREDITATION: Yes

Articulation: Associate to Baccalaureate

For Further Information Contact:

Mrs Migdalia Lopez Forty, Director
University of Puerto Rico-Arecibo Technical College
Box 1806
Arecibo, PR 00613-4010
(787) 878-2830

University of Puerto Rico at Mayaguez
—Mayaguez—

Full-Time Enrollments:	—	Evening Classes:	—
Part-Time Enrollments:	—	Weekend Classes:	—
Affiliation:	Public	Distance Learning:	—

NLN ACCREDITATION: Yes

Articulation: None

For Further Information Contact:

Dr Hayden Rios, Director
University of Puerto Rico at Mayaguez
PO Box 5000
Mayaguez, PR 00681-5000
(787) 832-4040

University of Puerto Rico-Humacao
—Humacao—

Full-Time Enrollments:	—	Evening Classes:	—
Part-Time Enrollments:	—	Weekend Classes:	—
Affiliation:	Public	Distance Learning:	—

NLN ACCREDITATION: Yes

Articulation: None

For Further Information Contact:

Prof Alida Santana Troche, Director
University of Puerto Rico-Humacao
Station
Humacao, PR 00790
(787) 850-9346

University of Sacred Heart
—Santurce—

Full-Time Enrollments:	26	Evening Classes:	Yes
Part-Time Enrollments:	—	Weekend Classes:	Yes
Affiliation:	Religious	Distance Learning:	No

NLN ACCREDITATION: No

Articulation: Associate to Baccalaureate
Diploma to Baccalaureate

For Further Information Contact:

Dr Amelia Yordan, Director
University of Sacred Heart
PO Box 12383, Loiza Sta
Santurce, PR 00914-2383
(787) 728-1515

Rhode Island

Community College of Rhode Island
(Flanagan Campus)
—Lincoln—

Full-Time Enrollments:	—	Evening Classes:	—
Part-Time Enrollments:	—	Weekend Classes:	—
Affiliation:	Public	Distance Learning:	—

NLN ACCREDITATION: Yes

Articulation: None

For Further Information Contact:

Ms Elizabeth A Murphy, Chair
Community College of Rhode Island (Flanagan
Campus)
Louisquisset Pike
Lincoln, RI 02865
(401) 825-1000

Community College of Rhode Island
(Knight Campus)
—Warwick—

Full-Time Enrollments:	216	Evening Classes:	—
Part-Time Enrollments:	200	Weekend Classes:	—
Affiliation:	Public	Distance Learning:	—

NLN ACCREDITATION: Yes

Articulation: None

For Further Information Contact:

Ms Elizabeth A Murphy, Chair
Community College of Rhode Island (Knight Campus)
400 East Ave
Warwick, RI 02886
(401) 333-7265

Salve Regina University
—Newport—

Full-Time Enrollments:	—	Evening Classes:	—
Part-Time Enrollments:	—	Weekend Classes:	—
Affiliation:	Religious	Distance Learning:	—

NLN ACCREDITATION: No

Articulation: None

For Further Information Contact:

Dr Eileen Donnelly, Chair
Salve Regina University
100 Ochre Point Ave
Newport, RI 02840-4192
(401) 847-6650

South Carolina

Aiken Regional Campus-University of South Carolina
—Aiken—

Full-Time Enrollments:	100	Evening Classes:	Yes
Part-Time Enrollments:	53	Weekend Classes:	No
Affiliation:	Public	Distance Learning:	Yes

NLN ACCREDITATION: Yes

Articulation: Associate to Baccalaureate

For Further Information Contact:

Dr Trudy Groves, Dept Head
Aiken Regional Campus-University of South Carolina
171 Univ Pkwy
Aiken, SC 29801
(803) 648-6851

Central Carolina Technical College
—Sumter—

Full-Time Enrollments:	79	Evening Classes:	No
Part-Time Enrollments:	—	Weekend Classes:	No
Affiliation:	Public	Distance Learning:	No

NLN ACCREDITATION: Yes

Articulation: None

For Further Information Contact:

Mrs Laurie Harden, Chair
Central Carolina Technical College
506 N Guignard
Sumter, SC 29150
(803) 778-1961

Florence-Darlington Technical College
—Florence—

Full-Time Enrollments:	97	Evening Classes:	Yes
Part-Time Enrollments:	78	Weekend Classes:	No
Affiliation:	Public	Distance Learning:	Yes

NLN ACCREDITATION: Yes

Articulation: Associate to Baccalaureate
LPN to Associate

For Further Information Contact:

Mrs Mary S Teal, Dept Head
Florence-Darlington Technical College
PO Box 100548
Florence, SC 29501-0548
(803) 661-8147

Greenville Technical College
—Greenville—

Full-Time Enrollments:	86	Evening Classes:	No
Part-Time Enrollments:	245	Weekend Classes:	No
Affiliation:	Public	Distance Learning:	No

NLN ACCREDITATION: Yes

Articulation: Associate to Baccalaureate
LPN to Associate

For Further Information Contact:

Ms Gayle Heller, Dept Chair
Greenville Technical College
Box 5616
Greenville, SC 29606
(864) 250-8288

Horry-Georgetown Technical College
—Conway—

Full-Time Enrollments:	103	Evening Classes:	No
Part-Time Enrollments:	—	Weekend Classes:	No
Affiliation:	Public	Distance Learning:	No

NLN ACCREDITATION: No

Articulation: LPN to Associate

For Further Information Contact:

Dr Wilma Vines, Dept Head
Horry-Georgetown Technical College
PO Box 1966 Hwy 501 East
Conway, SC 29526-1966
(803) 347-3186

Midlands Technical College
—Columbia—

Full-Time Enrollments:	201	Evening Classes:	Yes
Part-Time Enrollments:	129	Weekend Classes:	Yes
Affiliation:	Public	Distance Learning:	Yes

NLN ACCREDITATION: Yes

Articulation: Associate to Baccalaureate
LPN to Associate
RN to MSN

For Further Information Contact:

Dr Madelon Ceman, Dept Chair
Midlands Technical College
PO Box 2408
Columbia, SC 29202
(803) 822-3319

Orangeburg-Calhoun Technical College
—Orangeburg—

Full-Time Enrollments:	27	Evening Classes:	Yes
Part-Time Enrollments:	83	Weekend Classes:	No
Affiliation:	Public	Distance Learning:	Yes

NLN ACCREDITATION: Yes

Articulation: Associate to Baccalaureate

For Further Information Contact:

Mrs Delura Knight, Dept Head
Orangeburg-Calhoun Technical College
PO Box 1767
Orangeburg, SC 29115
(803) 535-0311

Piedmont Technical College
—Greenwood—

Full-Time Enrollments: 84
Part-Time Enrollments: —
Affiliation: Public
Evening Classes: Yes
Weekend Classes: Yes
Distance Learning: Yes

NLN ACCREDITATION: Yes

Articulation: Associate to Baccalaureate
LPN to Associate

For Further Information Contact:

Mrs Lena Wood Warren, Dean
Piedmont Technical College
Emerald Rd Drawer 1467
Greenwood, SC 29648
(864) 941-8536

Technical College of the Lowcountry
—Beaufort—

Full-Time Enrollments: 3
Part-Time Enrollments: 73
Affiliation: Public
Evening Classes: No
Weekend Classes: No
Distance Learning: Yes

NLN ACCREDITATION: Yes

Articulation: LPN to Associate

For Further Information Contact:

Dr Rose Kearney Nunnery, Dept Head
Technical College of the Lowcountry
PO Box 1288
Beaufort, SC 29902
(803) 525-8267

Tri-County Technical College
—Pendleton—

Full-Time Enrollments: 30
Part-Time Enrollments: 81
Affiliation: Public
Evening Classes: No
Weekend Classes: No
Distance Learning: No

NLN ACCREDITATION: No

Articulation: LPN to Associate

For Further Information Contact:

Ms Karen Sorrow, Chair
Tri-County Technical College
PO Box 587
Pendleton, SC 29670
(803) 646-8361

Trident Technical College
—Charleston—

Full-Time Enrollments: 24
Part-Time Enrollments: 210
Affiliation: Public
Evening Classes: No
Weekend Classes: No
Distance Learning: No

NLN ACCREDITATION: Yes

Articulation: LPN to Associate

For Further Information Contact:

Ms Anne Beck, Dept Head
Trident Technical College
PO Box 118067
Charleston, SC 29423
(803) 572-6041

University of South Carolina-Spartanburg
—Spartanburg—

Full-Time Enrollments: 46
Part-Time Enrollments: 82
Affiliation: Public
Evening Classes: Yes
Weekend Classes: No
Distance Learning: No

NLN ACCREDITATION: Yes

Articulation: Associate to Baccalaureate

For Further Information Contact:

Mrs Carol Rentz, Chair
University of South Carolina-Spartanburg
800 University Way
Spartanburg, SC 29303
(864) 503-5440

University of South Carolina-York Technical College
—Rock Hill—

Full-Time Enrollments: —
Part-Time Enrollments: —
Affiliation: Public
Evening Classes: —
Weekend Classes: —
Distance Learning: —

NLN ACCREDITATION: Yes

Articulation: None

For Further Information Contact:

Mrs Francine Manion, Director
University of South Carolina-York Technical College
452 S Anderson Rd
Rock Hill, SC 29730
(803) 822-3319

South Dakota

Dakota Wesleyan University
—Mitchell—

Full-Time Enrollments:	54	Evening Classes:	No
Part-Time Enrollments:	29	Weekend Classes:	No
Affiliation:	Religious	Distance Learning:	No

NLN ACCREDITATION: Yes

Articulation: Associate to Baccalaureate
LPN to Associate

For Further Information Contact:

Mrs Nancy Nelson, Chair
Dakota Wesleyan University
1200 W Univ Ave
Mitchell, SD 57301
(605) 995-2702

Huron University/Regional Medical Center
—Huron—

Full-Time Enrollments:	23	Evening Classes:	No
Part-Time Enrollments:	3	Weekend Classes:	No
Affiliation:	Private	Distance Learning:	No

NLN ACCREDITATION: Yes

Articulation: Associate to Baccalaureate

For Further Information Contact:

Mrs Joyce E Fjelland, Dean
Huron University/Regional Medical Center
333 9th St SW
Huron, SD 57350
(605) 352-8721

Oglala Lakota College
—Pine Ridge—

Full-Time Enrollments:	30	Evening Classes:	No
Part-Time Enrollments:	—	Weekend Classes:	No
Affiliation:	Public	Distance Learning:	Yes

NLN ACCREDITATION: No

Articulation: Associate to Baccalaureate
RN to MSN

For Further Information Contact:

Dr Donna Demarest, Director
Oglala Lakota College
Box 861
Pine Ridge, SD 57770
(605) 867-5857

Presentation College
—Aberdeen—

Full-Time Enrollments:	24	Evening Classes:	—
Part-Time Enrollments:	1	Weekend Classes:	—
Affiliation:	Religious	Distance Learning:	No

NLN ACCREDITATION: Yes

Articulation: Associate to Baccalaureate
Diploma to Baccalaureate

For Further Information Contact:

Mr Thomas Stenvig, Chair
Presentation College
1500 North Main St
Aberdeen, SD 57401
(605) 229-8472

Sisseton Wahpeton Community College
—Sisseton—

Full-Time Enrollments:	38	Evening Classes:	Yes
Part-Time Enrollments:	1	Weekend Classes:	No
Affiliation:	Private	Distance Learning:	No

NLN ACCREDITATION: No

Articulation: Associate to Baccalaureate

For Further Information Contact:

Mrs Susan Hardin Palmer, Director
Sisseton Wahpeton Community College
Old Agency Box 689
Sisseton, SD 57282
(605) 698-3621

University of South Dakota
—Vermillion—

Full-Time Enrollments:	223	Evening Classes:	Yes
Part-Time Enrollments:	71	Weekend Classes:	No
Affiliation:	Public	Distance Learning:	Yes

NLN ACCREDITATION: Yes

Articulation: Associate to Baccalaureate
LPN to Associate

For Further Information Contact:

Dr Susan Johnson, Chair
University of South Dakota
414 E Clark
Vermillion, SD 57069
(605) 677-5251

Tennessee

Aquinas College
—Nashville—

Full-Time Enrollments:	40	Evening Classes:	No
Part-Time Enrollments:	92	Weekend Classes:	No
Affiliation:	Religious	Distance Learning:	No

NLN ACCREDITATION: Yes

Articulation: None

For Further Information Contact:

Mrs Peggy Daniel, Director
Aquinas College
4210 Harding Pl
Nashville, TN 37205
(615) 297-7545

Chattanooga State Technical Community College
—Chattanooga—

Full-Time Enrollments:	263	Evening Classes:	Yes
Part-Time Enrollments:	—	Weekend Classes:	—
Affiliation:	Public	Distance Learning:	—

NLN ACCREDITATION: Yes

Articulation: Associate to Baccalaureate
LPN to Associate

For Further Information Contact:

Dr Cynthia W Swafford, Director
Chattanooga State Technical Community College
4501 Amnicola Hwy
Chattanooga, TN 37406
(423) 778-8080

Cleveland State Community College
—Cleveland—

Full-Time Enrollments:	111	Evening Classes:	No
Part-Time Enrollments:	—	Weekend Classes:	No
Affiliation:	Public	Distance Learning:	No

NLN ACCREDITATION: Yes

Articulation: None

For Further Information Contact:

Mrs Elizabeth Eiswerth, Director
Cleveland State Community College
Cleveland, TN 37311
(423) 478-7141

Columbia State Community College
—Columbia—

Full-Time Enrollments:	88	Evening Classes:	No
Part-Time Enrollments:	183	Weekend Classes:	No
Affiliation:	Public	Distance Learning:	Yes

NLN ACCREDITATION: Yes

Articulation: LPN to Associate

For Further Information Contact:

Dr Deanna J Naddy, Assistant Dean
Columbia State Community College
PO Box 3570
Columbia, TN 38401
(615) 540-2722

Dyersburg State Community College
—Dyersburg—

Full-Time Enrollments:	51	Evening Classes:	No
Part-Time Enrollments:	92	Weekend Classes:	No
Affiliation:	Public	Distance Learning:	No

NLN ACCREDITATION: Yes

Articulation: Associate to Baccalaureate
LPN to Associate

For Further Information Contact:

Ms Phyllis Koonce, Dean
Dyersburg State Community College
1510 Lake Rd
Dyersburg, TN 38024
(901) 286-3390

East Tennessee State University
—Johnson City—

Full-Time Enrollments:	40	Evening Classes:	Yes
Part-Time Enrollments:	26	Weekend Classes:	No
Affiliation:	Public	Distance Learning:	Yes

NLN ACCREDITATION: Yes

Articulation: Associate to Baccalaureate
Diploma to Baccalaureate

For Further Information Contact:

Dr Joellen Edwards, Dean
East Tennessee State University
PO Box 70617
Johnson City, TN 37614-0617
(423) 439-6752

No AD program any longer (handwritten note)

Jackson State Community College
—Jackson—

Full-Time Enrollments:	100	Evening Classes:	—
Part-Time Enrollments:	11	Weekend Classes:	—
Affiliation:	Public	Distance Learning:	—

NLN ACCREDITATION: Yes

Articulation: None

For Further Information Contact:

Dr Leslie West-Sands, Chair
Jackson State Community College
2046 North Parkway East
Jackson, TN 38301-3797
(901) 425-2622

Lincoln Memorial University
—Harrogate—

Full-Time Enrollments:	69	Evening Classes:	No
Part-Time Enrollments:	138	Weekend Classes:	No
Affiliation:	Private	Distance Learning:	No

NLN ACCREDITATION: Yes

Articulation: None

For Further Information Contact:

Mrs Elizabeth Yeary, Chair
Lincoln Memorial University
Harrogate, TN 37752
(423) 869-3611

Motlow State Community College
—Tullahoma—

Full-Time Enrollments:	46	Evening Classes:	Yes
Part-Time Enrollments:	96	Weekend Classes:	No
Affiliation:	Public	Distance Learning:	No

NLN ACCREDITATION: Yes

Articulation: Associate to Baccalaureate

For Further Information Contact:

Ms Susan Sanders, Director
Motlow State Community College
PO Box 88100
Tullahoma, TN 37388
(615) 393-1628

Roane State Community College
—Harriman—

Full-Time Enrollments:	220	Evening Classes:	No
Part-Time Enrollments:	—	Weekend Classes:	No
Affiliation:	Public	Distance Learning:	Yes

NLN ACCREDITATION: Yes

Articulation: Associate to Baccalaureate

For Further Information Contact:

Ms Karen Wilken, Chair
Roane State Community College
Harriman, TN 37748
(423) 354-3000

Shelby State Community College
—Memphis—

Full-Time Enrollments:	66	Evening Classes:	Yes
Part-Time Enrollments:	235	Weekend Classes:	Yes
Affiliation:	Public	Distance Learning:	No

NLN ACCREDITATION: Yes

Articulation: Associate to Baccalaureate
LPN to Associate

For Further Information Contact:

Mrs Carolyn Brown, Acting Head
Shelby State Community College
737 Union Ave
Memphis, TN 38174
(901) 528-6870

Southern Adventist University
—Collegedale—

Full-Time Enrollments:	108	Evening Classes:	No
Part-Time Enrollments:	45	Weekend Classes:	No
Affiliation:	Religious	Distance Learning:	No

NLN ACCREDITATION: Yes

Articulation: Associate to Baccalaureate

For Further Information Contact:

Mrs Katie A Lamb, Chair
Southern Adventist University
Collegedale, TN 37315
(423) 238-2942

Tennessee State University-School of Nursing
—Nashville—

Full-Time Enrollments:	263	Evening Classes:	—
Part-Time Enrollments:	—	Weekend Classes:	Yes
Affiliation:	Public	Distance Learning:	Yes

NLN ACCREDITATION: Yes

Articulation: LPN to Associate

For Further Information Contact:

Dr Christine Sharpe, Assistant Dean
Tennessee State University-School of Nursing
3500 John A Merritt Blvd
Nashville, TN 37209-1561
(615) 963-5266

Walters State Community College
—Morristown—

Full-Time Enrollments:	134	Evening Classes:	Yes
Part-Time Enrollments:	138	Weekend Classes:	Yes
Affiliation:	Public	Distance Learning:	No

NLN ACCREDITATION: Yes

Articulation: Associate to Baccalaureate
LPN to Associate

For Further Information Contact:

Mrs Mary L Apple, Chair
Walters State Community College
500 S Davy Crockett Pky
Morristown, TN 37813-6899
(423) 585-6983

Texas

Abilene Inter Collegiate School
—Abiline—

Full-Time Enrollments:	17	Evening Classes:	No
Part-Time Enrollments:	—	Weekend Classes:	No
Affiliation:	Religious	Distance Learning:	No

NLN ACCREDITATION: No

Articulation: Associate to Baccalaureate
Diploma to Baccalaureate

For Further Information Contact:

Dr Corine N Bonnet, Dean
Abilene Inter Collegiate School
2149 Hickory
Abiline, TX 79601
(915) 672-2441

Alvin Community College
—Alvin—

Full-Time Enrollments:	18	Evening Classes:	No
Part-Time Enrollments:	96	Weekend Classes:	No
Affiliation:	Public	Distance Learning:	No

NLN ACCREDITATION: Yes

Articulation: None

For Further Information Contact:

Ms Elizabeth J Oliver, Director
Alvin Community College
3110 Mustang Rd
Alvin, TX 77511-4898
(281) 331-6111

Amarillo College
—Amarillo—

Full-Time Enrollments:	306	Evening Classes:	No
Part-Time Enrollments:	20	Weekend Classes:	No
Affiliation:	Public	Distance Learning:	No

NLN ACCREDITATION: Yes

Articulation: Associate to Baccalaureate
LPN to Associate

For Further Information Contact:

Ms Sue McGee, Chair
Amarillo College
Box 447
Amarillo, TX 79178
(806) 354-6009

Angelina College
—Lufkin—

Full-Time Enrollments:	130	Evening Classes:	—
Part-Time Enrollments:	84	Weekend Classes:	—
Affiliation:	Public	Distance Learning:	—

NLN ACCREDITATION: No

Articulation: None

For Further Information Contact:

Ms Jere Hammer, Coordinator
Angelina College
PO Box 1768
Lufkin, TX 75901
(409) 639-1301

Angelo State University
—San Angelo—

Full-Time Enrollments:	140	Evening Classes:	No
Part-Time Enrollments:	154	Weekend Classes:	No
Affiliation:	Public	Distance Learning:	No

NLN ACCREDITATION: Yes

Articulation: LPN to Associate

For Further Information Contact:

Dr Leslie Mayrand, Dept Head
Angelo State University
PO Box 10902
San Angelo, TX 76909
(915) 942-2224

Austin Community College
—Austin—

Full-Time Enrollments:	148	Evening Classes:	Yes
Part-Time Enrollments:	33	Weekend Classes:	Yes
Affiliation:	Public	Distance Learning:	Yes

NLN ACCREDITATION: Yes

Articulation: Associate to Baccalaureate
RN to MSN

For Further Information Contact:

Ms Gail Snyder, Dept Head
Austin Community College
1020 Grove Blvd
Austin, TX 78741
(512) 223-6109

Blinn College
—Bryan—

Full-Time Enrollments:	49	Evening Classes:	No
Part-Time Enrollments:	31	Weekend Classes:	No
Affiliation:	Public	Distance Learning:	No

NLN ACCREDITATION: Yes

Articulation: Associate to Baccalaureate

For Further Information Contact:

Dr Linda Carpenter, Director
Blinn College
1905 South Texas Ave
Bryan, TX 77802
(409) 821-0204

Central Texas College
—Killeen—

Full-Time Enrollments:	198	Evening Classes:	No
Part-Time Enrollments:	2	Weekend Classes:	No
Affiliation:	Public	Distance Learning:	No

NLN ACCREDITATION: Yes

Articulation: LPN to Associate

For Further Information Contact:

Dr Elaine E Hayes, Chair
Central Texas College
6200 W Central Tx Expressway
Killeen, TX 76540-1800
(817) 526-1266

Cisco Jr College
—Abelene—

Full-Time Enrollments:	18	Evening Classes:	Yes
Part-Time Enrollments:	6	Weekend Classes:	No
Affiliation:	Public	Distance Learning:	No

NLN ACCREDITATION: No

Articulation: None

For Further Information Contact:

Dr Barbara McClurg, Director
Cisco Jr College
841 North Judge Ely
Abelene, TX 79601
(915) 673-4567

College of the Mainland
—Texas City—

Full-Time Enrollments:	8	Evening Classes:	No
Part-Time Enrollments:	84	Weekend Classes:	No
Affiliation:	Public	Distance Learning:	No

NLN ACCREDITATION: Yes

Articulation: Associate to Baccalaureate

For Further Information Contact:

Ms Pattie Tyler, Interim Director
College of the Mainland
1200 Amburn Rd
Texas City, TX 77591
(409) 938-1211

Collin County Community College
—McKinney—

Full-Time Enrollments:	2	Evening Classes:	—
Part-Time Enrollments:	62	Weekend Classes:	—
Affiliation:	Public	Distance Learning:	—

NLN ACCREDITATION: Yes

Articulation: Associate to Baccalaureate

For Further Information Contact:

Dr Vivian C Lilly, Associate Dean
Collin County Community College
2200 W Univ Dr
McKinney, TX 75070
(972) 548-6883

Del Mar College
—Corpus Christi—

Full-Time Enrollments:	8	Evening Classes:	Yes
Part-Time Enrollments:	270	Weekend Classes:	No
Affiliation:	Public	Distance Learning:	No

NLN ACCREDITATION: Yes

Articulation: LPN to Associate

For Further Information Contact:

Dr Blanca Rosa Garcia, Chair
Del Mar College
Baldwin & Ayers
Corpus Christi, TX 78404
(512) 886-1320

El Centro College
—Dallas—

Full-Time Enrollments:	510	Evening Classes:	No
Part-Time Enrollments:	—	Weekend Classes:	No
Affiliation:	Public	Distance Learning:	No

NLN ACCREDITATION: Yes

Articulation: Associate to Baccalaureate
LPN to Associate

For Further Information Contact:

Dr Kathryn Eggleston, Dean
El Centro College
Main & Lamar Sts
Dallas, TX 75202
(214) 860-2269

El Paso Community College
—El Paso—

Full-Time Enrollments:	97	Evening Classes:	No
Part-Time Enrollments:	62	Weekend Classes:	No
Affiliation:	Public	Distance Learning:	No

NLN ACCREDITATION: Yes

Articulation: Associate to Baccalaureate
LPN to Associate
RN to MSN

For Further Information Contact:

Dr Paula R Mitchell, Div Chair
El Paso Community College
PO Box 20500-Rio Grande Ctr
El Paso, TX 79998
(915) 534-4030

Galveston College
—Galveston—

Full-Time Enrollments:	135	Evening Classes:	No
Part-Time Enrollments:	—	Weekend Classes:	No
Affiliation:	Public	Distance Learning:	No

NLN ACCREDITATION: Yes

Articulation: Associate to Baccalaureate
LPN to Associate

For Further Information Contact:

Mrs Elizabeth Michel, Assistant Dean
Galveston College
4015 Ave Q
Galveston, TX 77550
(409) 763-6551

Grayson County College
—Denison—

Full-Time Enrollments:	181	Evening Classes:	No
Part-Time Enrollments:	—	Weekend Classes:	No
Affiliation:	Public	Distance Learning:	No

NLN ACCREDITATION: Yes

Articulation: Associate to Baccalaureate
LPN to Associate

For Further Information Contact:

Mrs Joann Bohm-Adair, Dean
Grayson County College
6101 Grayson Dr
Denison, TX 75020
(903) 463-8634

Houston Baptist University
—Houston—

Full-Time Enrollments:	55	Evening Classes:	No
Part-Time Enrollments:	—	Weekend Classes:	No
Affiliation:	Religious	Distance Learning:	No

NLN ACCREDITATION: Yes

Articulation: Associate to Baccalaureate

For Further Information Contact:

Dr Nancy C Yuill, Dean
Houston Baptist University
7202 Fondren Rd
Houston, TX 77074-3298
(713) 995-3300

Howard County Jr College District
—Big Spring—

Full-Time Enrollments:	42	Evening Classes:	No
Part-Time Enrollments:	—	Weekend Classes:	No
Affiliation:	Public	Distance Learning:	No

NLN ACCREDITATION: Yes

Articulation: Associate to Baccalaureate

For Further Information Contact:

Mrs Cindy Stokes, Dean
Howard County Jr College District
1001 Birdwell Lane
Big Spring, TX 79720
(915) 264-5071

Kilgore College
—Kilgore—

Full-Time Enrollments:	115	Evening Classes:	No
Part-Time Enrollments:	—	Weekend Classes:	No
Affiliation:	Public	Distance Learning:	No

NLN ACCREDITATION: Yes

Articulation: Associate to Baccalaureate

For Further Information Contact:

Miss Ida Riddle, Director
Kilgore College
1100 Broadway
Kilgore, TX 75662
(903) 983-8168

Lamar University
—Beaumont—

Full-Time Enrollments:	40	Evening Classes:	No
Part-Time Enrollments:	—	Weekend Classes:	No
Affiliation:	Public	Distance Learning:	No

NLN ACCREDITATION: Yes

Articulation: LPN to Associate

For Further Information Contact:

Ms Sandra Dickey, Director
Lamar University
PO Box 10081
Beaumont, TX 77710
(409) 880-8831

Lamar University-At Orange
—Orange—

Full-Time Enrollments:	40	Evening Classes:	No
Part-Time Enrollments:	—	Weekend Classes:	No
Affiliation:	Public	Distance Learning:	No

NLN ACCREDITATION: Yes

Articulation: LPN to Associate

For Further Information Contact:

Ms Sandra Dickey, Director
Lamar University-At Orange
410 Front St
Orange, TX 77630
(409) 882-3311

Lamar University-Port Arthur
—Port Arthur—

Full-Time Enrollments:	30	Evening Classes:	No
Part-Time Enrollments:	—	Weekend Classes:	No
Affiliation:	Public	Distance Learning:	No

NLN ACCREDITATION: Yes

Articulation: None

For Further Information Contact:

Ms Lino Chien, Director
Lamar University-Port Arthur
Box 310
Port Arthur, TX 77641
(409) 984-6354

Laredo Community College
—Laredo—

Full-Time Enrollments:	52	Evening Classes:	—
Part-Time Enrollments:	—	Weekend Classes:	—
Affiliation:	Public	Distance Learning:	—

NLN ACCREDITATION: Yes

Articulation: None

For Further Information Contact:

Ms Dianna Milles, Interim Director
Laredo Community College
West End Washington St
Laredo, TX 78040
(210) 721-5252

Lee College
—Baytown—

Full-Time Enrollments:	107	Evening Classes:	Yes
Part-Time Enrollments:	—	Weekend Classes:	No
Affiliation:	Public	Distance Learning:	No

NLN ACCREDITATION: Yes

Articulation: Associate to Baccalaureate
LPN to Associate

For Further Information Contact:

Dr Lorena Maher, Div Chair
Lee College
PO Box 818
Baytown, TX 77522
(713) 425-6449

McLennan Community College
—Waco—

Full-Time Enrollments:	214	Evening Classes:	Yes
Part-Time Enrollments:	—	Weekend Classes:	No
Affiliation:	Public	Distance Learning:	No

NLN ACCREDITATION: Yes

Articulation: None

For Further Information Contact:

Mrs Alice Myers, Director
McLennan Community College
1400 College Dr
Waco, TX 76708
(817) 750-3541

Midland College
—Midland—

Full-Time Enrollments:	86	Evening Classes:	No
Part-Time Enrollments:	—	Weekend Classes:	Yes
Affiliation:	Public	Distance Learning:	No

NLN ACCREDITATION: Yes

Articulation: Associate to Baccalaureate

For Further Information Contact:

Mrs Nancy Shaw, Chair
Midland College
3600 N Garfield
Midland, TX 79705
(915) 685-4600

Navarro College ADN Program
—Corsicana—

Full-Time Enrollments:	68	Evening Classes:	No
Part-Time Enrollments:	—	Weekend Classes:	No
Affiliation:	Public	Distance Learning:	No

NLN ACCREDITATION: Yes

Articulation: LPN to Associate

For Further Information Contact:

Dr Judy Howden, Director
Navarro College ADN Program
3200 W 7th Ave
Corsicana, TX 75110
(903) 874-6501

North Central Texas College
—Gainesville—

Full-Time Enrollments:	107	Evening Classes:	No
Part-Time Enrollments:	3	Weekend Classes:	No
Affiliation:	Public	Distance Learning:	No

NLN ACCREDITATION: Yes

Articulation: LPN to Associate

For Further Information Contact:

Mrs Maurice Robeson, Chair
North Central Texas College
1525 W California
Gainesville, TX 76240
(817) 668-7731

North Harris Montgomery Community College
—Houston—

Full-Time Enrollments:	225	Evening Classes:	No
Part-Time Enrollments:	—	Weekend Classes:	No
Affiliation:	Public	Distance Learning:	No

NLN ACCREDITATION: Yes

Articulation: Associate to Baccalaureate
LPN to Associate

For Further Information Contact:

Mrs Peggy Aalund, Director
North Harris Montgomery Community College
2700 W Thorne Dr
Houston, TX 77073
(281) 443-5751

Northeast Texas Community College
—Mt Pleasant—

Full-Time Enrollments:	8	Evening Classes:	No
Part-Time Enrollments:	39	Weekend Classes:	No
Affiliation:	Public	Distance Learning:	No

NLN ACCREDITATION: No

Articulation: LPN to Associate

For Further Information Contact:

Mrs Cynthia Amerson, Director
Northeast Texas Community College
PO Box 1307
Mt Pleasant, TX 75455
(903) 572-1911

Odessa College
—Odessa—

Full-Time Enrollments:	106	Evening Classes:	Yes
Part-Time Enrollments:	48	Weekend Classes:	No
Affiliation:	Public	Distance Learning:	Yes

NLN ACCREDITATION: Yes

Articulation: Associate to Baccalaureate

For Further Information Contact:

Dr Carol Boswell, Chair
Odessa College
201 W University
Odessa, TX 79764
(915) 335-6672

Panola College
—Carthage—

Full-Time Enrollments:	—	Evening Classes:	No
Part-Time Enrollments:	89	Weekend Classes:	No
Affiliation:	Public	Distance Learning:	No

NLN ACCREDITATION: No

Articulation: None

For Further Information Contact:

Ms Jerri Faircloth, Director
Panola College
820 W Panola
Carthage, TX 75633
(903) 694-4000

75633

Paris Jr College
—Paris—

Full-Time Enrollments:	67	Evening Classes:	No
Part-Time Enrollments:	—	Weekend Classes:	No
Affiliation:	Public	Distance Learning:	No

NLN ACCREDITATION: Yes

Articulation: Associate to Baccalaureate
                LPN to Associate

For Further Information Contact:

Mrs Virginia Holmes, Director
Paris Jr College
2400 Clarksville St
Paris, TX 75460
(903) 784-9467

San Antonio College
—San Antonio—

Full-Time Enrollments:	439	Evening Classes:	Yes
Part-Time Enrollments:	—	Weekend Classes:	No
Affiliation:	Public	Distance Learning:	No

NLN ACCREDITATION: Yes

Articulation: Associate to Baccalaureate
                LPN to Associate

For Further Information Contact:

Ms Leana Revell, Chair
San Antonio College
1300 San Pedro Ave
San Antonio, TX 78212
(210) 733-2365

San Jacinto College Central
—Pasadena—

Full-Time Enrollments:	311	Evening Classes:	Yes
Part-Time Enrollments:	—	Weekend Classes:	No
Affiliation:	Public	Distance Learning:	No

NLN ACCREDITATION: Yes

Articulation: Associate to Baccalaureate
                LPN to Associate

For Further Information Contact:

Dr Marlene Luna, Chair
San Jacinto College Central
Box 2007 8060 Spencer Hwy
Pasadena, TX 77501-2007
(281) 476-1842

San Jacinto College South
—Houston—

Full-Time Enrollments:	—	Evening Classes:	Yes
Part-Time Enrollments:	30	Weekend Classes:	No
Affiliation:	Public	Distance Learning:	No

NLN ACCREDITATION: Yes

Articulation: Associate to Baccalaureate

For Further Information Contact:

Dr Joyce Adams, Chair
San Jacinto College South
13735 Beamer Rd
Houston, TX 77089
(281) 922-3468

South Plains College
—Levelland—

Full-Time Enrollments:	98	Evening Classes:	No
Part-Time Enrollments:	—	Weekend Classes:	No
Affiliation:	Public	Distance Learning:	No

NLN ACCREDITATION: Yes

Articulation: Associate to Baccalaureate

For Further Information Contact:

Mrs Marla K Cottenoir, Chair
South Plains College
1400 College Ave
Levelland, TX 79336
(806) 894-9611

Southwestern Adventist College
—Keene—

Full-Time Enrollments:	53	Evening Classes:	No
Part-Time Enrollments:	34	Weekend Classes:	No
Affiliation:	Religious	Distance Learning:	No

NLN ACCREDITATION: Yes

Articulation: None

For Further Information Contact:

Dr Catherine Turner, Chair
Southwestern Adventist College
PO Box 58
Keene, TX 76059
(817) 645-3921

Tarleton State University
—Stephenville—

Full-Time Enrollments:	57	Evening Classes:	—
Part-Time Enrollments:	38	Weekend Classes:	—
Affiliation:	Public	Distance Learning:	—

NLN ACCREDITATION: No

Articulation: None

For Further Information Contact:

Dr Elaine Evans, Director
Tarleton State University
Box T-500
Stephenville, TX 76402
(817) 968-9139

Tarrant County Jr College District
—Fort Worth—

Full-Time Enrollments:	322	Evening Classes:	Yes
Part-Time Enrollments:	—	Weekend Classes:	No
Affiliation:	Public	Distance Learning:	No

NLN ACCREDITATION: Yes

Articulation: LPN to Associate

For Further Information Contact:

Dr Sue E Ochsner, Director
Tarrant County Jr College District
5301 Campus Dr
Fort Worth, TX 76119
(817) 531-4549

Temple College
—Temple—

Full-Time Enrollments:	59	Evening Classes:	No
Part-Time Enrollments:	—	Weekend Classes:	No
Affiliation:	Public	Distance Learning:	No

NLN ACCREDITATION: Yes

Articulation: None

For Further Information Contact:

Mrs Virginia Leak, Director
Temple College
2600 South First St
Temple, TX 76504
(817) 773-9961

Texarkana Community College
—Texarkana—

Full-Time Enrollments:	183	Evening Classes:	Yes
Part-Time Enrollments:	—	Weekend Classes:	No
Affiliation:	Public	Distance Learning:	No

NLN ACCREDITATION: Yes

Articulation: LPN to Associate

For Further Information Contact:

Mrs Carol Hodgson, Chair
Texarkana Community College
2500 N Robinson Rd
Texarkana, TX 75599
(903) 838-4541

The Houston Community College System
—Houston—

Full-Time Enrollments:	377	Evening Classes:	Yes
Part-Time Enrollments:	—	Weekend Classes:	No
Affiliation:	Public	Distance Learning:	No

NLN ACCREDITATION: No

Articulation: None

For Further Information Contact:

Dr Jane Perez, Director
The Houston Community College System
7000 Fannin Suite 2600
Houston, TX 77030
(713) 718-7300

The University of Texas Brownsville
—Brownsville—

Full-Time Enrollments:	137	Evening Classes:	No
Part-Time Enrollments:	—	Weekend Classes:	No
Affiliation:	Public	Distance Learning:	No

NLN ACCREDITATION: Yes

Articulation: Associate to Baccalaureate
LPN to Associate

For Further Information Contact:

Dr Edna Garza-Escobedo, Chair
The University of Texas Brownsville
80 Fort Brown
Brownsville, TX 78520
(210) 544-8924

Trinity Valley Community College
—Kaufman—

Full-Time Enrollments:	101	Evening Classes:	No
Part-Time Enrollments:	66	Weekend Classes:	Yes
Affiliation:	Public	Distance Learning:	No

NLN ACCREDITATION: Yes

Articulation: Associate to Baccalaureate
LPN to Associate

For Further Information Contact:

Mrs Helen Reid, Dean
Trinity Valley Community College
800 Hwy 243 W
Kaufman, TX 75142
(214) 932-4309

Tyler Jr College
—Tyler—

Full-Time Enrollments:	155	Evening Classes:	No
Part-Time Enrollments:	—	Weekend Classes:	No
Affiliation:	Public	Distance Learning:	No

NLN ACCREDITATION: No

Articulation: LPN to Associate

For Further Information Contact:

Mrs Marie Jackson, Director
Tyler Jr College
P O Box 9020
Tyler, TX 75711
(903) 510-2869

University of Texas-Pan American
—Edinburg—

Full-Time Enrollments:	90	Evening Classes:	No
Part-Time Enrollments:	—	Weekend Classes:	No
Affiliation:	Public	Distance Learning:	No

NLN ACCREDITATION: Yes

Articulation: None

For Further Information Contact:

Dr Carolina Huerta, Chair
University of Texas-Pan American
1201 W Univ Dr
Edinburg, TX 78504
(210) 381-3491

Vernon Region Jr College
—Vernon—

Full-Time Enrollments:	81	Evening Classes:	—
Part-Time Enrollments:	—	Weekend Classes:	—
Affiliation:	Public	Distance Learning:	—

NLN ACCREDITATION: No

Articulation: None

For Further Information Contact:

Ms Cathy Bolton, Director
Vernon Region Jr College
4400 College Dr
Vernon, TX 76384
(817) 552-6291

Victoria College
—Victoria—

Full-Time Enrollments:	130	Evening Classes:	No
Part-Time Enrollments:	—	Weekend Classes:	No
Affiliation:	Public	Distance Learning:	No

NLN ACCREDITATION: Yes

Articulation: Associate to Baccalaureate
LPN to Associate

For Further Information Contact:

Mrs LeAnn Wagner, Director
Victoria College
2200 E Red River
Victoria, TX 77901-4494
(512) 573-3291

Wharton Co Junior College
—Wharton—

Full-Time Enrollments:	36	Evening Classes:	No
Part-Time Enrollments:	24	Weekend Classes:	No
Affiliation:	Public	Distance Learning:	Yes

NLN ACCREDITATION: No

Articulation: LPN to Associate

For Further Information Contact:

Mrs Netha O'Meara, Director
Wharton Co Junior College
911 Boling Hwy
Wharton, TX 77488
(409) 532-4560

Utah

College of Eastern Utah
—Price—

Full-Time Enrollments:	52	Evening Classes:	No
Part-Time Enrollments:	—	Weekend Classes:	No
Affiliation:	Public	Distance Learning:	No

NLN ACCREDITATION: Yes

Articulation: Associate to Baccalaureate
LPN to Associate
RN to MSN

For Further Information Contact:

Ms Diana Talbot, Director
College of Eastern Utah
Price, UT 84501
(801) 637-2120

Salt Lake Community College
—Salt Lake City—

Full-Time Enrollments:	278	Evening Classes:	Yes
Part-Time Enrollments:	—	Weekend Classes:	Yes
Affiliation:	Public	Distance Learning:	—

NLN ACCREDITATION: Yes

Articulation: Associate to Baccalaureate
LPN to Baccalaureate

For Further Information Contact:

Ms Marilyn Little, Coordinator
Salt Lake Community College
PO Box 31808
Salt Lake City, UT 84131
(801) 957-4164

Utah Valley State College
—Orem—

Full-Time Enrollments:	70	Evening Classes:	No
Part-Time Enrollments:	—	Weekend Classes:	No
Affiliation:	Public	Distance Learning:	No

NLN ACCREDITATION: Yes

Articulation: LPN to Associate

For Further Information Contact:

Mrs Karin L Swendsen, Director
Utah Valley State College
800 West 1200 South
Orem, UT 84058
(801) 222-8000

Weber State University
—Ogden—

Full-Time Enrollments:	272	Evening Classes:	Yes
Part-Time Enrollments:	—	Weekend Classes:	—
Affiliation:	Public	Distance Learning:	Yes

NLN ACCREDITATION: Yes

Articulation: Associate to Baccalaureate
LPN to Baccalaureate
LPN to Associate

For Further Information Contact:

Dr Gerry Hansen, Director
Weber State University
3750 Harrison Blvd, 1602
Ogden, UT 84403
(801) 626-6125

Vermont

Castleton State College
—Castleton—

Full-Time Enrollments:	44	Evening Classes:	No
Part-Time Enrollments:	25	Weekend Classes:	No
Affiliation:	Public	Distance Learning:	No

NLN ACCREDITATION: Yes

Articulation: None

For Further Information Contact:

Mrs Susan Farrell, Chair
Castleton State College
Castleton, VT 05735
(802) 468-5611

Norwich University
—Northfield—

Full-Time Enrollments:	10	Evening Classes:	—
Part-Time Enrollments:	56	Weekend Classes:	—
Affiliation:	Private	Distance Learning:	—

NLN ACCREDITATION: Yes

Articulation: None

For Further Information Contact:

Dr Linda Ellis, Div Head
Norwich University
Northfield, VT 05663
(802) 485-2600

Southern Vermont College
—Bennington—

Full-Time Enrollments:	9	Evening Classes:	Yes
Part-Time Enrollments:	34	Weekend Classes:	Yes
Affiliation:	Private	Distance Learning:	Yes

NLN ACCREDITATION: Yes

Articulation: Associate to Baccalaureate
LPN to Associate

For Further Information Contact:

Ms Wendy Lafage, Director
Southern Vermont College
Monument Ave Ext
Bennington, VT 05201
(802) 442-5427

Virgin Islands

University of the Virgin Islands
—Kingshill-St Croix—

Full-Time Enrollments:	37	Evening Classes:	No
Part-Time Enrollments:	24	Weekend Classes:	No
Affiliation:	Public	Distance Learning:	Yes

NLN ACCREDITATION: Yes

Articulation: Associate to Baccalaureate

For Further Information Contact:

Dr Edith Ramsay-Johnson, Chair
University of the Virgin Islands
2 John Brawers Bay
Kingshill-St Croix, VI 00802-9990
(809) 776-9200

Virginia

Blue Ridge Community College
—Weyers Cave—

Full-Time Enrollments:	2	Evening Classes:	Yes
Part-Time Enrollments:	56	Weekend Classes:	No
Affiliation:	Public	Distance Learning:	Yes

NLN ACCREDITATION: Yes

Articulation: Associate to Baccalaureate
LPN to Associate

For Further Information Contact:

Ms Lori Wack, Coordinator
Blue Ridge Community College
PO Box 80
Weyers Cave, VA 24431
(540) 234-9261 Ext 321

CHRV College of Health Sciences
—Roanoke—

Full-Time Enrollments:	59	Evening Classes:	Yes
Part-Time Enrollments:	36	Weekend Classes:	No
Affiliation:	Private	Distance Learning:	No

NLN ACCREDITATION: Yes

Articulation: LPN to Associate

For Further Information Contact:

Ms Linda R Rickabaugh, Director
CHRV College of Health Sciences
PO Box 13186
Roanoke, VA 24031
(540) 985-8260

Dabney S Lancaster Community College
—Clifton Forge—

Full-Time Enrollments:	61	Evening Classes:	No
Part-Time Enrollments:	—	Weekend Classes:	No
Affiliation:	Public	Distance Learning:	No

NLN ACCREDITATION: Yes

Articulation: None

For Further Information Contact:

Ms Lisa Allison-Jones, Head
Dabney S Lancaster Community College
PO Box 1000
Clifton Forge, VA 24422
(540) 862-4246

Germanna Community College
—Locust Grove—

Full-Time Enrollments:	28	Evening Classes:	Yes
Part-Time Enrollments:	52	Weekend Classes:	—
Affiliation:	Public	Distance Learning:	Yes

NLN ACCREDITATION: Yes

Articulation: Associate to Baccalaureate
LPN to Associate

For Further Information Contact:

Dr Jane Ingalls, Director
Germanna Community College
PO Box 339
Locust Grove, VA 22508
(703) 727-3000

J Sargeant Reynolds Community College
—Richmond—

Full-Time Enrollments:	192	Evening Classes:	No
Part-Time Enrollments:	123	Weekend Classes:	No
Affiliation:	Public	Distance Learning:	Yes

NLN ACCREDITATION: Yes

Articulation: LPN to Associate

For Further Information Contact:

Mrs Fran Stanley, Prog Head
J Sargeant Reynolds Community College
PO Box 85622
Richmond, VA 23285-5622
(804) 786-1371

John Tyler Community College
—Chester—

Full-Time Enrollments:	10	Evening Classes:	Yes
Part-Time Enrollments:	136	Weekend Classes:	Yes
Affiliation:	Public	Distance Learning:	No

NLN ACCREDITATION: Yes

Articulation: LPN to Associate

For Further Information Contact:

Dr Shelley Conroy, Head
John Tyler Community College
13101 Jefferson Davis Highway
Chester, VA 23831
(804) 796-4077

Marymount University
—Arlington—

Full-Time Enrollments:	120	Evening Classes:	Yes
Part-Time Enrollments:	177	Weekend Classes:	Yes
Affiliation:	Religious	Distance Learning:	No

NLN ACCREDITATION: Yes

Articulation: Associate to Baccalaureate
LPN to Associate

For Further Information Contact:

Dr Shirley Jarecki, Acting Dean
Marymount University
2807 N Glebe Rd
Arlington, VA 22207
(703) 284-1580

Norfolk State University
—Norfolk—

Full-Time Enrollments:	49	Evening Classes:	—
Part-Time Enrollments:	31	Weekend Classes:	—
Affiliation:	Public	Distance Learning:	—

NLN ACCREDITATION: Yes

Articulation: None

For Further Information Contact:

Candace Rogers, Acting Dept Head
Norfolk State University
2401 Corprew Ave
Norfolk, VA 23504
(804) 683-8525

Northern Virginia Community College
—Annandale—

Full-Time Enrollments:	—	Evening Classes:	No
Part-Time Enrollments:	262	Weekend Classes:	No
Affiliation:	Public	Distance Learning:	No

NLN ACCREDITATION: Yes

Articulation: Associate to Baccalaureate
LPN to Associate

For Further Information Contact:

Dr Evelyn C Atchison, Prog Head
Northern Virginia Community College
8333 Little River Tpk
Annandale, VA 22003
(703) 323-3405

Patrick Henry Community College
—Martinsville—

Full-Time Enrollments:	93	Evening Classes:	No
Part-Time Enrollments:	—	Weekend Classes:	No
Affiliation:	Public	Distance Learning:	No

NLN ACCREDITATION: Yes

Articulation: Associate to Baccalaureate

For Further Information Contact:

Mrs Mildred G Owings, Head
Patrick Henry Community College
PO Box 5311
Martinsville, VA 24115
(540) 638-8777

Piedmont Virginia Community College
—Charlottesville—

Full-Time Enrollments:	2	Evening Classes:	Yes
Part-Time Enrollments:	100	Weekend Classes:	Yes
Affiliation:	Public	Distance Learning:	Yes

NLN ACCREDITATION: Yes

Articulation: Associate to Baccalaureate
RN to MSN

For Further Information Contact:

Ms Mary Wayland, Head
Piedmont Virginia Community College
501 College Dr
Charlottesville, VA 22902
(804) 977-3900

Shenandoah University-School of Nursing
—Winchester—

Full-Time Enrollments:	114	Evening Classes:	No
Part-Time Enrollments:	89	Weekend Classes:	No
Affiliation:	Religious	Distance Learning:	No

NLN ACCREDITATION: Yes

Articulation: LPN to Associate

For Further Information Contact:

Dr Pamela B Webber, Chair
Shenandoah University-School of Nursing
1775 N Selter Court
Winchester, VA 22601
(540) 665-5500

Thomas Nelson Community College
—Hampton—

Full-Time Enrollments:	90	Evening Classes:	Yes
Part-Time Enrollments:	—	Weekend Classes:	No
Affiliation:	Public	Distance Learning:	No

NLN ACCREDITATION: Yes

Articulation: LPN to Associate

For Further Information Contact:

Mrs Sandra Marcuson, Head
Thomas Nelson Community College
PO Box 9407
Hampton, VA 23670
(757) 825-2808

Tidewater Community College-Portsmouth Campus
—Portsmouth—

Full-Time Enrollments:	126	Evening Classes:	Yes
Part-Time Enrollments:	81	Weekend Classes:	No
Affiliation:	Public	Distance Learning:	Yes

NLN ACCREDITATION: Yes

Articulation: Associate to Baccalaureate
LPN to Associate

For Further Information Contact:

Mrs Denise Bell Artis, Dept Head
Tidewater Community College-Portsmouth Campus
7001 College Dr
Portsmouth, VA 23703
(787) 484-2121

Virginia Appalachian Tri College
—Abingdon—

Full-Time Enrollments:	361	Evening Classes:	No
Part-Time Enrollments:	—	Weekend Classes:	No
Affiliation:	Public	Distance Learning:	No

NLN ACCREDITATION: Yes

Articulation: Associate to Baccalaureate
LPN to Associate

For Further Information Contact:

Ms Lois S Caldwell, Director
Virginia Appalachian Tri College
PO Box 828
Abingdon, VA 24210
(540) 628-6094

Virginia Western Community College
—Roanoke—

Full-Time Enrollments:	95	Evening Classes:	No
Part-Time Enrollments:	—	Weekend Classes:	No
Affiliation:	Public	Distance Learning:	No

NLN ACCREDITATION: Yes

Articulation: Associate to Baccalaureate
LPN to Associate

For Further Information Contact:

Mrs Martha Barnas, Head
Virginia Western Community College
3095 Colonial Ave SW
Roanoke, VA 24038
(540) 857-7306

Wytheville Community College/New River Community College
—Wytheville—

Full-Time Enrollments:	74	Evening Classes:	No
Part-Time Enrollments:	137	Weekend Classes:	No
Affiliation:	Public	Distance Learning:	No

NLN ACCREDITATION: Yes

Articulation: LPN to Associate

For Further Information Contact:

Ms Grace Johnson, Head
Wytheville Community College/New River Community College
1000 E Main St
Wytheville, VA 24382
(703) 228-5541

Washington

Bellevue Community College
—Bellevue—

Full-Time Enrollments:	90	Evening Classes:	No
Part-Time Enrollments:	—	Weekend Classes:	No
Affiliation:	Public	Distance Learning:	No

NLN ACCREDITATION: Yes

Articulation: Associate to Baccalaureate
LPN to Associate

For Further Information Contact:

Ms Cheryl Becker, Chair
Bellevue Community College
3000 Landerholm Circle SE
Bellevue, WA 98007
(206) 641-2012

Clark College
—Vancouver—

Full-Time Enrollments:	156	Evening Classes:	Yes
Part-Time Enrollments:	—	Weekend Classes:	No
Affiliation:	Public	Distance Learning:	No

NLN ACCREDITATION: Yes

Articulation: Associate to Baccalaureate
LPN to Associate

For Further Information Contact:

Ms Linda E Hein, Director
Clark College
1800 E McLoughlin Blvd
Vancouver, WA 98663
(360) 992-2192

Columbia Basin College
—Pasco—

Full-Time Enrollments:	90	Evening Classes:	Yes
Part-Time Enrollments:	—	Weekend Classes:	Yes
Affiliation:	Public	Distance Learning:	Yes

NLN ACCREDITATION: No

Articulation: Associate to Baccalaureate

For Further Information Contact:

Mrs Donna E Campbell, Dean
Columbia Basin College
2600 N 20th
Pasco, WA 99301
(509) 547-0511

Everett Community College
—Everett—

Full-Time Enrollments:	114	Evening Classes:	No
Part-Time Enrollments:	—	Weekend Classes:	No
Affiliation:	Public	Distance Learning:	No

NLN ACCREDITATION: Yes

Articulation: LPN to Associate

For Further Information Contact:

Mr Stuart Barger, Director
Everett Community College
801 Wetmore Ave
Everett, WA 98201
(206) 388-9399

Grays Harbor College
—Aberdeen—

Full-Time Enrollments:	38	Evening Classes:	No
Part-Time Enrollments:	—	Weekend Classes:	No
Affiliation:	Public	Distance Learning:	No

NLN ACCREDITATION: Yes

Articulation: LPN to Associate

For Further Information Contact:

Ms Candice Burchett, Chair
Grays Harbor College
1620 Edward P Smith Dr
Aberdeen, WA 98520
(360) 532-9020

Highline Community College
—Des Moines—

Full-Time Enrollments:	—	Evening Classes:	—
Part-Time Enrollments:	90	Weekend Classes:	—
Affiliation:	Public	Distance Learning:	—

NLN ACCREDITATION: Yes

Articulation: None

For Further Information Contact:

Ms Christine Henshaw, Coordinator
Highline Community College
PO Box 98000
Des Moines, WA 98198-9800
(206) 878-3710 Ext 3467

Lower Columbia College
—Longview—

Full-Time Enrollments:	117	Evening Classes:	No
Part-Time Enrollments:	—	Weekend Classes:	No
Affiliation:	Public	Distance Learning:	No

NLN ACCREDITATION: Yes

Articulation: Associate to Baccalaureate
LPN to Associate

For Further Information Contact:

Ms Helen Kuebel, Director
Lower Columbia College
1600 Maple St Box 3010
Longview, WA 98632-0310
(360) 577-2316

Olympic College
—Bremerton—

Full-Time Enrollments:	73	Evening Classes:	No
Part-Time Enrollments:	—	Weekend Classes:	No
Affiliation:	Public	Distance Learning:	No

NLN ACCREDITATION: Yes

Articulation: Associate to Baccalaureate

For Further Information Contact:

Mrs Margaret Herzog, Coordinator
Olympic College
1600 and Chester Ave
Bremerton, WA 98310-1699
(360) 478-4604

Peninsula College
—Port Angeles—

Full-Time Enrollments:	40	Evening Classes:	—
Part-Time Enrollments:	—	Weekend Classes:	—
Affiliation:	Public	Distance Learning:	—

NLN ACCREDITATION: No

Articulation: None

For Further Information Contact:

Ms Marca Davies, Coordinator
Peninsula College
1502 E Lauridsen
Port Angeles, WA 98362
(360) 452-9277 Ext 265

Seattle Central Community College
—Seattle—

Full-Time Enrollments:	37	Evening Classes:	No
Part-Time Enrollments:	—	Weekend Classes:	No
Affiliation:	Public	Distance Learning:	No

NLN ACCREDITATION: Yes

Articulation: None

For Further Information Contact:

Ms Maria Azpitarte, Director
Seattle Central Community College
1701 Broadway 2BE3210
Seattle, WA 98122
(206) 587-6956

Shoreline Community College
—Seattle—

Full-Time Enrollments:	142	Evening Classes:	No
Part-Time Enrollments:	—	Weekend Classes:	No
Affiliation:	Public	Distance Learning:	No

NLN ACCREDITATION: Yes

Articulation: None

For Further Information Contact:

Dr Janice Ellis, Director
Shoreline Community College
16101 Greenwood Ave, N
Seattle, WA 98133
(206) 546-4756

Skagit Valley College
—Mt Vernon—

Full-Time Enrollments:	74	Evening Classes:	Yes
Part-Time Enrollments:	23	Weekend Classes:	No
Affiliation:	Public	Distance Learning:	Yes

NLN ACCREDITATION: Yes

Articulation: Associate to Baccalaureate
LPN to Associate

For Further Information Contact:

Mrs Flora Adams, Chair
Skagit Valley College
2405 College Way
Mt Vernon, WA 98273
(360) 428-1136

South Puget Sound Community College
—Olympia—

Full-Time Enrollments:	21	Evening Classes:	—
Part-Time Enrollments:	14	Weekend Classes:	—
Affiliation:	Public	Distance Learning:	—

NLN ACCREDITATION: Yes

Articulation: None

For Further Information Contact:

Mrs Ruby S Flesner, Director
South Puget Sound Community College
2011 Mottman Rd NW
Olympia, WA 98502
(206) 754-7711 Ext 285

Spokane Community College
—Spokane—

Full-Time Enrollments:	160	Evening Classes:	No
Part-Time Enrollments:	10	Weekend Classes:	No
Affiliation:	Public	Distance Learning:	No

NLN ACCREDITATION: Yes

Articulation: LPN to Associate

For Further Information Contact:

Mrs Carol Nelson, Director
Spokane Community College
N 1810 Greene St
Spokane, WA 99207
(509) 533-7311

Tacoma Community College
—Tacoma—

Full-Time Enrollments:	101	Evening Classes:	No
Part-Time Enrollments:	6	Weekend Classes:	No
Affiliation:	Public	Distance Learning:	No

NLN ACCREDITATION: Yes

Articulation: LPN to Associate

For Further Information Contact:

Ms Kim Nichols Rzeszewicz, Coordinator
Tacoma Community College
5900 S 12th St
Tacoma, WA 98407
(206) 566-5162

Walla Walla Community College
—Walla Walla—

Full-Time Enrollments:	149	Evening Classes:	Yes
Part-Time Enrollments:	—	Weekend Classes:	—
Affiliation:	Public	Distance Learning:	—

NLN ACCREDITATION: Yes

Articulation: LPN to Associate

For Further Information Contact:

Mrs Marilyn Galusha, Director
Walla Walla Community College
500 Tausick Way
Walla Walla, WA 99362
(509) 527-4241

Wenatchee Valley College
—Wenatchee—

Full-Time Enrollments:	84	Evening Classes:	—
Part-Time Enrollments:	—	Weekend Classes:	—
Affiliation:	Public	Distance Learning:	—

NLN ACCREDITATION: Yes

Articulation: None

For Further Information Contact:

Mrs Connie Barnes, Director
Wenatchee Valley College
1300 5th St
Wenatchee, WA 98801
(509) 662-1651

Yakima Valley College
—Yakima—

Full-Time Enrollments:	127	Evening Classes:	Yes
Part-Time Enrollments:	—	Weekend Classes:	No
Affiliation:	Public	Distance Learning:	No

NLN ACCREDITATION: Yes

Articulation: LPN to Associate

For Further Information Contact:

Dr Bronwynne Evans, Dept Head
Yakima Valley College
16th & North Hill Blvd
Yakima, WA 98901
(509) 574-4902

West Virginia

Bluefield State College
—Bluefield—

Full-Time Enrollments:	94	Evening Classes:	No
Part-Time Enrollments:	28	Weekend Classes:	No
Affiliation:	Public	Distance Learning:	No

NLN ACCREDITATION: Yes

Articulation: Associate to Baccalaureate

For Further Information Contact:

Ms Carol Cofer, Director
Bluefield State College
219 Rock St
Bluefield, WV 24701
(304) 327-4136

Davis & Elkins College
—Elkins—

Full-Time Enrollments:	42	Evening Classes:	No
Part-Time Enrollments:	26	Weekend Classes:	No
Affiliation:	Religious	Distance Learning:	No

NLN ACCREDITATION: Yes

Articulation: LPN to Associate

For Further Information Contact:

Dr Carol Cochran, Director
Davis & Elkins College
100 Sycamore St
Elkins, WV 26241
(304) 637-1900

Fairmont State College
—Fairmont—

Full-Time Enrollments:	95	Evening Classes:	No
Part-Time Enrollments:	21	Weekend Classes:	No
Affiliation:	Public	Distance Learning:	No

NLN ACCREDITATION: Yes

Articulation: Associate to Baccalaureate
LPN to Associate

For Further Information Contact:

Dr Deborah M Kisner, Director
Fairmont State College
1201 Locust Ave
Fairmont, WV 26554
(304) 367-4767

Northern West Virginia Community College
—Wheeling—

Full-Time Enrollments:	68	Evening Classes:	Yes
Part-Time Enrollments:	171	Weekend Classes:	—
Affiliation:	Public	Distance Learning:	Yes

NLN ACCREDITATION: Yes

Articulation: Associate to Baccalaureate
LPN to Associate

For Further Information Contact:

Dr M Regina Jennette, Director
Northern West Virginia Community College
College Sq
Wheeling, WV 26003
(304) 233-5900

Shepherd College
—Shepherdstown—

Full-Time Enrollments:	54	Evening Classes:	No
Part-Time Enrollments:	—	Weekend Classes:	No
Affiliation:	Public	Distance Learning:	No

NLN ACCREDITATION: Yes

Articulation: Associate to Baccalaureate
LPN to Associate

For Further Information Contact:

Dr Charlotte Anderson, Chair
Shepherd College
Shepherdstown, WV 25443
(304) 876-2511

Southern West Virginia Community College
—Logan—

Full-Time Enrollments:	108	Evening Classes:	Yes
Part-Time Enrollments:	5	Weekend Classes:	—
Affiliation:	Public	Distance Learning:	Yes

NLN ACCREDITATION: Yes

Articulation: Associate to Baccalaureate

No longer there

For Further Information Contact:

Ms Barbara Donahue, Director
Southern West Virginia Community College
PO Box 2900
Logan, WV 25601
(304) 792-7098

St Mary's/ Marshall University
—Huntington—

Full-Time Enrollments:	101	Evening Classes:	No
Part-Time Enrollments:	1	Weekend Classes:	No
Affiliation:	Religious	Distance Learning:	No

NLN ACCREDITATION: No

Articulation: None

For Further Information Contact:

Mrs Barbara Stevens, Director
St Mary's/ Marshall University
2900 First Ave
Huntington, WV 25702
(304) 526-1415

University of Charleston
—Charleston—

Full-Time Enrollments:	82	Evening Classes:	—
Part-Time Enrollments:	27	Weekend Classes:	—
Affiliation:	Private	Distance Learning:	—

NLN ACCREDITATION: Yes

Articulation: None

For Further Information Contact:

Dr Sandra S Bowles, Dean
University of Charleston
2300 Mccorkle Ave, Se
Charleston, WV 25304
(304) 357-4835

West Virginia University Institute of Technology
—Montgomery—

Full-Time Enrollments: 108   Evening Classes: —
Part-Time Enrollments: —   Weekend Classes: —
Affiliation: Public   Distance Learning: —

NLN ACCREDITATION: Yes

Articulation: None

For Further Information Contact:

Ms Jean Hoff, Interim Chair
West Virginia University Institute of Technology
Box 64 Orndurff Hall
Montgomery, WV 25136
(304) 442-3221

West Virginia University at Parkersburg
—Parkersburg—

Full-Time Enrollments: 106   Evening Classes: No
Part-Time Enrollments: —   Weekend Classes: No
Affiliation: Public   Distance Learning: No

NLN ACCREDITATION: Yes

Articulation: LPN to Associate

For Further Information Contact:

Dr Alita Sellers, Chair
West Virginia University at Parkersburg
Route 5, Box 167A
Parkersburg, WV 26101-9577
(304) 424-8300

Wisconsin

Blackhawk Technical College
—Janesville—

Full-Time Enrollments: —   Evening Classes: Yes
Part-Time Enrollments: 97   Weekend Classes: No
Affiliation: Public   Distance Learning: No

NLN ACCREDITATION: Yes

Articulation: Associate to Baccalaureate
LPN to Associate

For Further Information Contact:

Mr Richard McKnight, Associate Dean
Blackhawk Technical College
6004 Prairie Rd
Janesville, WI 53547
(608) 757-7711

Cardinal Stritch College
—Milwaukee—

Full-Time Enrollments: 96   Evening Classes: Yes
Part-Time Enrollments: 89   Weekend Classes: No
Affiliation: Religious   Distance Learning: No

NLN ACCREDITATION: Yes

Articulation: Associate to Baccalaureate
Diploma to Baccalaureate
LPN to Baccalaureate
LPN to Associate

For Further Information Contact:

Dr Zaiga G Kalnins, Chair
Cardinal Stritch College
6801 North Yates Rd
Milwaukee, WI 53217
(414) 351-7514

Chippewa Valley Technical College
—Eau Claire—

Full-Time Enrollments: —   Evening Classes: —
Part-Time Enrollments: —   Weekend Classes: —
Affiliation: Public   Distance Learning: —

NLN ACCREDITATION: Yes

Articulation: None

For Further Information Contact:

Ms Margaret D Grosskopf, Director
Chippewa Valley Technical College
620 W Clairemont Ave
Eau Claire, WI 54701
(715) 833-6417

Fox Valley Technical College
—Appleton—

Full-Time Enrollments: 25   Evening Classes: Yes
Part-Time Enrollments: 85   Weekend Classes: No
Affiliation: Public   Distance Learning: Yes

NLN ACCREDITATION: Yes

Articulation: Associate to Baccalaureate
LPN to Associate

For Further Information Contact:

Mrs Ardythe Korpela, Coordinator
Fox Valley Technical College
1825 N Bluemound Dr Box 2277
Appleton, WI 54913
(414) 735-5664

Gateway Technical College
—Kenosha—

Full-Time Enrollments:	—	Evening Classes:	No
Part-Time Enrollments:	216	Weekend Classes:	No
Affiliation:	Public	Distance Learning:	No

NLN ACCREDITATION: Yes

Articulation: Associate to Baccalaureate
LPN to Associate
RN to MSN

For Further Information Contact:

Ms Diane Skewes, Chair
Gateway Technical College
3520 30th Ave
Kenosha, WI 53144
(414) 656-6934

Lakeshore Technical College
—Cleveland—

Full-Time Enrollments:	51	Evening Classes:	Yes
Part-Time Enrollments:	53	Weekend Classes:	No
Affiliation:	Public	Distance Learning:	Yes

NLN ACCREDITATION: Yes

Articulation: Associate to Baccalaureate
LPN to Associate

For Further Information Contact:

Ms Nancy Kaprelian, Dean
Lakeshore Technical College
1290 North Ave
Cleveland, WI 53015
(414) 458-4183

Madison Area Technical College
—Madison—

Full-Time Enrollments:	133	Evening Classes:	Yes
Part-Time Enrollments:	82	Weekend Classes:	No
Affiliation:	Public	Distance Learning:	—

NLN ACCREDITATION: Yes

Articulation: Associate to Baccalaureate

For Further Information Contact:

Ms Kathleen Koegel, Director
Madison Area Technical College
3550 Anderson St
Madison, WI 53704-2599
(608) 246-6877

Mid State Technical College
—Wisconsin Rapids—

Full-Time Enrollments:	56	Evening Classes:	—
Part-Time Enrollments:	—	Weekend Classes:	No
Affiliation:	Public	Distance Learning:	—

NLN ACCREDITATION: Yes

Articulation: Associate to Baccalaureate
LPN to Associate

For Further Information Contact:

Miss Vickie Gukenberger, Dean
Mid State Technical College
500 32nd North
Wisconsin Rapids, WI 54494
(715) 422-5310

Milwaukee Area Technical College
—Milwaukee—

Full-Time Enrollments:	179	Evening Classes:	No
Part-Time Enrollments:	111	Weekend Classes:	No
Affiliation:	Public	Distance Learning:	No

NLN ACCREDITATION: Yes

Articulation: Associate to Baccalaureate
LPN to Associate

For Further Information Contact:

Dr Mary E Eiche, Assoc Dean
Milwaukee Area Technical College
700 West State St
Milwaukee, WI 53233
(414) 297-6241

Moraine Park Technical College
—West Bend—

Full-Time Enrollments:	56	Evening Classes:	Yes
Part-Time Enrollments:	59	Weekend Classes:	Yes
Affiliation:	Public	Distance Learning:	No

NLN ACCREDITATION: Yes

Articulation: Associate to Baccalaureate

For Further Information Contact:

Mrs Wendy McCulloch, Director
Moraine Park Technical College
2151 N Main St
West Bend, WI 53095
(414) 334-3413

Nicolet Area Technical College
—Rhinelander—

Full-Time Enrollments:	3	Evening Classes:	Yes
Part-Time Enrollments:	39	Weekend Classes:	No
Affiliation:	Public	Distance Learning:	No

NLN ACCREDITATION: Yes

Articulation: Associate to Baccalaureate
LPN to Associate

For Further Information Contact:

Ms Clemetta Evenson, Director
Nicolet Area Technical College
Box 518
Rhinelander, WI 54501
(715) 365-4473

North Central Technical College
—Wausau—

Full-Time Enrollments:	43	Evening Classes:	Yes
Part-Time Enrollments:	78	Weekend Classes:	No
Affiliation:	Public	Distance Learning:	Yes

NLN ACCREDITATION: Yes

Articulation: Associate to Baccalaureate
LPN to Associate

For Further Information Contact:

Mrs Ellen Kafka, Educ Admin
North Central Technical College
1000 W Campus Dr
Wausau, WI 54401
(715) 675-3331

Northeast Wisconsin Technical College
—Green Bay—

Full-Time Enrollments:	136	Evening Classes:	Yes
Part-Time Enrollments:	—	Weekend Classes:	—
Affiliation:	Public	Distance Learning:	Yes

NLN ACCREDITATION: Yes

Articulation: LPN to Associate

For Further Information Contact:

Dr Judith A Mix, Associate Dean
Northeast Wisconsin Technical College
2740 W Mason St Box 19042
Green Bay, WI 54307
(414) 498-5482

Southwest Wisconsin Technical College
—Fennimore—

Full-Time Enrollments:	59	Evening Classes:	Yes
Part-Time Enrollments:	38	Weekend Classes:	—
Affiliation:	Public	Distance Learning:	Yes

NLN ACCREDITATION: Yes

Articulation: LPN to Associate

For Further Information Contact:

Ms S Selleck-Lehman, Dean
Southwest Wisconsin Technical College
1800 Bronson Blvd
Fennimore, WI 53809
(608) 822-3262

Waukesha County Technical College
—Pewaukee—

Full-Time Enrollments:	—	Evening Classes:	Yes
Part-Time Enrollments:	149	Weekend Classes:	No
Affiliation:	Public	Distance Learning:	No

NLN ACCREDITATION: Yes

Articulation: Associate to Baccalaureate

For Further Information Contact:

Dr Kitty Gotham, Associate Dean
Waukesha County Technical College
800 Main St
Pewaukee, WI 53072
(414) 691-5368

Western Wisconsin Technical College
—La Crosse—

Full-Time Enrollments:	62	Evening Classes:	—
Part-Time Enrollments:	40	Weekend Classes:	—
Affiliation:	Public	Distance Learning:	—

NLN ACCREDITATION: Yes

Articulation: None

For Further Information Contact:

Ms Donna M Haggard, Chair
Western Wisconsin Technical College
304 N 6th St
La Crosse, WI 54602
(608) 785-9186

Wisconsin Indianhead Technical College
—Shell Lake—

Full-Time Enrollments:	18	Evening Classes:	—
Part-Time Enrollments:	94	Weekend Classes:	—
Affiliation:	Public	Distance Learning:	Yes

NLN ACCREDITATION: Yes

Articulation: Associate to Baccalaureate

For Further Information Contact:

Ms Piper Larson, Dean
Wisconsin Indianhead Technical College
Hcr 61 Box 10B
Shell Lake, WI 54871
(715) 468-2815

Wyoming

Casper College
—Casper—

Full-Time Enrollments:	61	Evening Classes:	Yes
Part-Time Enrollments:	28	Weekend Classes:	No
Affiliation:	Public	Distance Learning:	No

NLN ACCREDITATION: Yes

Articulation: Associate to Baccalaureate
LPN to Associate

For Further Information Contact:

Mrs Judith S Turner, Chair
Casper College
125 College Dr
Casper, WY 82601
(307) 268-2233

Central Wyoming Community College
—Riverton—

Full-Time Enrollments:	24	Evening Classes:	Yes
Part-Time Enrollments:	16	Weekend Classes:	—
Affiliation:	Public	Distance Learning:	Yes

NLN ACCREDITATION: Yes

Articulation: None

For Further Information Contact:

Dr Janice L McCoy, Chair
Central Wyoming Community College
2660 Peck Ave
Riverton, WY 82501
(307) 856-9291

Gillette Campus of Northern Wyoming College
—Gillette—

Full-Time Enrollments:	—	Evening Classes:	No
Part-Time Enrollments:	—	Weekend Classes:	No
Affiliation:	Public	Distance Learning:	No

NLN ACCREDITATION: Yes

Articulation: LPN to Associate

For Further Information Contact:

Mrs Nancy Larmer, Director
Gillette Campus of Northern Wyoming College
720 West 8th St Suite 1
Gillette, WY 82716
(307) 686-1358

Laramie County Community College
—Cheyenne—

Full-Time Enrollments:	—	Evening Classes:	No
Part-Time Enrollments:	80	Weekend Classes:	No
Affiliation:	Public	Distance Learning:	No

NLN ACCREDITATION: Yes

Articulation: LPN to Associate

For Further Information Contact:

Ms Jan Freudenthal, Coordinator
Laramie County Community College
1400 E College Dr
Cheyenne, WY 82007
(307) 778-1267

Northwest College
—Powell—

Full-Time Enrollments:	33	Evening Classes:	No
Part-Time Enrollments:	14	Weekend Classes:	No
Affiliation:	Public	Distance Learning:	No

NLN ACCREDITATION: Yes

Articulation: Associate to Baccalaureate
RN to MSN

For Further Information Contact:

Mr William Clinton, Director
Northwest College
231 West 6th
Powell, WY 82435
(307) 754-6479

Sheridan College
—Sheridan—

Full-Time Enrollments: 36   **Evening Classes:** —
Part-Time Enrollments: —   **Weekend Classes:** —
Affiliation: Public   **Distance Learning:** —

NLN ACCREDITATION: Yes

Articulation: None

For Further Information Contact:

Dr Carol McFadyen, Director
Sheridan College
Sheridan, WY 82801
(800) 913-9139

Western Wyoming Community College
—Rock Spring—

Full-Time Enrollments: 24   **Evening Classes:** —
Part-Time Enrollments: 16   **Weekend Classes:** —
Affiliation: Public   **Distance Learning:** —

NLN ACCREDITATION: Yes

Articulation: None

For Further Information Contact:

Mrs Karen Medina, Director
Western Wyoming Community College
2500 College Dr
Rock Spring, WY 82901
(307) 382-1600

Section 2
Baccalaureate Degree
Programs by State

BACCALAUREATE DEGREE

Alabama

Auburn University
—Auburn—

Full-Time Enrollments:	140	Evening Classes:	No
Part-Time Enrollments:	—	Weekend Classes:	No
Affiliation:	Public	Distance Learning:	No

NLN ACCREDITATION: Yes

BSN for non-RNs w/degree in other field: No

Articulation: None

For Further Information Contact:

Dr Charlotte Pitts, Interim Dean
Auburn University
Auburn, AL 36849
(334) 844-5665

Auburn University at Montgomery
—Montgomery—

Full-Time Enrollments:	125	Evening Classes:	No
Part-Time Enrollments:	6	Weekend Classes:	No
Affiliation:	Public	Distance Learning:	No

NLN ACCREDITATION: Yes

BSN for non-RNs w/degree in other field: No

Articulation: None

For Further Information Contact:

Dr Sharon Farley, Interim Dean
Auburn University at Montgomery
73000 University Dr
Montgomery, AL 36117-3596
(334) 244-3658

Capstone College of Nursing-University of Alabama
—Tuscaloosa—

Full-Time Enrollments:	430	Evening Classes:	No
Part-Time Enrollments:	108	Weekend Classes:	No
Affiliation:	Public	Distance Learning:	Yes

NLN ACCREDITATION: Yes

BSN for non-RNs w/degree in other field: No

Articulation: None

For Further Information Contact:

Dr Sara Barger, Dean
Capstone College of Nursing-University of Alabama
PO Box 870358
Tuscaloosa, AL 35487-0358
(205) 348-1040

Ida V Moffett School-Samford University
—Birmingham—

Full-Time Enrollments:	—	Evening Classes:	—
Part-Time Enrollments:	—	Weekend Classes:	—
Affiliation:	Religious	Distance Learning:	—

NLN ACCREDITATION: Yes

BSN for non-RNs w/degree in other field: —

Articulation: —

For Further Information Contact:

Dr Marian K Baur, Dean
Ida V Moffett School-Samford University
820 Moutclair Rd
Birmingham, AL 35213
(205) 870-2861

Jacksonville State University-L B Wallace College
—Jacksonville—

Full-Time Enrollments:	315	Evening Classes:	No
Part-Time Enrollments:	—	Weekend Classes:	No
Affiliation:	Public	Distance Learning:	Yes

NLN ACCREDITATION: Yes

BSN for non-RNs w/degree in other field: Yes

Articulation: Associate to Baccalaureate
LPN to Baccalaureate

For Further Information Contact:

Dr Martha Lavender, Acting Dean
Jacksonville State University-L B Wallace College
Jacksonville, AL 36265
(205) 782-5428

Spring Hill College
—Mobile—

Full-Time Enrollments:	53	Evening Classes:	—
Part-Time Enrollments:	—	Weekend Classes:	—
Affiliation:	Religious	Distance Learning:	—

NLN ACCREDITATION: No

BSN for non-RNs w/degree in other field: No

Articulation: None

For Further Information Contact:

Dr Carol Henderson, Chair
Spring Hill College
4000 Dauphin St
Mobile, AL 36608
(334) 380-2267

Troy State University
—Troy—

Full-Time Enrollments:	90	Evening Classes:	Yes
Part-Time Enrollments:	10	Weekend Classes:	No
Affiliation:	Public	Distance Learning:	Yes

NLN ACCREDITATION: Yes

BSN for non-RNs w/degree in other field:　No

Articulation:　Associate to Baccalaureate

For Further Information Contact:

Dr Sandra Greniewicki, Dean
Troy State University
Collegeview Bldg
Troy, AL 36082
(334) 670-3712

Tuskegee University
—Tuskegee—

Full-Time Enrollments:	146	Evening Classes:	No
Part-Time Enrollments:	—	Weekend Classes:	No
Affiliation:	Private	Distance Learning:	Yes

NLN ACCREDITATION: Yes

BSN for non-RNs w/degree in other field:　No

Articulation:　None

For Further Information Contact:

Dr Margie N Johnson, Dean
Tuskegee University
Tuskegee, AL 36088
(334) 727-8130

University of Alabama at Birmingham
—Birmingham—

Full-Time Enrollments:	321	Evening Classes:	No
Part-Time Enrollments:	50	Weekend Classes:	No
Affiliation:	Public	Distance Learning:	No

NLN ACCREDITATION: Yes

BSN for non-RNs w/degree in other field:　No

Articulation:　RN to MSN

For Further Information Contact:

Dr Rachel Z Booth, Dean
University of Alabama at Birmingham
University Station
Birmingham, AL 35294-1210
(205) 934-5490

University of Alabama in Huntsville
—Huntsville—

Full-Time Enrollments:	155	Evening Classes:	Yes
Part-Time Enrollments:	64	Weekend Classes:	Yes
Affiliation:	Public	Distance Learning:	No

NLN ACCREDITATION: Yes

BSN for non-RNs w/degree in other field:　No

Articulation:　Associate to Baccalaureate
Diploma to Baccalaureate

For Further Information Contact:

Dr C Fay Raines, Dean
University of Alabama in Huntsville
Huntsville, AL 35899
(205) 890-6345

University of Mobile
—Mobile—

Full-Time Enrollments:	220	Evening Classes:	Yes
Part-Time Enrollments:	53	Weekend Classes:	No
Affiliation:	Religious	Distance Learning:	No

NLN ACCREDITATION: Yes

BSN for non-RNs w/degree in other field:　No

Articulation:　None

For Further Information Contact:

Dr Rosemary Adams, Dean
University of Mobile
PO Box 13220
Mobile, AL 36663-0220
(334) 675-5990

University of North Alabama
—Florence—

Full-Time Enrollments:	—	Evening Classes:	—
Part-Time Enrollments:	—	Weekend Classes:	—
Affiliation:	Public	Distance Learning:	—

NLN ACCREDITATION: Yes

BSN for non-RNs w/degree in other field:　—

Articulation:　None

For Further Information Contact:

Dr Frenesi Wilson, Dean
University of North Alabama
PO Box 5054
Florence, AL 35632
(205) 760-4311

University of South Alabama
—Mobile—

Full-Time Enrollments: 531
Part-Time Enrollments: 184
Affiliation: Public
Evening Classes: Yes
Weekend Classes: Yes
Distance Learning: —

NLN ACCREDITATION: Yes

BSN for non-RNs w/degree in other field: No

Articulation: None

For Further Information Contact:

Dr Amanda Baker, Dean
University of South Alabama
USA Springhill Ave
Mobile, AL 36688
(334) 434-3415

Alaska

University of Alaska Anchorage
—Anchorage—

Full-Time Enrollments: 137
Part-Time Enrollments: 70
Affiliation: Public
Evening Classes: Yes
Weekend Classes: Yes
Distance Learning: Yes

NLN ACCREDITATION: Yes

BSN for non-RNs w/degree in other field: No

Articulation: Associate to Baccalaureate

For Further Information Contact:

Dr Tina Delapp, Associate Dean
University of Alaska Anchorage
3211 Providence Drive
Anchorage, AK 99508-8030
(907) 786-4571

Arizona

Arizona State University
—Tempe—

Full-Time Enrollments: 278
Part-Time Enrollments: 109
Affiliation: Public
Evening Classes: Yes
Weekend Classes: No
Distance Learning: No

NLN ACCREDITATION: Yes

BSN for non-RNs w/degree in other field: Yes

Articulation: Associate to Baccalaureate

For Further Information Contact:

Dr Mary Killeen, Associate Dean
Arizona State University
College of Nursing
Tempe, AZ 85287-2602
(602) 965-6531

Northern Arizona University
—Flagstaff—

Full-Time Enrollments: 110
Part-Time Enrollments: —
Affiliation: Public
Evening Classes: Yes
Weekend Classes: Yes
Distance Learning: Yes

NLN ACCREDITATION: Yes

BSN for non-RNs w/degree in other field: No

Articulation: Associate to Baccalaureate

For Further Information Contact:

Dr Eileen Breslin, Chair
Northern Arizona University
Box 15035
Flagstaff, AZ 86011-5015
(520) 523-2671

Samaritan College of Nursing-Grand Canyon University
—Phoenix—

Full-Time Enrollments: 133
Part-Time Enrollments: —
Affiliation: Religious
Evening Classes: No
Weekend Classes: No
Distance Learning: No

NLN ACCREDITATION: Yes

BSN for non-RNs w/degree in other field: No

Articulation: None

For Further Information Contact:

Dr Jennifer Wilson, Dean
Samaritan College of Nursing-Grand Canyon University
PO Box 11097
Phoenix, AZ 85061
(602) 589-2730

University of Arizona
—Tucson—

Full-Time Enrollments: 206
Part-Time Enrollments: 30
Affiliation: Public
Evening Classes: No
Weekend Classes: No
Distance Learning: No

NLN ACCREDITATION: Yes

BSN for non-RNs w/degree in other field: Yes

Articulation: Associate to Baccalaureate
Diploma to Baccalaureate

For Further Information Contact:

Dr Suzanne Van Ort, Dean
University of Arizona
1305 N Martin St
Tucson, AZ 85721
(520) 626-6152

Arkansas

Arkansas State University
—State University—

Full-Time Enrollments:	172	Evening Classes:	No
Part-Time Enrollments:	—	Weekend Classes:	No
Affiliation:	Public	Distance Learning:	Yes

NLN ACCREDITATION: Yes

BSN for non-RNs w/degree in other field: No

Articulation: Associate to Baccalaureate
Diploma to Baccalaureate
LPN to Baccalaureate
LPN to Associate
RN to MSN

For Further Information Contact:

Dr Elizabeth Stokes, Interim Chair
Arkansas State University
PO Box 69
State University, AR 72437
(501) 972-3074

Arkansas Technical University
—Russellville—

Full-Time Enrollments:	52	Evening Classes:	Yes
Part-Time Enrollments:	6	Weekend Classes:	No
Affiliation:	Public	Distance Learning:	Yes

NLN ACCREDITATION: Yes

BSN for non-RNs w/degree in other field: No

Articulation: Associate to Baccalaureate
Diploma to Baccalaureate
LPN to Baccalaureate

For Further Information Contact:

Dr Audrey R Owens, Dept Head
Arkansas Technical University
Dean Hall
Russellville, AR 72801
(501) 968-0384

Harding University
—Searcy—

Full-Time Enrollments:	103	Evening Classes:	No
Part-Time Enrollments:	—	Weekend Classes:	No
Affiliation:	Religious	Distance Learning:	No

NLN ACCREDITATION: Yes

BSN for non-RNs w/degree in other field: Yes

Articulation: Associate to Baccalaureate
Diploma to Baccalaureate
LPN to Baccalaureate

For Further Information Contact:

Dr Cathleen M Shultz, Dean
Harding University
Box 2265
Searcy, AR 72149-0001
(501) 279-4476

Henderson State University
—Arkadelphia—

Full-Time Enrollments:	68	Evening Classes:	Yes
Part-Time Enrollments:	29	Weekend Classes:	No
Affiliation:	Public	Distance Learning:	No

NLN ACCREDITATION: Yes

BSN for non-RNs w/degree in other field: No

Articulation: Associate to Baccalaureate
Diploma to Baccalaureate
LPN to Baccalaureate

For Further Information Contact:

Dr Rita Black Monsen, Chair
Henderson State University
PO Box 7803
Arkadelphia, AR 71999
(501) 230-5000

University of Arkansas at Fayetteville
—Fayetteville—

Full-Time Enrollments:	64	Evening Classes:	Yes
Part-Time Enrollments:	3	Weekend Classes:	No
Affiliation:	Public	Distance Learning:	No

NLN ACCREDITATION: Yes

BSN for non-RNs w/degree in other field: No

Articulation: Associate to Baccalaureate

For Further Information Contact:

Dr Margaret Sullivan, Director
University of Arkansas at Fayetteville
217 Ozark Hall
Fayetteville, AR 72701
(501) 575-3904

University of Arkansas at Monticello
—Monticello—

Full-Time Enrollments:	53	Evening Classes:	No
Part-Time Enrollments:	—	Weekend Classes:	No
Affiliation:	Public	Distance Learning:	No

NLN ACCREDITATION: No

BSN for non-RNs w/degree in other field: No

Articulation: Associate to Baccalaureate
Diploma to Baccalaureate
LPN to Baccalaureate

For Further Information Contact:

Dr Brenda Wright, Chair
University of Arkansas at Monticello
PO Box 3606
Monticello, AR 71655
(501) 460-1069

University of Arkansas at Pine Bluff
—Pine Bluff—

Full-Time Enrollments:	43	Evening Classes:	No
Part-Time Enrollments:	—	Weekend Classes:	No
Affiliation:	Public	Distance Learning:	No

NLN ACCREDITATION: Yes

BSN for non-RNs w/degree in other field: No

Articulation: Associate to Baccalaureate
Diploma to Baccalaureate
LPN to Baccalaureate

For Further Information Contact:

Dr Irene Henderson, Chair
University of Arkansas at Pine Bluff
Box 44 Univ Dr
Pine Bluff, AR 71601
(501) 543-8220

University of Arkansas for Medical Sciences
—Little Rock—

Full-Time Enrollments:	130	Evening Classes:	No
Part-Time Enrollments:	6	Weekend Classes:	No
Affiliation:	Public	Distance Learning:	Yes

NLN ACCREDITATION: Yes

BSN for non-RNs w/degree in other field: No

Articulation: Associate to Baccalaureate
Diploma to Baccalaureate
LPN to Baccalaureate

For Further Information Contact:

Dr Linda C Hodges, Dean
University of Arkansas for Medical Sciences
4301 W Markham Slot 529
Little Rock, AR 72205
(501) 686-5375

University of Central Arkansas
—Conway—

Full-Time Enrollments:	148	Evening Classes:	No
Part-Time Enrollments:	9	Weekend Classes:	No
Affiliation:	Public	Distance Learning:	—

NLN ACCREDITATION: Yes

BSN for non-RNs w/degree in other field: No

Articulation: Associate to Baccalaureate
Diploma to Baccalaureate
LPN to Baccalaureate
RN to MSN

For Further Information Contact:

Dr Barbara G Williams, Chair
University of Central Arkansas
Donaghey & Bruce Sts
Conway, AR 72035
(501) 450-3119

California

Azusa Pacific University
—Azusa—

Full-Time Enrollments:	179	Evening Classes:	Yes
Part-Time Enrollments:	22	Weekend Classes:	No
Affiliation:	Religious	Distance Learning:	No

NLN ACCREDITATION: Yes

BSN for non-RNs w/degree in other field: No

Articulation: RN to MSN

For Further Information Contact:

Dr Rose Liegler, Dean
Azusa Pacific University
901 E Alosta Ave
Azusa, CA 91702
(818) 815-5381

Biola University
—La Mirada—

Full-Time Enrollments:	84	Evening Classes:	No
Part-Time Enrollments:	—	Weekend Classes:	No
Affiliation:	Religious	Distance Learning:	No

NLN ACCREDITATION: Yes

BSN for non-RNs w/degree in other field: Yes

Articulation: Associate to Baccalaureate

For Further Information Contact:

Dr Rebekah L Fleeger, Chair
Biola University
13800 Biola Ave
La Mirada, CA 90639
(310) 903-4850

California State University at San Bernadino
—San Bernadino—

Full-Time Enrollments:	—	Evening Classes:	—
Part-Time Enrollments:	—	Weekend Classes:	—
Affiliation:	Public	Distance Learning:	—

NLN ACCREDITATION: Yes

BSN for non-RNs w/degree in other field: —

Articulation: None

For Further Information Contact:

Dr Elizabeth Barfield, Chair
California State University at San Bernadino
5500 Univ Parkway
San Bernadino, CA 92407
(909) 880-5000

California State University-Bakersfield
—Bakersfield—

Full-Time Enrollments:	213	Evening Classes:	Yes
Part-Time Enrollments:	—	Weekend Classes:	Yes
Affiliation:	Public	Distance Learning:	No

NLN ACCREDITATION: Yes

BSN for non-RNs w/degree in other field: No

Articulation: Associate to Baccalaureate

For Further Information Contact:

Dr Peggy Leapley, Chair
California State University-Bakersfield
9001 Stockdale Hwy
Bakersfield, CA 93311-1099
(805) 664-3102

California State University-Chico
—Chico—

Full-Time Enrollments:	149	Evening Classes:	Yes
Part-Time Enrollments:	—	Weekend Classes:	No
Affiliation:	Public	Distance Learning:	No

NLN ACCREDITATION: Yes

BSN for non-RNs w/degree in other field: No

Articulation: Associate to Baccalaureate
LPN to Baccalaureate

For Further Information Contact:

Dr Sherry Fox, Director
California State University-Chico
Holt Hall Rm 369
Chico, CA 95929-2000
(916) 898-5183

California State University-Fresno
—Fresno—

Full-Time Enrollments:	201	Evening Classes:	Yes
Part-Time Enrollments:	33	Weekend Classes:	Yes
Affiliation:	Public	Distance Learning:	Yes

NLN ACCREDITATION: Yes

BSN for non-RNs w/degree in other field: No

Articulation: Associate to Baccalaureate

For Further Information Contact:

Dr Ruth Willmington, Chair
California State University-Fresno
2345 E San Ramon Ave
Fresno, CA 93740-8031
(209) 278-2041

California State University-Hayward
—Hayward—

Full-Time Enrollments:	184	Evening Classes:	No
Part-Time Enrollments:	—	Weekend Classes:	No
Affiliation:	Public	Distance Learning:	Yes

NLN ACCREDITATION: Yes

BSN for non-RNs w/degree in other field: No

Articulation: Associate to Baccalaureate

For Further Information Contact:

Dr Arlene Kahn, Chair
California State University-Hayward
Dept Of Nursing
Hayward, CA 94542-3086
(510) 885-3481

California State University-Long Beach
—Long Beach—

Full-Time Enrollments:	200	Evening Classes:	Yes
Part-Time Enrollments:	12	Weekend Classes:	Yes
Affiliation:	Public	Distance Learning:	Yes

NLN ACCREDITATION: Yes

BSN for non-RNs w/degree in other field: No

Articulation: Associate to Baccalaureate
LPN to Baccalaureate
RN to MSN

For Further Information Contact:

Dr Christine Talmadge, Chair
California State University-Long Beach
1250 Bellflower
Long Beach, CA 90840
(310) 985-8242

California State University-Los Angeles
—Los Angeles—

Full-Time Enrollments:	112	Evening Classes:	Yes
Part-Time Enrollments:	19	Weekend Classes:	No
Affiliation:	Public	Distance Learning:	No

NLN ACCREDITATION: Yes

BSN for non-RNs w/degree in other field: No

Articulation: Associate to Baccalaureate
Diploma to Associate
Diploma to Baccalaureate
LPN to Baccalaureate
RN to MSN

For Further Information Contact:

Dr Judith Papenhausen, Chair
California State University-Los Angeles
5151 State Univ Dr
Los Angeles, CA 90032
(213) 343-4700

California State University-Sacramento
—Sacramento—

Full-Time Enrollments:	197	Evening Classes:	Yes
Part-Time Enrollments:	19	Weekend Classes:	Yes
Affiliation:	Public	Distance Learning:	No

NLN ACCREDITATION: Yes

BSN for non-RNs w/degree in other field:　No

Articulation:　Associate to Baccalaureate

For Further Information Contact:

Dr Annita B Watson, Chair
California State University-Sacramento
6000 J St
Sacramento, CA 95819
(916) 278-6525

Dominican College of San Rafael
—San Rafael—

Full-Time Enrollments:	178	Evening Classes:	Yes
Part-Time Enrollments:	74	Weekend Classes:	No
Affiliation:	Private	Distance Learning:	No

NLN ACCREDITATION: Yes

BSN for non-RNs w/degree in other field:　No

Articulation:　Associate to Baccalaureate

For Further Information Contact:

Dr Martha Nelson, Dean
Dominican College of San Rafael
50 Acacia Ave
San Rafael, CA 94901
(415) 485-3295

Humboldt State University
—Arcata—

Full-Time Enrollments:	112	Evening Classes:	No
Part-Time Enrollments:	—	Weekend Classes:	No
Affiliation:	Public	Distance Learning:	Yes

NLN ACCREDITATION: Yes

BSN for non-RNs w/degree in other field:　Yes

Articulation:　Associate to Baccalaureate

For Further Information Contact:

Dr Wendy Woodward, Chair
Humboldt State University
Arcata, CA 95521
(707) 826-3215

Loma Linda University
—Loma Linda—

Full-Time Enrollments:	263	Evening Classes:	No
Part-Time Enrollments:	18	Weekend Classes:	No
Affiliation:	Religious	Distance Learning:	No

NLN ACCREDITATION: Yes

BSN for non-RNs w/degree in other field:　Yes

Articulation:　None

For Further Information Contact:

Dr Helen Emori King, Dean
Loma Linda University
School of Nsg-West Hall
Loma Linda, CA 92350
(909) 824-4360

Mt St Mary's College
—Los Angeles—

Full-Time Enrollments:	222	Evening Classes:	No
Part-Time Enrollments:	—	Weekend Classes:	No
Affiliation:	Religious	Distance Learning:	No

NLN ACCREDITATION: Yes

BSN for non-RNs w/degree in other field:　Yes

Articulation:　Associate to Baccalaureate
　　　　　　　Diploma to Baccalaureate
　　　　　　　LPN to Baccalaureate

For Further Information Contact:

Dr Marjorie Dobratz, Chair
Mt St Mary's College
12001 Chalon Rd
Los Angeles, CA 90049
(310) 471-9521

Point Loma Nazarene College
—San Diego—

Full-Time Enrollments:	121	Evening Classes:	No
Part-Time Enrollments:	—	Weekend Classes:	No
Affiliation:	Religious	Distance Learning:	No

NLN ACCREDITATION: Yes

BSN for non-RNs w/degree in other field:　No

Articulation:　None

For Further Information Contact:

Dr Margaret Stevenson, Chair
Point Loma Nazarene College
3900 Lomaland Dr
San Diego, CA 92106-2899
(619) 849-2425

Samuel Merritt College-St Mary College
—Oakland—

Full-Time Enrollments:	270	Evening Classes:	Yes
Part-Time Enrollments:	15	Weekend Classes:	Yes
Affiliation:	Private	Distance Learning:	No

NLN ACCREDITATION: Yes

BSN for non-RNs w/degree in other field: No

Articulation: None

For Further Information Contact:

Ms Gail Deboer, Coordinator
Samuel Merritt College-St Mary College
370 Hawthorne Ave
Oakland, CA 94609
(510) 869-6129

San Diego State University
—San Diego—

Full-Time Enrollments:	304	Evening Classes:	Yes
Part-Time Enrollments:	—	Weekend Classes:	No
Affiliation:	Public	Distance Learning:	No

NLN ACCREDITATION: Yes

BSN for non-RNs w/degree in other field: No

Articulation: Associate to Baccalaureate

For Further Information Contact:

Dr Patricia R Wahl, Director
San Diego State University
5300 Campanile Dr
San Diego, CA 92182
(619) 594-6384

San Francisco State University-Nursing Department
—San Francisco—

Full-Time Enrollments:	183	Evening Classes:	Yes
Part-Time Enrollments:	2	Weekend Classes:	No
Affiliation:	Public	Distance Learning:	No

NLN ACCREDITATION: Yes

BSN for non-RNs w/degree in other field: Yes

Articulation: Associate to Baccalaureate
RN to MSN

For Further Information Contact:

Dr Shannon Perry, Director
San Francisco State University-Nursing Department
1600 Holloway Ave
San Francisco, CA 94132
(415) 338-1801

San Jose State University
—San Jose—

Full-Time Enrollments:	323	Evening Classes:	Yes
Part-Time Enrollments:	41	Weekend Classes:	No
Affiliation:	Public	Distance Learning:	Yes

NLN ACCREDITATION: Yes

BSN for non-RNs w/degree in other field: No

Articulation: Associate to Baccalaureate

For Further Information Contact:

Dr Bobbye Gorenberg, Director
San Jose State University
One Washington Sq
San Jose, CA 95192-0057
(408) 924-3131

Sonoma State University
—Rohnert Park—

Full-Time Enrollments:	57	Evening Classes:	No
Part-Time Enrollments:	—	Weekend Classes:	No
Affiliation:	Public	Distance Learning:	No

NLN ACCREDITATION: Yes

BSN for non-RNs w/degree in other field: No

Articulation: None

For Further Information Contact:

Dr Janice Hitchcook, Acting Chair
Sonoma State University
1801 E Contati Ave
Rohnert Park, CA 94928-3609
(707) 664-2654

UCLA Center for the Health Sciences
—Los Angeles—

Full-Time Enrollments:	28	Evening Classes:	No
Part-Time Enrollments:	3	Weekend Classes:	No
Affiliation:	Public	Distance Learning:	No

NLN ACCREDITATION: Yes

BSN for non-RNs w/degree in other field: No

Articulation: None

For Further Information Contact:

Dr Adeline Nyamathi, Associate Dean
UCLA Center for the Health Sciences
700 Tiverton Ave Box 951702
Los Angeles, CA 90095-1702
(310) 825-5654

University of California-San Francisco
—San Francisco—

Full-Time Enrollments: —   Evening Classes: —
Part-Time Enrollments: —   Weekend Classes: —
Affiliation: Public   Distance Learning: —

NLN ACCREDITATION: Yes

BSN for non-RNs w/degree in other field: No

Articulation: None

For Further Information Contact:

Dr Marilyn Flood, Associate Dean
University of California-San Francisco
School of Nursing
San Francisco, CA 94143-0604
(415) 476-1435

University of San Francisco
—San Francisco—

Full-Time Enrollments: 577   Evening Classes: —
Part-Time Enrollments: 86   Weekend Classes: —
Affiliation: Religious   Distance Learning: —

NLN ACCREDITATION: Yes

BSN for non-RNs w/degree in other field: No

Articulation: None

For Further Information Contact:

To be named
University of San Francisco
2130 Fulton St
San Francisco, CA 94117
(415) 422-6681

University of Southern California
—Los Angeles—

Full-Time Enrollments: 252   Evening Classes: No
Part-Time Enrollments: —   Weekend Classes: No
Affiliation: Private   Distance Learning: No

NLN ACCREDITATION: Yes

BSN for non-RNs w/degree in other field: No

Articulation: None

For Further Information Contact:

Dr Adele Pillitteri, Chair
University of Southern California
1540 Alcazar St Ste 222
Los Angeles, CA 90033
(213) 342-1999

Colorado

Beth El College of Nursing
—Colorado Spring—

Full-Time Enrollments: —   Evening Classes: —
Part-Time Enrollments: —   Weekend Classes: —
Affiliation: Public   Distance Learning: —

NLN ACCREDITATION: Yes

BSN for non-RNs w/degree in other field: —

Articulation: None

For Further Information Contact:

Dr Carole Schoffstall, Dean
Beth El College of Nursing
2790 N Academy Blvd
Colorado Spring, CO 80917-5338
(719) 475-5170

Mesa State College
—Grand Junction—

Full-Time Enrollments: 68   Evening Classes: No
Part-Time Enrollments: 5   Weekend Classes: No
Affiliation: Public   Distance Learning: No

NLN ACCREDITATION: Yes

BSN for non-RNs w/degree in other field: No

Articulation: Associate to Baccalaureate
Diploma to Baccalaureate

For Further Information Contact:

Dr Sandy Forrest, Chair
Mesa State College
PO Box 2647
Grand Junction, CO 81502
(970) 248-1398

Regis University
—Denver—

Full-Time Enrollments: 186   Evening Classes: Yes
Part-Time Enrollments: 2   Weekend Classes: Yes
Affiliation: Religious   Distance Learning: No

NLN ACCREDITATION: Yes

BSN for non-RNs w/degree in other field: Yes

Articulation: Associate to Baccalaureate
Diploma to Baccalaureate

For Further Information Contact:

Dr Nancy Kiernan Case, Director
Regis University
West 50th Ave Lowell Blvd
Denver, CO 80221
(303) 458-4168

University of Colorado
—Denver—

Full-Time Enrollments:	158	Evening Classes:	Yes
Part-Time Enrollments:	8	Weekend Classes:	—
Affiliation:	Public	Distance Learning:	Yes

NLN ACCREDITATION: Yes

BSN for non-RNs w/degree in other field: No

Articulation: RN to MSN

For Further Information Contact:

Dr Bonita Cavanaugh, Director
University of Colorado
4200 East 9th Ave Box C 288
Denver, CO 80262
(303) 270-7754

University of Northern Colorado
—Greeley—

Full-Time Enrollments:	143	Evening Classes:	No
Part-Time Enrollments:	1	Weekend Classes:	No
Affiliation:	Public	Distance Learning:	No

NLN ACCREDITATION: Yes

BSN for non-RNs w/degree in other field: No

Articulation: Associate to Baccalaureate
Diploma to Associate
Diploma to Baccalaureate
LPN to Baccalaureate
RN to MSN

For Further Information Contact:

Dr Sandra Baird, Director
University of Northern Colorado
Greeley, CO 80639
(970) 351-2293

University of Southern Colorado
—Pueblo—

Full-Time Enrollments:	98	Evening Classes:	No
Part-Time Enrollments:	—	Weekend Classes:	No
Affiliation:	Public	Distance Learning:	No

NLN ACCREDITATION: Yes

BSN for non-RNs w/degree in other field: No

Articulation: Associate to Baccalaureate
Diploma to Baccalaureate

For Further Information Contact:

Dr Melva Steen, Chair
University of Southern Colorado
2200 Bonforte Blvd
Pueblo, CO 81001
(719) 549-2401

Connecticut

Fairfield University-School of Nursing
—Fairfield—

Full-Time Enrollments:	195	Evening Classes:	Yes
Part-Time Enrollments:	33	Weekend Classes:	No
Affiliation:	Religious	Distance Learning:	No

NLN ACCREDITATION: Yes

BSN for non-RNs w/degree in other field: Yes

Articulation: Diploma to Baccalaureate

For Further Information Contact:

Dr Theresa M Valiga, Dean
Fairfield University-School of Nursing
N Benson Rd
Fairfield, CT 06430-5195
(203) 254-4150

Quinnipiac College
—Hamden—

Full-Time Enrollments:	245	Evening Classes:	Yes
Part-Time Enrollments:	8	Weekend Classes:	—
Affiliation:	Private	Distance Learning:	—

NLN ACCREDITATION: Yes

BSN for non-RNs w/degree in other field: No

Articulation: Associate to Baccalaureate

For Further Information Contact:

Dr Rita Hammer, Chair
Quinnipiac College
Mount Carmel Ave
Hamden, CT 06518
(203) 281-8686

Sacred Heart University
—Fairfield—

Full-Time Enrollments:	61	Evening Classes:	Yes
Part-Time Enrollments:	9	Weekend Classes:	No
Affiliation:	Private	Distance Learning:	No

NLN ACCREDITATION: Yes

BSN for non-RNs w/degree in other field: No

Articulation: Associate to Baccalaureate
Diploma to Baccalaureate
RN to MSN

For Further Information Contact:

Dr Anne Barker, Director
Sacred Heart University
5151 Park Ave
Fairfield, CT 06432
(203) 371-7844

Southern Connecticut State University
—New Haven—

Full-Time Enrollments:	110	Evening Classes:	Yes
Part-Time Enrollments:	18	Weekend Classes:	No
Affiliation:	Public	Distance Learning:	Yes

NLN ACCREDITATION: Yes

BSN for non-RNs w/degree in other field: No

Articulation: Associate to Baccalaureate
Diploma to Baccalaureate

For Further Information Contact:

Dr Cesarina Thompson, Chair
Southern Connecticut State University
Jennings Hall, 501 Crescent St
New Haven, CT 06515
(203) 392-6487

St Joseph College
—West Hartford—

Full-Time Enrollments:	121	Evening Classes:	Yes
Part-Time Enrollments:	73	Weekend Classes:	Yes
Affiliation:	Religious	Distance Learning:	No

NLN ACCREDITATION: Yes

BSN for non-RNs w/degree in other field: Yes

Articulation: Associate to Baccalaureate
Diploma to Baccalaureate

For Further Information Contact:

Dr Esther P Haloburdo, Chair
St Joseph College
1678 Asylum Ave
West Hartford, CT 06117
(860) 232-4571

University of Connecticut
—Storrs—

Full-Time Enrollments:	320	Evening Classes:	No
Part-Time Enrollments:	45	Weekend Classes:	No
Affiliation:	Public	Distance Learning:	No

NLN ACCREDITATION: Yes

BSN for non-RNs w/degree in other field: No

Articulation: Associate to Baccalaureate
Diploma to Baccalaureate

For Further Information Contact:

Dr Barbara Redman, Dean
University of Connecticut
231 Glenbrook Rd
Storrs, CT 06269
(860) 486-4730

Western Connecticut State University
—Danbury—

Full-Time Enrollments:	91	Evening Classes:	Yes
Part-Time Enrollments:	43	Weekend Classes:	No
Affiliation:	Public	Distance Learning:	Yes

NLN ACCREDITATION: Yes

BSN for non-RNs w/degree in other field: No

Articulation: Associate to Baccalaureate

For Further Information Contact:

Dr Barbara Piscopo, Chair
Western Connecticut State University
181 White St
Danbury, CT 06810
(203) 797-4359

Yale University
—New Haven—

Full-Time Enrollments:	49	Evening Classes:	No
Part-Time Enrollments:	—	Weekend Classes:	No
Affiliation:	Private	Distance Learning:	No

NLN ACCREDITATION: Yes

BSN for non-RNs w/degree in other field: No

Articulation: None

For Further Information Contact:

Ms Judith B Krauss, Dean
Yale University
100 Church St South
New Haven, CT 06536-0740
(203) 785-2393

Delaware

Delaware State University
—Dover—

Full-Time Enrollments:	187	Evening Classes:	Yes
Part-Time Enrollments:	29	Weekend Classes:	No
Affiliation:	Public	Distance Learning:	No

NLN ACCREDITATION: Yes

BSN for non-RNs w/degree in other field: No

Articulation: Associate to Baccalaureate
Diploma to Baccalaureate

For Further Information Contact:

Dr Mary Watkins, Chair
Delaware State University
1200 N DuPont Hwy
Dover, DE 19901-2277
(302) 739-4933

University of Delaware
—Newark—

Full-Time Enrollments:	418	Evening Classes:	Yes
Part-Time Enrollments:	18	Weekend Classes:	Yes
Affiliation:	Public	Distance Learning:	Yes

NLN ACCREDITATION: Yes

BSN for non-RNs w/degree in other field: Yes

Articulation: None

For Further Information Contact:

Dr Betty Paulanka, Dean
University of Delaware
Newark, DE 19716
(302) 831-2381

District of Columbia

Catholic University of America
—Washington—

Full-Time Enrollments:	212	Evening Classes:	Yes
Part-Time Enrollments:	10	Weekend Classes:	No
Affiliation:	Religious	Distance Learning:	No

NLN ACCREDITATION: Yes

BSN for non-RNs w/degree in other field: Yes

Articulation: Associate to Baccalaureate

For Further Information Contact:

Sr Mary J Flaherty, Dean
Catholic University of America
3800 Brookland Ave, NE
Washington, DC 20064
(202) 319-5403

Georgetown University
—Washington—

Full-Time Enrollments:	277	Evening Classes:	No
Part-Time Enrollments:	3	Weekend Classes:	No
Affiliation:	Religious	Distance Learning:	—

NLN ACCREDITATION: Yes

BSN for non-RNs w/degree in other field: No

Articulation: None

For Further Information Contact:

Dr Elaine Larson, Dean
Georgetown University
3700 Reservoir Rd, NW
Washington, DC 20007
(202) 687-3118

Howard University
—Washington—

Full-Time Enrollments:	258	Evening Classes:	Yes
Part-Time Enrollments:	43	Weekend Classes:	Yes
Affiliation:	Private	Distance Learning:	No

NLN ACCREDITATION: Yes

BSN for non-RNs w/degree in other field: No

Articulation: Associate to Baccalaureate

For Further Information Contact:

Dr Dorothy Powell, Dean
Howard University
2400 6th St, NW
Washington, DC 20059
(202) 806-7459

University of District of Columbia
—Washington—

Full-Time Enrollments:	30	Evening Classes:	No
Part-Time Enrollments:	—	Weekend Classes:	No
Affiliation:	Public	Distance Learning:	No

NLN ACCREDITATION: Yes

BSN for non-RNs w/degree in other field: No

Articulation: Associate to Baccalaureate
Diploma to Baccalaureate
LPN to Associate

For Further Information Contact:

Dr Hazel Marshall, Interim Director
University of District of Columbia
4200 Conn Ave NW, Bldg 44
Washington, DC 20008
(202) 274-5685

Florida

Barry University
—Miami Shore—

Full-Time Enrollments:	153	Evening Classes:	Yes
Part-Time Enrollments:	50	Weekend Classes:	No
Affiliation:	Religious	Distance Learning:	No

NLN ACCREDITATION: Yes

BSN for non-RNs w/degree in other field: Yes

Articulation: None

For Further Information Contact:

Dr Judith A Balcerski, Dean
Barry University
11300 Second Ave NE
Miami Shore, FL 33161
(305) 899-3800

Bethune-Cookman College
—Daytona Beach—

Full-Time Enrollments:	54	Evening Classes:	No
Part-Time Enrollments:	—	Weekend Classes:	No
Affiliation:	Private	Distance Learning:	No

NLN ACCREDITATION: Yes

BSN for non-RNs w/degree in other field: No

Articulation: None

For Further Information Contact:

Dr B J Primus-Cotton, Director
Bethune-Cookman College
Dr Mcleod Bethune Blvd
Daytona Beach, FL 32114-3099
(904) 255-1401

Florida Agricultural and Mechanical University
—Tallahassee—

Full-Time Enrollments:	381	Evening Classes:	Yes
Part-Time Enrollments:	—	Weekend Classes:	No
Affiliation:	Public	Distance Learning:	No

NLN ACCREDITATION: Yes

BSN for non-RNs w/degree in other field: No

Articulation: Associate to Baccalaureate

For Further Information Contact:

Dr Margaret W Lewis, Dean
Florida Agricultural and Mechanical University
Box 136-FAMU
Tallahassee, FL 32307-3500
(904) 599-3017

Florida Atlantic University-College of Nursing
—Boca Raton—

Full-Time Enrollments:	80	Evening Classes:	Yes
Part-Time Enrollments:	37	Weekend Classes:	Yes
Affiliation:	Public	Distance Learning:	Yes

NLN ACCREDITATION: Yes

BSN for non-RNs w/degree in other field: No

Articulation: Associate to Baccalaureate

For Further Information Contact:

Dr Anne Boykin, Dean
Florida Atlantic University-College of Nursing
777 Glades Rd
Boca Raton, FL 33431
(561) 367-3260

Florida International University
—No Miami—

Full-Time Enrollments:	190	Evening Classes:	Yes
Part-Time Enrollments:	—	Weekend Classes:	—
Affiliation:	Public	Distance Learning:	Yes

NLN ACCREDITATION: Yes

BSN for non-RNs w/degree in other field: No

Articulation: Associate to Baccalaureate

For Further Information Contact:

Dr Linda Simunek, Dean
Florida International University
NE 151st Biscayne Blvd
No Miami, FL 33181
(305) 919-5915

Florida State University
—Tallahassee—

Full-Time Enrollments:	252	Evening Classes:	Yes
Part-Time Enrollments:	5	Weekend Classes:	No
Affiliation:	Public	Distance Learning:	Yes

NLN ACCREDITATION: Yes

BSN for non-RNs w/degree in other field: No

Articulation: Associate to Baccalaureate
                Diploma to Baccalaureate

For Further Information Contact:

Dr Evelyn T Singer, Dean
Florida State University
School of Nursing
Tallahassee, FL 32306-3051
(904) 644-3299

Jacksonville University
—Jacksonville—

Full-Time Enrollments:	106	Evening Classes:	—
Part-Time Enrollments:	—	Weekend Classes:	Yes
Affiliation:	Private	Distance Learning:	No

NLN ACCREDITATION: Yes

BSN for non-RNs w/degree in other field: No

Articulation: None

For Further Information Contact:

Dr Linda Miller, Director
Jacksonville University
2800 Univ Blvd N
Jacksonville, FL 32277
(904) 744-3950

Pensacola Christian College
—Pensacola—

Full-Time Enrollments:	—	Evening Classes:	—
Part-Time Enrollments:	—	Weekend Classes:	—
Affiliation:	Private	Distance Learning:	—

NLN ACCREDITATION: No

BSN for non-RNs w/degree in other field: —

Articulation: None

For Further Information Contact:

Mrs Teresa Haughton, Director
Pensacola Christian College
250 Brent Ln
Pensacola, FL 32503
(904) 478-8496

University of Central Florida
—Orlando—

Full-Time Enrollments:	135	Evening Classes:	Yes
Part-Time Enrollments:	1	Weekend Classes:	Yes
Affiliation:	Public	Distance Learning:	Yes

NLN ACCREDITATION: Yes

BSN for non-RNs w/degree in other field: No

Articulation: Associate to Baccalaureate

For Further Information Contact:

Dr Elizabeth Stullenbarger, Director
University of Central Florida
PO Box 162210
Orlando, FL 32816-2210
(407) 823-2744

University of Florida-J H Miller Health Center
—Gainesville—

Full-Time Enrollments:	265	Evening Classes:	No
Part-Time Enrollments:	—	Weekend Classes:	No
Affiliation:	Public	Distance Learning:	No

NLN ACCREDITATION: Yes

BSN for non-RNs w/degree in other field: No

Articulation: Associate to Baccalaureate

For Further Information Contact:

Dr Kathleen Long, Dean
University of Florida-J H Miller Health Center
Box 100197 JHMC
Gainesville, FL 32610
(904) 392-3752

University of Miami
—Coral Gables—

Full-Time Enrollments:	182	Evening Classes:	Yes
Part-Time Enrollments:	8	Weekend Classes:	—
Affiliation:	Private	Distance Learning:	—

NLN ACCREDITATION: Yes

BSN for non-RNs w/degree in other field: Yes

Articulation: Associate to Baccalaureate
Diploma to Baccalaureate

For Further Information Contact:

Dr Marydelle Polk, Assistant Dean
University of Miami
5801 Red Rd
Coral Gables, FL 33124-3850
(305) 284-3666

University of North Florida
—Jacksonville—

Full-Time Enrollments:	128	Evening Classes:	Yes
Part-Time Enrollments:	—	Weekend Classes:	No
Affiliation:	Public	Distance Learning:	No

NLN ACCREDITATION: Yes

BSN for non-RNs w/degree in other field: No

Articulation: Associate to Baccalaureate

For Further Information Contact:

Dr Helene Krouse, Acting Chair
University of North Florida
4567 St John's Bluff Rd South
Jacksonville, FL 32224-2645
(904) 646-2684

University of South Florida
—Tampa—

Full-Time Enrollments:	107	Evening Classes:	Yes
Part-Time Enrollments:	—	Weekend Classes:	No
Affiliation:	Public	Distance Learning:	Yes

NLN ACCREDITATION: Yes

BSN for non-RNs w/degree in other field: No

Articulation: Associate to Baccalaureate

For Further Information Contact:

Dr Patricia Burns, Dean
University of South Florida
Box 22 12901 Bruce Downs Blvd
Tampa, FL 33612-4799
(813) 974-2191

Georgia

Albany State University
—Albany—

Full-Time Enrollments:	99	Evening Classes:	Yes
Part-Time Enrollments:	—	Weekend Classes:	No
Affiliation:	Public	Distance Learning:	No

NLN ACCREDITATION: Yes

BSN for non-RNs w/degree in other field: Yes

Articulation: Associate to Baccalaureate
Diploma to Baccalaureate

For Further Information Contact:

Dr Lucille B Wilson, Dean
Albany State University
Albany, GA 31705
(912) 430-5106

Armstrong Atlantic State University
—Savannah—

Full-Time Enrollments:	110	Evening Classes:	Yes
Part-Time Enrollments:	2	Weekend Classes:	Yes
Affiliation:	Public	Distance Learning:	Yes

NLN ACCREDITATION: Yes

BSN for non-RNs w/degree in other field: No

Articulation: Associate to Baccalaureate
Diploma to Baccalaureate
RN to MSN

For Further Information Contact:

Dr Carole Massey, Coordinator
Armstrong Atlantic State University
Savannah, GA 31419-1997
(912) 927-5302

Brenau University-Department of Nursing
—Gainesville—

Full-Time Enrollments:	120	Evening Classes:	Yes
Part-Time Enrollments:	3	Weekend Classes:	Yes
Affiliation:	Private	Distance Learning:	No

NLN ACCREDITATION: Yes

BSN for non-RNs w/degree in other field: No

Articulation: Associate to Baccalaureate
Diploma to Baccalaureate

For Further Information Contact:

Dr Veta Massey, Chair
Brenau University-Department of Nursing
One Centennial Circle
Gainesville, GA 30501
(770) 534-6261

Clayton College and State University
—Morrow—

Full-Time Enrollments:	—	Evening Classes:	—
Part-Time Enrollments:	—	Weekend Classes:	—
Affiliation:	Public	Distance Learning:	—

NLN ACCREDITATION: Yes

BSN for non-RNs w/degree in other field: —

Articulation: —

For Further Information Contact:

Dr Linda Samson, Dean
Clayton College and State University
PO Box 285
Morrow, GA 30260
(770) 961-3701

Columbus State University
—Columbus—

Full-Time Enrollments:	68	Evening Classes:	Yes
Part-Time Enrollments:	—	Weekend Classes:	—
Affiliation:	Public	Distance Learning:	—

NLN ACCREDITATION: Yes

BSN for non-RNs w/degree in other field: No

Articulation: Associate to Baccalaureate

For Further Information Contact:

Dr Marlene Mitchell-Tibbs, Director
Columbus State University
4225 University Ave
Columbus, GA 31907-5645
(706) 568-2243

Georgia Baptist College of Nursing
—Atlanta—

Full-Time Enrollments:	297	Evening Classes:	No
Part-Time Enrollments:	21	Weekend Classes:	No
Affiliation:	Religious	Distance Learning:	No

NLN ACCREDITATION: Yes

BSN for non-RNs w/degree in other field: No

Articulation: Associate to Baccalaureate
Diploma to Baccalaureate

For Further Information Contact:

Dr Susan Gunby, President
Georgia Baptist College of Nursing
274 Boulevard NE Box 411
Atlanta, GA 30312
(404) 265-4795

Georgia College
—Milledgeville—

Full-Time Enrollments:	138	Evening Classes:	Yes
Part-Time Enrollments:	—	Weekend Classes:	—
Affiliation:	Public	Distance Learning:	Yes

NLN ACCREDITATION: Yes

BSN for non-RNs w/degree in other field: No

Articulation: Associate to Baccalaureate
Diploma to Baccalaureate

For Further Information Contact:

Dr Pamela C Levi, Dean
Georgia College
PO Box 64
Milledgeville, GA 31062
(912) 453-4004

Georgia Southern University
—Statesboro—

Full-Time Enrollments:	171	Evening Classes:	Yes
Part-Time Enrollments:	—	Weekend Classes:	No
Affiliation:	Public	Distance Learning:	Yes

NLN ACCREDITATION: Yes

BSN for non-RNs w/degree in other field: No

Articulation: Associate to Baccalaureate
Diploma to Baccalaureate

For Further Information Contact:

Dr Kaye A Herth, Chair
Georgia Southern University
Landrum Box 8158
Statesboro, GA 30460-8158
(912) 681-5455

Georgia State University
—Atlanta—

Full-Time Enrollments:	50	Evening Classes:	Yes
Part-Time Enrollments:	86	Weekend Classes:	No
Affiliation:	Public	Distance Learning:	Yes

NLN ACCREDITATION: Yes

BSN for non-RNs w/degree in other field: No

Articulation: Associate to Baccalaureate
Diploma to Baccalaureate
RN to MSN

For Further Information Contact:

Dr Judith Lupo Wold, Director
Georgia State University
PO Box 4019
Atlanta, GA 30302-4019
(404) 651-2000

Kennesaw State University
—Marietta—

Full-Time Enrollments:	125	Evening Classes:	No
Part-Time Enrollments:	100	Weekend Classes:	No
Affiliation:	Public	Distance Learning:	No

NLN ACCREDITATION: Yes

BSN for non-RNs w/degree in other field: No

Articulation: Associate to Baccalaureate

For Further Information Contact:

Dr David Bennett, Chair
Kennesaw State University
Marietta, GA 30061
(770) 423-6061

La Grange College
—La Grange—

Full-Time Enrollments:	22	Evening Classes:	Yes
Part-Time Enrollments:	6	Weekend Classes:	No
Affiliation:	Private	Distance Learning:	No

NLN ACCREDITATION: No

BSN for non-RNs w/degree in other field: No

Articulation: Associate to Baccalaureate
Diploma to Baccalaureate

For Further Information Contact:

Dr Sandra Kratina, Chair
La Grange College
601 Broad St
La Grange, GA 30240-2999
(706) 812-7220

Medical College of Georgia
—Augusta—

Full-Time Enrollments:	291	Evening Classes:	Yes
Part-Time Enrollments:	5	Weekend Classes:	—
Affiliation:	Public	Distance Learning:	Yes

NLN ACCREDITATION: Yes

BSN for non-RNs w/degree in other field: No

Articulation: Associate to Baccalaureate

For Further Information Contact:

Dr Vickie A Lambert, Dean
Medical College of Georgia
Augusta, GA 30912-4200
(706) 721-2651

Nell Hodgson Woodruff School-Emory University
—Atlanta—

Full-Time Enrollments:	195	Evening Classes:	No
Part-Time Enrollments:	15	Weekend Classes:	No
Affiliation:	Private	Distance Learning:	No

NLN ACCREDITATION: Yes

BSN for non-RNs w/degree in other field: No

Articulation: None

For Further Information Contact:

Dr Dyanne Affonso, Dean
Nell Hodgson Woodruff School-Emory University
531 Asbury Circle
Atlanta, GA 30322
(404) 727-7981

Valdosta State University
—Valdosta—

Full-Time Enrollments:	—	Evening Classes:	—
Part-Time Enrollments:	—	Weekend Classes:	—
Affiliation:	Public	Distance Learning:	—

NLN ACCREDITATION: Yes

BSN for non-RNs w/degree in other field: —

Articulation: None

For Further Information Contact:

Dr Frances Brown, Acting Dean
Valdosta State University
Valdosta, GA 31601
(912) 333-5959

Guam

University of Guam
—Mangilao—

Full-Time Enrollments:	80	Evening Classes:	Yes
Part-Time Enrollments:	—	Weekend Classes:	No
Affiliation:	Public	Distance Learning:	Yes

NLN ACCREDITATION: Yes

BSN for non-RNs w/degree in other field: No

Articulation: None

For Further Information Contact:

Dr Maureen M Fochtman, Dean
University of Guam
UOG Station
Mangilao, GU 96923
(671) 735-2650

Hawaii

Hawaii Pacific University
—Kaneohe—

Full-Time Enrollments:	442	Evening Classes:	Yes
Part-Time Enrollments:	131	Weekend Classes:	Yes
Affiliation:	Private	Distance Learning:	No

NLN ACCREDITATION: Yes

BSN for non-RNs w/degree in other field: No

Articulation: None

For Further Information Contact:

Dr Carol E Winters-Maloney, Dean
Hawaii Pacific University
45-045 Kamehameha Hwy
Kaneohe, HI 96744
(808) 233-3252

University of Hawaii
—Honolulu—

Full-Time Enrollments:	153	Evening Classes:	No
Part-Time Enrollments:	5	Weekend Classes:	No
Affiliation:	Public	Distance Learning:	Yes

NLN ACCREDITATION: Yes

BSN for non-RNs w/degree in other field: No

Articulation: Associate to Baccalaureate
Diploma to Baccalaureate

For Further Information Contact:

Dr Rosanne Harrigan, Dean
University of Hawaii
2538 The Mall
Honolulu, HI 96822
(808) 956-8939

University of Hawaii at Hilo
—Hilo—

Full-Time Enrollments:	31	Evening Classes:	—
Part-Time Enrollments:	—	Weekend Classes:	—
Affiliation:	Public	Distance Learning:	—

NLN ACCREDITATION: No

BSN for non-RNs w/degree in other field: No

Articulation: None

For Further Information Contact:

Dr G Lehua Kinney, Director
University of Hawaii at Hilo
Dept of Nursing
Hilo, HI 96720-4091
(808) 933-3764

Idaho

Boise State University
—Boise—

Full-Time Enrollments:	115	Evening Classes:	No
Part-Time Enrollments:	—	Weekend Classes:	No
Affiliation:	Public	Distance Learning:	Yes

NLN ACCREDITATION: Yes

BSN for non-RNs w/degree in other field:　No

Articulation:　Associate to Baccalaureate
Diploma to Baccalaureate
LPN to Associate

For Further Information Contact:

Dr Anne Payne, Chair
Boise State University
1910 Univ Dr
Boise, ID 83725
(208) 385-1768

Idaho State University
—Pocatello—

Full-Time Enrollments:	96	Evening Classes:	Yes
Part-Time Enrollments:	—	Weekend Classes:	No
Affiliation:	Public	Distance Learning:	Yes

NLN ACCREDITATION: Yes

BSN for non-RNs w/degree in other field:　No

Articulation:　Associate to Baccalaureate
LPN to Baccalaureate
RN to MSN

For Further Information Contact:

Dr Pamela Clarke, Chair
Idaho State University
Box 8101
Pocatello, ID 83209
(208) 236-3085

Lewis Clark State University
—Lewiston—

Full-Time Enrollments:	76	Evening Classes:	Yes
Part-Time Enrollments:	—	Weekend Classes:	Yes
Affiliation:	Public	Distance Learning:	Yes

NLN ACCREDITATION: Yes

BSN for non-RNs w/degree in other field:　No

Articulation:　Associate to Baccalaureate
LPN to Baccalaureate

For Further Information Contact:

Dr Mary McFarland, Chair
Lewis Clark State University
500 8th Ave
Lewiston, ID 83501
(208) 799-2402

Illinois

Aurora University School of Nursing & Health
—Aurora—

Full-Time Enrollments:	138	Evening Classes:	Yes
Part-Time Enrollments:	115	Weekend Classes:	No
Affiliation:	Private	Distance Learning:	No

NLN ACCREDITATION: Yes

BSN for non-RNs w/degree in other field:　No

Articulation:　None

For Further Information Contact:

Dr Mary Miller, Dean
Aurora University School of Nursing & Health
347 S Gladstone
Aurora, IL 60506
(630) 844-5130

Bradley University
—Peoria—

Full-Time Enrollments:	201	Evening Classes:	Yes
Part-Time Enrollments:	19	Weekend Classes:	No
Affiliation:	Private	Distance Learning:	Yes

NLN ACCREDITATION: Yes

BSN for non-RNs w/degree in other field:　No

Articulation:　Associate to Baccalaureate

For Further Information Contact:

Dr Francesca Armmer, Chair
Bradley University
Peoria, IL 61625
(309) 677-2528

Chicago State University-Department of Nursing
—Chicago—

Full-Time Enrollments:	190	Evening Classes:	—
Part-Time Enrollments:	—	Weekend Classes:	—
Affiliation:	Public	Distance Learning:	—

NLN ACCREDITATION: Yes

BSN for non-RNs w/degree in other field:　No

Articulation:　None

For Further Information Contact:

Dr Linda Hureston, Chair
Chicago State University-Department of Nursing
9501 S King Dr
Chicago, IL 60628-1598
(773) 995-3987

Concordia University-West Suburban College of Nursing
—Oak Park—

Full-Time Enrollments:	194	Evening Classes:	Yes
Part-Time Enrollments:	19	Weekend Classes:	No
Affiliation:	Private	Distance Learning:	No

NLN ACCREDITATION: Yes

BSN for non-RNs w/degree in other field: No

Articulation: Associate to Baccalaureate

For Further Information Contact:

Dr Donna Ipema, Provost
Concordia University-West Suburban College of Nursing
Erie at Austin
Oak Park, IL 60302
(708) 383-3901

Culver-Stockton College & Blessing-Rieman College
—Quincy—

Full-Time Enrollments:	153	Evening Classes:	Yes
Part-Time Enrollments:	12	Weekend Classes:	No
Affiliation:	Private	Distance Learning:	No

NLN ACCREDITATION: Yes

BSN for non-RNs w/degree in other field: No

Articulation: Associate to Baccalaureate

For Further Information Contact:

Dr Carole Piles, President
Culver-Stockton College & Blessing-Rieman College
Broadway at 11th St Ecx 7005
Quincy, IL 62305-7005
(217) 228-5520

Elmhurst College-Deicke Center for Nursing Education
—Elmhurst—

Full-Time Enrollments:	112	Evening Classes:	Yes
Part-Time Enrollments:	30	Weekend Classes:	Yes
Affiliation:	Religious	Distance Learning:	No

NLN ACCREDITATION: Yes

BSN for non-RNs w/degree in other field: Yes

Articulation: None

For Further Information Contact:

Dr Jean E Lytle, Director
Elmhurst College-Deicke Center for Nursing Education
190 Prospect Ave
Elmhurst, IL 60126-3296
(630) 617-3503

Illinois Wesleyan University-School of Nursing
—Bloomington—

Full-Time Enrollments:	98	Evening Classes:	No
Part-Time Enrollments:	1	Weekend Classes:	No
Affiliation:	Private	Distance Learning:	No

NLN ACCREDITATION: Yes

BSN for non-RNs w/degree in other field: No

Articulation: Diploma to Baccalaureate

For Further Information Contact:

Dr Donna L Hartweg, Director
Illinois Wesleyan University-School of Nursing
1312 N Park St Box 2900
Bloomington, IL 61702
(309) 556-3051

Lakeview College
—Danville—

Full-Time Enrollments:	69	Evening Classes:	Yes
Part-Time Enrollments:	29	Weekend Classes:	Yes
Affiliation:	Private	Distance Learning:	Yes

NLN ACCREDITATION: No

BSN for non-RNs w/degree in other field: No

Articulation: None

For Further Information Contact:

Dr Joyce Atchison, Dean
Lakeview College
903 North Logan Ave
Danville, IL 61832
(217) 443-5238

Lewis University-College of Nursing
—Romeoville—

Full-Time Enrollments:	335	Evening Classes:	—
Part-Time Enrollments:	—	Weekend Classes:	—
Affiliation:	Religious	Distance Learning:	—

NLN ACCREDITATION: Yes

BSN for non-RNs w/degree in other field: No

Articulation: None

For Further Information Contact:

Dr Marilyn M Bunt, Dean
Lewis University-College of Nursing
Route 53
Romeoville, IL 60446
(815) 838-0500

MacMurray College
—Jacksonville—

Full-Time Enrollments:	47	Evening Classes:	No
Part-Time Enrollments:	—	Weekend Classes:	No
Affiliation:	Religious	Distance Learning:	No

NLN ACCREDITATION: Yes

BSN for non-RNs w/degree in other field: No

Articulation: Associate to Baccalaureate
Diploma to Baccalaureate

For Further Information Contact:

Dr Margaret Boudreau, Director
MacMurray College
446 E State St
Jacksonville, IL 62650
(217) 479-7083

Marcella Niehoff School of nursing-Loyola University
—Chicago—

Full-Time Enrollments:	378	Evening Classes:	Yes
Part-Time Enrollments:	11	Weekend Classes:	Yes
Affiliation:	Religious	Distance Learning:	—

NLN ACCREDITATION: Yes

BSN for non-RNs w/degree in other field: Yes

Articulation: Associate to Baccalaureate
RN to MSN

For Further Information Contact:

Dr Shirley Dooling, Dean
Marcella Niehoff School of nursing-Loyola University
6525 N Sheridan Rd
Chicago, IL 60626
(773) 508-3264

Mennonite College of Nursing
—Bloomington—

Full-Time Enrollments:	158	Evening Classes:	No
Part-Time Enrollments:	6	Weekend Classes:	No
Affiliation:	Private	Distance Learning:	No

NLN ACCREDITATION: Yes

BSN for non-RNs w/degree in other field: No

Articulation: Associate to Baccalaureate

For Further Information Contact:

Dr Jerry Durham, Dean
Mennonite College of Nursing
804 North East St
Bloomington, IL 61701
(309) 829-0715

Millikin University School of Nursing
—Decatur—

Full-Time Enrollments:	—	Evening Classes:	—
Part-Time Enrollments:	—	Weekend Classes:	—
Affiliation:	Religious	Distance Learning:	—

NLN ACCREDITATION: Yes

BSN for non-RNs w/degree in other field: —

Articulation: None

For Further Information Contact:

Dr Linda Niedringhaus, Dean
Millikin University School of Nursing
1184 W Main
Decatur, IL 62522
(217) 424-6348

North Park College
—Chicago—

Full-Time Enrollments:	191	Evening Classes:	Yes
Part-Time Enrollments:	22	Weekend Classes:	No
Affiliation:	Religious	Distance Learning:	No

NLN ACCREDITATION: Yes

BSN for non-RNs w/degree in other field: No

Articulation: None

For Further Information Contact:

Dr Alma Labunski, Chair
North Park College
3225 W Foster Ave
Chicago, IL 60625
(312) 244-5691

Northern Illinois University
—DeKalb—

Full-Time Enrollments:	334	Evening Classes:	Yes
Part-Time Enrollments:	95	Weekend Classes:	Yes
Affiliation:	Public	Distance Learning:	Yes

NLN ACCREDITATION: Yes

BSN for non-RNs w/degree in other field: No

Articulation: None

For Further Information Contact:

Dr Marilyn Stromborg, Chair
Northern Illinois University
1240 Normal Rd
DeKalb, IL 60115
(815) 753-1231

Olivet Nazarene University
—Kankakee—

Full-Time Enrollments:	140	Evening Classes:	Yes
Part-Time Enrollments:	—	Weekend Classes:	—
Affiliation:	Religious	Distance Learning:	—

NLN ACCREDITATION: Yes

BSN for non-RNs w/degree in other field: No

Articulation: None

For Further Information Contact:

Dr Norma Wood, Chair
Olivet Nazarene University
240 Marsiles
Kankakee, IL 60901
(815) 939-5340

Rockford College
—Rockford—

Full-Time Enrollments:	100	Evening Classes:	Yes
Part-Time Enrollments:	32	Weekend Classes:	No
Affiliation:	Private	Distance Learning:	No

NLN ACCREDITATION: Yes

BSN for non-RNs w/degree in other field: No

Articulation: Associate to Baccalaureate
Diploma to Baccalaureate

For Further Information Contact:

Ms Marilyn Hartinger, Interim Chair
Rockford College
5050 East State St
Rockford, IL 61108-2393
(815) 226-4054

Rush University
—Chicago—

Full-Time Enrollments:	227	Evening Classes:	—
Part-Time Enrollments:	14	Weekend Classes:	—
Affiliation:	Private	Distance Learning:	—

NLN ACCREDITATION: Yes

BSN for non-RNs w/degree in other field: No

Articulation: None

For Further Information Contact:

Dr Kathleen G Andreoli, Dean
Rush University
1743 W Harrison
Chicago, IL 60612
(312) 942-2165

Southern Illinois University School of Nursing
—Edwardsville—

Full-Time Enrollments:	258	Evening Classes:	Yes
Part-Time Enrollments:	—	Weekend Classes:	Yes
Affiliation:	Public	Distance Learning:	Yes

NLN ACCREDITATION: Yes

BSN for non-RNs w/degree in other field: Yes

Articulation: Associate to Baccalaureate

For Further Information Contact:

Dr Felissa Cohen, Dean
Southern Illinois University School of Nursing
Rm 2333 Bldg 111
Edwardsville, IL 62026-1066
(618) 692-3959

St Anthony College of Nursing
—Rockford—

Full-Time Enrollments:	76	Evening Classes:	Yes
Part-Time Enrollments:	3	Weekend Classes:	—
Affiliation:	Religious	Distance Learning:	—

NLN ACCREDITATION: Yes

BSN for non-RNs w/degree in other field: Yes

Articulation: None

For Further Information Contact:

Dr Terese Burch, Dean
St Anthony College of Nursing
5658 East State St
Rockford, IL 61108-2468
(815) 395-5091

St Francis Medical Center-College of Nursing
—Peoria—

Full-Time Enrollments:	103	Evening Classes:	Yes
Part-Time Enrollments:	34	Weekend Classes:	No
Affiliation:	Religious	Distance Learning:	No

NLN ACCREDITATION: Yes

BSN for non-RNs w/degree in other field: No

Articulation: None

For Further Information Contact:

Sr Mary L Pieperbeck, Dean
St Francis Medical Center-College of Nursing
511 NE Greenleaf St
Peoria, IL 61603
(309) 655-2086

St John's College-Department of Nursing
—Springfield—

Full-Time Enrollments:	109	Evening Classes:	No
Part-Time Enrollments:	4	Weekend Classes:	No
Affiliation:	Religious	Distance Learning:	No

NLN ACCREDITATION: Yes

BSN for non-RNs w/degree in other field:　No

Articulation:　None

For Further Information Contact:

Dr Kay O'Neil, Dean
St John's College-Department of Nursing
421 N 9th St
Springfield, IL 62702
(217) 544-6464

St Joseph College of Nursing
—Joliet—

Full-Time Enrollments:	124	Evening Classes:	Yes
Part-Time Enrollments:	40	Weekend Classes:	No
Affiliation:	Religious	Distance Learning:	Yes

NLN ACCREDITATION: Yes

BSN for non-RNs w/degree in other field:　No

Articulation:　Associate to Baccalaureate
　　　　　　　Diploma to Baccalaureate

For Further Information Contact:

Dr Albertta David, Dean
St Joseph College of Nursing
290 N Springfield Ave
Joliet, IL 60435
(815) 741-7123

St Xavier University
—Chicago—

Full-Time Enrollments:	295	Evening Classes:	Yes
Part-Time Enrollments:	143	Weekend Classes:	Yes
Affiliation:	Religious	Distance Learning:	Yes

NLN ACCREDITATION: Yes

BSN for non-RNs w/degree in other field:　No

Articulation:　Associate to Baccalaureate

For Further Information Contact:

Dr Mary Lebold, Dean
St Xavier University
3700 W 103rd St
Chicago, IL 60655
(312) 298-3300

Trinity Christian College
—Palos Heights—

Full-Time Enrollments:	53	Evening Classes:	No
Part-Time Enrollments:	4	Weekend Classes:	No
Affiliation:	Religious	Distance Learning:	No

NLN ACCREDITATION: Yes

BSN for non-RNs w/degree in other field:　No

Articulation:　None

For Further Information Contact:

Dr Cynthia Sander, Chair
Trinity Christian College
6601 West College Dr
Palos Heights, IL 60463
(708) 597-3000

Trinity College of Nursing
—Moline—

Full-Time Enrollments:	—	Evening Classes:	—
Part-Time Enrollments:	—	Weekend Classes:	—
Affiliation:	Private	Distance Learning:	—

NLN ACCREDITATION: No

BSN for non-RNs w/degree in other field:　—

Articulation:　None

For Further Information Contact:

Ms Jo Ellen Sharer, President
Trinity College of Nursing
501 10th Ave
Moline, IL 61265
(309) 757-2910

University of Illinois-College of Nursing
—Chicago—

Full-Time Enrollments:	573	Evening Classes:	No
Part-Time Enrollments:	37	Weekend Classes:	No
Affiliation:	Public	Distance Learning:	No

NLN ACCREDITATION: Yes

BSN for non-RNs w/degree in other field:　No

Articulation:　None

For Further Information Contact:

Dr Joan Shaver, Dean
University of Illinois-College of Nursing
MC/802 845 S Damen
Chicago, IL 60612-7350
(312) 996-7805

Indiana

Anderson University
—Anderson—

Full-Time Enrollments:	77	Evening Classes:	Yes
Part-Time Enrollments:	12	Weekend Classes:	Yes
Affiliation:	Religious	Distance Learning:	No

NLN ACCREDITATION: Yes

BSN for non-RNs w/degree in other field: No

Articulation: Associate to Baccalaureate

For Further Information Contact:

Dr Patricia Bennett, Director
Anderson University
1100 East 5th St
Anderson, IN 46012
(317) 641-4380

Ball State University
—Muncie—

Full-Time Enrollments:	135	Evening Classes:	No
Part-Time Enrollments:	2	Weekend Classes:	No
Affiliation:	Public	Distance Learning:	Yes

NLN ACCREDITATION: Yes

BSN for non-RNs w/degree in other field: No

Articulation: Associate to Baccalaureate
LPN to Associate
RN to MSN

For Further Information Contact:

Dr Phyllis Irvine, Director
Ball State University
2000 Univ Ave
Muncie, IN 47306
(317) 285-5571

Bethel College
—Mishawaka—

Full-Time Enrollments:	30	Evening Classes:	Yes
Part-Time Enrollments:	24	Weekend Classes:	Yes
Affiliation:	Religious	Distance Learning:	—

NLN ACCREDITATION: Yes

BSN for non-RNs w/degree in other field: No

Articulation: Associate to Baccalaureate

For Further Information Contact:

Dr Ruth Davidhizar, Dean
Bethel College
1001 West McKinley Ave
Mishawaka, IN 46545
(219) 259-8511

Goshen College
—Goshen—

Full-Time Enrollments:	50	Evening Classes:	Yes
Part-Time Enrollments:	4	Weekend Classes:	No
Affiliation:	Religious	Distance Learning:	No

NLN ACCREDITATION: Yes

BSN for non-RNs w/degree in other field: No

Articulation: Associate to Baccalaureate
Diploma to Baccalaureate

For Further Information Contact:

Dr Miriam Martin, Director
Goshen College
Goshen, IN 46526
(219) 535-7000

Indiana State University School of Nursing
—Terre Haute—

Full-Time Enrollments:	96	Evening Classes:	Yes
Part-Time Enrollments:	37	Weekend Classes:	No
Affiliation:	Public	Distance Learning:	No

NLN ACCREDITATION: Yes

BSN for non-RNs w/degree in other field: No

Articulation: Associate to Baccalaureate

For Further Information Contact:

Dr Ann Tomey, Dean
Indiana State University School of Nursing
Terre Haute, IN 47809
(812) 237-2323

Indiana University
—Indianapolis—

Full-Time Enrollments:	491	Evening Classes:	No
Part-Time Enrollments:	30	Weekend Classes:	No
Affiliation:	Public	Distance Learning:	No

NLN ACCREDITATION: Yes

BSN for non-RNs w/degree in other field: Yes

Articulation: Associate to Baccalaureate
LPN to Associate
RN to MSN

For Further Information Contact:

Dr Angela McBride, Univ Dean
Indiana University
1111 Middle Dr
Indianapolis, IN 46202-5107
(317) 274-1486

Indiana University East
—Richmond—

Full-Time Enrollments:	50	Evening Classes:	Yes
Part-Time Enrollments:	—	Weekend Classes:	Yes
Affiliation:	Public	Distance Learning:	Yes

NLN ACCREDITATION: Yes

BSN for non-RNs w/degree in other field: No

Articulation: Associate to Baccalaureate
Diploma to Baccalaureate
LPN to Associate

For Further Information Contact:

Dr Joanne Rains, Dean
Indiana University East
2325 Chester Blvd
Richmond, IN 47374
(317) 973-8257

Indiana University Kokomo
—Kokomo—

Full-Time Enrollments:	64	Evening Classes:	Yes
Part-Time Enrollments:	—	Weekend Classes:	Yes
Affiliation:	Public	Distance Learning:	Yes

NLN ACCREDITATION: Yes

BSN for non-RNs w/degree in other field: No

Articulation: Associate to Baccalaureate
Diploma to Baccalaureate
LPN to Associate

For Further Information Contact:

Dr Penny Cass, Dean
Indiana University Kokomo
2300 S Washington St Box 9003
Kokomo, IN 46904-9003
(317) 455-9288

Indiana University Northwest
—Gary—

Full-Time Enrollments:	55	Evening Classes:	Yes
Part-Time Enrollments:	7	Weekend Classes:	Yes
Affiliation:	Public	Distance Learning:	Yes

NLN ACCREDITATION: Yes

BSN for non-RNs w/degree in other field: No

Articulation: Associate to Baccalaureate
Diploma to Baccalaureate
LPN to Associate

For Further Information Contact:

Dr Doris R Blaney, Dean
Indiana University Northwest
3400 Broadway
Gary, IN 46408
(219) 980-6449

Indiana University South Bend
—South Bend—

Full-Time Enrollments:	51	Evening Classes:	Yes
Part-Time Enrollments:	5	Weekend Classes:	Yes
Affiliation:	Public	Distance Learning:	Yes

NLN ACCREDITATION: Yes

BSN for non-RNs w/degree in other field: No

Articulation: None

For Further Information Contact:

Dr Marian Pettengill, Dean
Indiana University South Bend
1700 Mishawaka PO Box 7111
South Bend, IN 46634
(219) 237-4111

Indiana University Southeast
—New Albany—

Full-Time Enrollments:	93	Evening Classes:	No
Part-Time Enrollments:	—	Weekend Classes:	No
Affiliation:	Public	Distance Learning:	—

NLN ACCREDITATION: Yes

BSN for non-RNs w/degree in other field: No

Articulation: Associate to Baccalaureate
Diploma to Baccalaureate

For Further Information Contact:

Dr Anita Hufft, Dean
Indiana University Southeast
4201 Grant Line Rd
New Albany, IN 47150
(812) 941-2000

Indiana Wesleyan University
—Marion—

Full-Time Enrollments:	133	Evening Classes:	Yes
Part-Time Enrollments:	28	Weekend Classes:	Yes
Affiliation:	Religious	Distance Learning:	Yes

NLN ACCREDITATION: Yes

BSN for non-RNs w/degree in other field: No

Articulation: None

For Further Information Contact:

Dr Susan Stranahan, Chair
Indiana Wesleyan University
4201 S Washington St
Marion, IN 46953
(317) 677-2269

Marian College
—Indianapolis—

Full-Time Enrollments: 140 Evening Classes: Yes
Part-Time Enrollments: 41 Weekend Classes: No
Affiliation: Religious Distance Learning: No

NLN ACCREDITATION: Yes

BSN for non-RNs w/degree in other field: Yes

Articulation: Associate to Baccalaureate
Diploma to Baccalaureate
LPN to Associate

For Further Information Contact:

Dr Esther O'Dea, Chair
Marian College
3200 Cold Spring Rd
Indianapolis, IN 46222
(317) 929-0311

Purdue University
—West Lafayette—

Full-Time Enrollments: 440 Evening Classes: Yes
Part-Time Enrollments: 10 Weekend Classes: Yes
Affiliation: Public Distance Learning: No

NLN ACCREDITATION: Yes

BSN for non-RNs w/degree in other field: No

Articulation: None

For Further Information Contact:

Dr Jo Brooks, Dept Head
Purdue University
West Lafayette, IN 47907-1337
(317) 494-4008

St Francis College
—Fort Wayne—

Full-Time Enrollments: 111 Evening Classes: Yes
Part-Time Enrollments: 4 Weekend Classes: Yes
Affiliation: Religious Distance Learning: Yes

NLN ACCREDITATION: Yes

BSN for non-RNs w/degree in other field: Yes

Articulation: LPN to Baccalaureate

For Further Information Contact:

Dr Nightingale Gillespie, Chair
St Francis College
2701 Spring St
Fort Wayne, IN 46808
(219) 434-3239

St Mary's College
—Notre Dame—

Full-Time Enrollments: 65 Evening Classes: No
Part-Time Enrollments: — Weekend Classes: No
Affiliation: Religious Distance Learning: No

NLN ACCREDITATION: Yes

BSN for non-RNs w/degree in other field: Yes

Articulation: None

For Further Information Contact:

Dr M Regan-Kubinski, Chair
St Mary's College
Havican Hall
Notre Dame, IN 46556
(219) 284-4680

University of Evansville
—Evansville—

Full-Time Enrollments: 135 Evening Classes: No
Part-Time Enrollments: — Weekend Classes: No
Affiliation: Private Distance Learning: No

NLN ACCREDITATION: Yes

BSN for non-RNs w/degree in other field: No

Articulation: None

For Further Information Contact:

Dr Rita K Behnke, Chair
University of Evansville
1800 Lincoln Ave
Evansville, IN 47722
(812) 479-2343

University of Indianapolis
—Indianapolis—

Full-Time Enrollments: 84 Evening Classes: No
Part-Time Enrollments: 93 Weekend Classes: No
Affiliation: Religious Distance Learning: No

NLN ACCREDITATION: Yes

BSN for non-RNs w/degree in other field: No

Articulation: None

For Further Information Contact:

Mrs Anita H Siccardi, Coordinator
University of Indianapolis
1400 E Hanna Ave
Indianapolis, IN 46227
(317) 788-3206

University of Southern Indiana-School of Nursing
—Evansville—

Full-Time Enrollments:	124	Evening Classes:	Yes
Part-Time Enrollments:	63	Weekend Classes:	No
Affiliation:	Public	Distance Learning:	Yes

NLN ACCREDITATION: Yes

BSN for non-RNs w/degree in other field: No

Articulation: Associate to Baccalaureate
Diploma to Baccalaureate

For Further Information Contact:

Dr Nadine A Coudret, Dean
University of Southern Indiana-School of Nursing
8600 University Blvd
Evansville, IN 47710
(812) 464-1708

Valparaiso University
—Valparaiso—

Full-Time Enrollments:	207	Evening Classes:	Yes
Part-Time Enrollments:	32	Weekend Classes:	—
Affiliation:	Religious	Distance Learning:	—

NLN ACCREDITATION: Yes

BSN for non-RNs w/degree in other field: Yes

Articulation: Associate to Baccalaureate

For Further Information Contact:

Dr Cynthia Russell, Acting Dean
Valparaiso University
Valparaiso, IN 46383
(219) 464-5289

Iowa

Allen College of Nursing
—Waterloo—

Full-Time Enrollments:	145	Evening Classes:	Yes
Part-Time Enrollments:	51	Weekend Classes:	—
Affiliation:	Private	Distance Learning:	—

NLN ACCREDITATION: Yes

BSN for non-RNs w/degree in other field: No

Articulation: Associate to Baccalaureate
Diploma to Baccalaureate

For Further Information Contact:

Dr Jane Hasek, Chancellor
Allen College of Nursing
1825 Logan Ave
Waterloo, IA 50703
(319) 235-3649

Briar Cliff College
—Sioux City—

Full-Time Enrollments:	42	Evening Classes:	Yes
Part-Time Enrollments:	7	Weekend Classes:	Yes
Affiliation:	Religious	Distance Learning:	Yes

NLN ACCREDITATION: Yes

BSN for non-RNs w/degree in other field: No

Articulation: Associate to Baccalaureate
Diploma to Baccalaureate

For Further Information Contact:

Sr Patricia Miller, Chair
Briar Cliff College
3303 Rebecca St
Sioux City, IA 51104
(712) 279-5497

Clarke College
—Dubuque—

Full-Time Enrollments:	61	Evening Classes:	Yes
Part-Time Enrollments:	2	Weekend Classes:	Yes
Affiliation:	Religious	Distance Learning:	No

NLN ACCREDITATION: Yes

BSN for non-RNs w/degree in other field: No

Articulation: Associate to Baccalaureate
Diploma to Baccalaureate

For Further Information Contact:

Dr D Hames Wertenberger, Chair
Clarke College
1550 Clarke Dr
Dubuque, IA 52001
(319) 588-6406

Coe College
—Cedar Rapids—

Full-Time Enrollments:	37	Evening Classes:	Yes
Part-Time Enrollments:	5	Weekend Classes:	No
Affiliation:	Private	Distance Learning:	No

NLN ACCREDITATION: Yes

BSN for non-RNs w/degree in other field: No

Articulation: Associate to Baccalaureate

For Further Information Contact:

Dr Evelyn J Benda, Chair
Coe College
1220 First Ave NE
Cedar Rapids, IA 52402
(319) 369-8120

Grand View College
—Des Moines—

Full-Time Enrollments:	152	Evening Classes:	Yes
Part-Time Enrollments:	23	Weekend Classes:	No
Affiliation:	Religious	Distance Learning:	Yes

NLN ACCREDITATION: Yes

BSN for non-RNs w/degree in other field: Yes

Articulation: Associate to Baccalaureate
Diploma to Baccalaureate
LPN to Baccalaureate

For Further Information Contact:

Dr Ellen M Strachota, Head
Grand View College
1200 Grandview Ave
Des Moines, IA 50316
(515) 263-2850

Iowa Wesleyan College
—Mount Pleasant—

Full-Time Enrollments:	45	Evening Classes:	Yes
Part-Time Enrollments:	2	Weekend Classes:	No
Affiliation:	Private	Distance Learning:	No

NLN ACCREDITATION: Yes

BSN for non-RNs w/degree in other field: No

Articulation: Associate to Baccalaureate

For Further Information Contact:

Ms Judith Hausner, Chair
Iowa Wesleyan College
601 N Main
Mount Pleasant, IA 52641
(319) 385-6346

Luther College
—Decorah—

Full-Time Enrollments:	146	Evening Classes:	No
Part-Time Enrollments:	4	Weekend Classes:	No
Affiliation:	Religious	Distance Learning:	No

NLN ACCREDITATION: Yes

BSN for non-RNs w/degree in other field: No

Articulation: Associate to Baccalaureate

For Further Information Contact:

Dr Donna Kubesh, Chair
Luther College
700 College Dr
Decorah, IA 52101
(319) 387-1057

Marycrest University International
—Davenport—

Full-Time Enrollments:	59	Evening Classes:	—
Part-Time Enrollments:	—	Weekend Classes:	—
Affiliation:	Private	Distance Learning:	—

NLN ACCREDITATION: Yes

BSN for non-RNs w/degree in other field: No

Articulation: None

For Further Information Contact:

Dr Dolores Hilden, Chair
Marycrest University International
1607 W 12th St
Davenport, IA 52804
(319) 326-9279

Morningside College
—Sioux City—

Full-Time Enrollments:	41	Evening Classes:	Yes
Part-Time Enrollments:	7	Weekend Classes:	No
Affiliation:	Religious	Distance Learning:	No

NLN ACCREDITATION: Yes

BSN for non-RNs w/degree in other field: No

Articulation: Associate to Baccalaureate
Diploma to Baccalaureate

For Further Information Contact:

Dr Kathy Buchheit, Chair
Morningside College
1501 Morningside Ave
Sioux City, IA 51106
(712) 274-5156

Mount Mercy College
—Cedar Rapids—

Full-Time Enrollments:	37	Evening Classes:	Yes
Part-Time Enrollments:	27	Weekend Classes:	Yes
Affiliation:	Religious	Distance Learning:	No

NLN ACCREDITATION: Yes

BSN for non-RNs w/degree in other field: No

Articulation: Associate to Baccalaureate
Diploma to Baccalaureate

For Further Information Contact:

Dr Mary P Tarbox, Chair
Mount Mercy College
1330 Elmhurst Dr, NE
Cedar Rapids, IA 52402
(319) 368-6471

University of Iowa
—Iowa City—

Full-Time Enrollments:	226	Evening Classes:	No
Part-Time Enrollments:	147	Weekend Classes:	No
Affiliation:	Public	Distance Learning:	Yes

NLN ACCREDITATION: Yes

BSN for non-RNs w/degree in other field: No

Articulation: Associate to Baccalaureate
Diploma to Baccalaureate

For Further Information Contact:

Dr Geraldene Felton, Dean
University of Iowa
101 Nursing Bldg
Iowa City, IA 52242-1121
(319) 335-7018

Kansas

Baker University
—Topeka—

Full-Time Enrollments:	99	Evening Classes:	No
Part-Time Enrollments:	9	Weekend Classes:	—
Affiliation:	Public	Distance Learning:	No

NLN ACCREDITATION: Yes

BSN for non-RNs w/degree in other field: No

Articulation: None

For Further Information Contact:

Dr Mary Turley, Dean
Baker University
1500 W 10th
Topeka, KS 66604
(913) 354-5854

Bethel College
—North Newton—

Full-Time Enrollments:	—	Evening Classes:	—
Part-Time Enrollments:	—	Weekend Classes:	—
Affiliation:	Religious	Distance Learning:	—

NLN ACCREDITATION: Yes

BSN for non-RNs w/degree in other field: —

Articulation: None

For Further Information Contact:

Dr J Unruh Davidson, Chair
Bethel College
300 E 27th St
North Newton, KS 67117
(316) 283-2500

Emporia State University
—Emporia—

Full-Time Enrollments:	80	Evening Classes:	No
Part-Time Enrollments:	—	Weekend Classes:	No
Affiliation:	Public	Distance Learning:	No

NLN ACCREDITATION: Yes

BSN for non-RNs w/degree in other field: No

Articulation: Diploma to Baccalaureate
LPN to Baccalaureate

For Further Information Contact:

Dr Merle Bolz, Chair
Emporia State University
1127 Chestnut St
Emporia, KS 66801
(316) 343-6800

Fort Hays State University
—Hays—

Full-Time Enrollments:	88	Evening Classes:	Yes
Part-Time Enrollments:	—	Weekend Classes:	Yes
Affiliation:	Public	Distance Learning:	Yes

NLN ACCREDITATION: Yes

BSN for non-RNs w/degree in other field: No

Articulation: Associate to Baccalaureate
Diploma to Baccalaureate

For Further Information Contact:

Dr Mary Hassett, Chair
Fort Hays State University
600 Park St Stroup Hall
Hays, KS 67601
(913) 628-4498

Kansas Newman College
—Wichita—

Full-Time Enrollments:	91	Evening Classes:	No
Part-Time Enrollments:	6	Weekend Classes:	No
Affiliation:	Religious	Distance Learning:	No

NLN ACCREDITATION: Yes

BSN for non-RNs w/degree in other field: No

Articulation: None

For Further Information Contact:

Dr Joan Felts, Chair
Kansas Newman College
3100 McCormick
Wichita, KS 67213
(316) 942-4291

BACCALAUREATE DEGREE

Kansas University-School of Nursing
—Kansas City—

Full-Time Enrollments: 229   Evening Classes: No
Part-Time Enrollments: 22   Weekend Classes: No
Affiliation: Public   Distance Learning: No

NLN ACCREDITATION: Yes

BSN for non-RNs w/degree in other field: No

Articulation: Associate to Baccalaureate
Diploma to Baccalaureate
RN to MSN

For Further Information Contact:

Dr Karen Miller, Dean
Kansas University-School of Nursing
3901 Rainbow Blvd
Kansas City, KS 66160-7500
(913) 588-1619

Mid-America Nazarene College
—Olathe—

Full-Time Enrollments: 115   Evening Classes: No
Part-Time Enrollments: 12   Weekend Classes: No
Affiliation: Religious   Distance Learning: No

NLN ACCREDITATION: Yes

BSN for non-RNs w/degree in other field: Yes

Articulation: None

For Further Information Contact:

Dr Palma Smith, Chair
Mid-America Nazarene College
2030 E College Way
Olathe, KS 66062-1899
(913) 782-3750

Pittsburg State University
—Pittsburg—

Full-Time Enrollments: 140   Evening Classes: —
Part-Time Enrollments: —   Weekend Classes: —
Affiliation: Public   Distance Learning: —

NLN ACCREDITATION: Yes

BSN for non-RNs w/degree in other field: No

Articulation: None

For Further Information Contact:

Dr Jo-Ann Marrs, Chair
Pittsburg State University
Pittsburg, KS 66762
(316) 235-4431

Southwestern College
—Winfield—

Full-Time Enrollments: —   Evening Classes: —
Part-Time Enrollments: —   Weekend Classes: —
Affiliation: Religious   Distance Learning: —

NLN ACCREDITATION: Yes

BSN for non-RNs w/degree in other field: —

Articulation: None

For Further Information Contact:

Dr Martha R Butler, Director
Southwestern College
100 College St
Winfield, KS 67156
(316) 221-4150

Washburn University of Topeka
—Topeka—

Full-Time Enrollments: 200   Evening Classes: Yes
Part-Time Enrollments: 31   Weekend Classes: No
Affiliation: Public   Distance Learning: Yes

NLN ACCREDITATION: Yes

BSN for non-RNs w/degree in other field: No

Articulation: Associate to Baccalaureate
Diploma to Baccalaureate
LPN to Baccalaureate

For Further Information Contact:

Dr Alice Adam Young, Dean
Washburn University of Topeka
1700 College St
Topeka, KS 66621
(913) 231-1010

Wichita State University
—Wichita—

Full-Time Enrollments: 154   Evening Classes: Yes
Part-Time Enrollments: 1   Weekend Classes: Yes
Affiliation: Public   Distance Learning: Yes

NLN ACCREDITATION: Yes

BSN for non-RNs w/degree in other field: No

Articulation: Associate to Baccalaureate
Diploma to Baccalaureate
LPN to Baccalaureate
RN to MSN

For Further Information Contact:

Dr Bonnie Holaday, Chair
Wichita State University
1845 Fairmount
Wichita, KS 67208
(316) 978-3610

Kentucky

Bellarmine College
—Louisville—

Full-Time Enrollments:	145	Evening Classes:	Yes
Part-Time Enrollments:	87	Weekend Classes:	Yes
Affiliation:	Private	Distance Learning:	Yes

NLN ACCREDITATION: Yes

BSN for non-RNs w/degree in other field: No

Articulation: Associate to Baccalaureate
Diploma to Baccalaureate

For Further Information Contact:

Dr Susan Hockenberger, Dean
Bellarmine College
2001 Newburg Rd
Louisville, KY 40205-0671
(502) 452-8414

Berea College
—Berea—

Full-Time Enrollments:	37	Evening Classes:	No
Part-Time Enrollments:	—	Weekend Classes:	No
Affiliation:	Religious	Distance Learning:	No

NLN ACCREDITATION: Yes

BSN for non-RNs w/degree in other field: No

Articulation: None

For Further Information Contact:

Dr Cora Newell-Withrow, Chair
Berea College
2290 College Sta
Berea, KY 40404
(606) 986-9341

Eastern Kentucky University
—Richmond—

Full-Time Enrollments:	160	Evening Classes:	—
Part-Time Enrollments:	81	Weekend Classes:	—
Affiliation:	Public	Distance Learning:	—

NLN ACCREDITATION: Yes

BSN for non-RNs w/degree in other field: No

Articulation: None

For Further Information Contact:

Dr D McNeil Whitehouse, Chair
Eastern Kentucky University
Rowlett Bldg Rm 220
Richmond, KY 40475-0956
(606) 622-1956

Morehead State University
—Morehead—

Full-Time Enrollments:	92	Evening Classes:	Yes
Part-Time Enrollments:	—	Weekend Classes:	No
Affiliation:	Public	Distance Learning:	Yes

NLN ACCREDITATION: Yes

BSN for non-RNs w/degree in other field: No

Articulation: Associate to Baccalaureate

For Further Information Contact:

Dr Betty Porter, Chair
Morehead State University
234 Reed Hall
Morehead, KY 40351
(606) 783-2639

Murray State University
—Murray—

Full-Time Enrollments:	154	Evening Classes:	Yes
Part-Time Enrollments:	22	Weekend Classes:	No
Affiliation:	Public	Distance Learning:	Yes

NLN ACCREDITATION: Yes

BSN for non-RNs w/degree in other field: No

Articulation: None

For Further Information Contact:

Dr Marcia Blix Hobbs, Chair
Murray State University
PO Box 9
Murray, KY 42071
(502) 762-2193

Spalding University
—Louisville—

Full-Time Enrollments:	177	Evening Classes:	Yes
Part-Time Enrollments:	—	Weekend Classes:	Yes
Affiliation:	Private	Distance Learning:	—

NLN ACCREDITATION: Yes

BSN for non-RNs w/degree in other field: No

Articulation: Associate to Baccalaureate

For Further Information Contact:

Dr Marjorie Perrin, Dean
Spalding University
851 S 4th St
Louisville, KY 40203
(502) 585-9911

Thomas More College
—Crestview Hills—

Full-Time Enrollments:	—	Evening Classes:	—
Part-Time Enrollments:	—	Weekend Classes:	—
Affiliation:	Religious	Distance Learning:	—

NLN ACCREDITATION: Yes

BSN for non-RNs w/degree in other field: —

Articulation: None

For Further Information Contact:

Mrs Mary E Kelley, Chair
Thomas More College
333 Thomas More Pkwy
Crestview Hills, KY 41017

Thomas More College (2 Campuses)
—Crestview Hills—

Full-Time Enrollments:	70	Evening Classes:	—
Part-Time Enrollments:	—	Weekend Classes:	—
Affiliation:	Religious	Distance Learning:	—

NLN ACCREDITATION: Yes

BSN for non-RNs w/degree in other field: No

Articulation: None

For Further Information Contact:

Mrs Mary E Kelley, Chair
Thomas More College (2 Campuses)
2771 Turkeyfoot Rd
Crestview Hills, KY 41017
(606) 344-3412

University of Kentucky-College of Nursing
—Lexington—

Full-Time Enrollments:	284	Evening Classes:	Yes
Part-Time Enrollments:	23	Weekend Classes:	Yes
Affiliation:	Public	Distance Learning:	Yes

NLN ACCREDITATION: Yes

BSN for non-RNs w/degree in other field: No

Articulation: Associate to Baccalaureate
Diploma to Baccalaureate
RN to MSN

For Further Information Contact:

Dr Carolyn Williams, Dean
University of Kentucky-College of Nursing
760 Rose Street, Room 315
Lexington, KY 40536-0232
(606) 323-6533

University of Louisville
—Louisville—

Full-Time Enrollments:	187	Evening Classes:	Yes
Part-Time Enrollments:	120	Weekend Classes:	—
Affiliation:	Public	Distance Learning:	—

NLN ACCREDITATION: Yes

BSN for non-RNs w/degree in other field: No

Articulation: Associate to Baccalaureate
Diploma to Baccalaureate
RN to MSN

For Further Information Contact:

Dr Paulette Adams, Acting Dean
University of Louisville
Hlth Science Center
Louisville, KY 40292
(502) 852-5366

Western Kentucky University (2 Campuses)
—Bowling Green—

Full-Time Enrollments:	102	Evening Classes:	—
Part-Time Enrollments:	—	Weekend Classes:	—
Affiliation:	Public	Distance Learning:	—

NLN ACCREDITATION: Yes

BSN for non-RNs w/degree in other field: No

Articulation: None

For Further Information Contact:

Dr Kay Carr, Interim Head
Western Kentucky University (2 Campuses)
Dept of Nursing
Bowling Green, KY 42101
(502) 745-3791

Louisiana

Dillard University
—New Orleans—

Full-Time Enrollments:	150	Evening Classes:	No
Part-Time Enrollments:	6	Weekend Classes:	No
Affiliation:	Religious	Distance Learning:	No

NLN ACCREDITATION: Yes

BSN for non-RNs w/degree in other field: No

Articulation: Associate to Baccalaureate
LPN to Baccalaureate

For Further Information Contact:

Dr Enrica K Singleton, Chair
Dillard University
2601 Gentilly Blvd
New Orleans, LA 70122-3097
(504) 283-8822

Grambling State University
—Grambling—

Full-Time Enrollments:	249	Evening Classes:	Yes
Part-Time Enrollments:	—	Weekend Classes:	No
Affiliation:	Public	Distance Learning:	No

NLN ACCREDITATION: Yes

BSN for non-RNs w/degree in other field:　No

Articulation:　Diploma to Baccalaureate
　　　　　　　LPN to Baccalaureate

For Further Information Contact:

Dr Betty E Smith, Dean
Grambling State University
Box 4272
Grambling, LA 71245
(318) 274-2672

Louisiana College
—Pineville—

Full-Time Enrollments:	66	Evening Classes:	No
Part-Time Enrollments:	—	Weekend Classes:	No
Affiliation:	Religious	Distance Learning:	No

NLN ACCREDITATION: Yes

BSN for non-RNs w/degree in other field:　No

Articulation:　Associate to Baccalaureate
　　　　　　　Diploma to Baccalaureate

For Further Information Contact:

Dr Anne Fortenberry, Div Chair
Louisiana College
PO Box 556 CS
Pineville, LA 71359
(318) 487-7127

Louisiana State University Medical Center
—New Orleans—

Full-Time Enrollments:	377	Evening Classes:	No
Part-Time Enrollments:	35	Weekend Classes:	No
Affiliation:	Public	Distance Learning:	No

NLN ACCREDITATION: Yes

BSN for non-RNs w/degree in other field:　No

Articulation:　Associate to Baccalaureate
　　　　　　　Diploma to Baccalaureate

For Further Information Contact:

Dr Elizabeth Humphrey, Acting Dean
Louisiana State University Medical Center
1900 Gravier St
New Orleans, LA 70112-2262
(504) 568-4114

McNeese State University
—Lake Charles—

Full-Time Enrollments:	276	Evening Classes:	No
Part-Time Enrollments:	158	Weekend Classes:	No
Affiliation:	Public	Distance Learning:	Yes

NLN ACCREDITATION: Yes

BSN for non-RNs w/degree in other field:　No

Articulation:　Associate to Baccalaureate
　　　　　　　LPN to Baccalaureate

For Further Information Contact:

Dr Anita Fields, Dean
McNeese State University
PO Box 90415
Lake Charles, LA 70609
(318) 475-5822

Nicholls State University Department of Nursing
—Thibodaux—

Full-Time Enrollments:	155	Evening Classes:	Yes
Part-Time Enrollments:	—	Weekend Classes:	Yes
Affiliation:	Public	Distance Learning:	—

NLN ACCREDITATION: Yes

BSN for non-RNs w/degree in other field:　No

Articulation:　Associate to Baccalaureate
　　　　　　　Diploma to Baccalaureate
　　　　　　　LPN to Baccalaureate

For Further Information Contact:

Dr Demetrius Porche, Director
Nicholls State University Department of Nursing
College Sta, PO Box 2143
Thibodaux, LA 70310
(504) 448-4696

Northeast Louisiana University
—Monroe—

Full-Time Enrollments:	198	Evening Classes:	No
Part-Time Enrollments:	12	Weekend Classes:	No
Affiliation:	Public	Distance Learning:	No

NLN ACCREDITATION: Yes

BSN for non-RNs w/degree in other field:　Yes

Articulation:　Associate to Baccalaureate
　　　　　　　Diploma to Baccalaureate
　　　　　　　LPN to Baccalaureate

For Further Information Contact:

Dr Barbara Heil-Foss, Director
Northeast Louisiana University
700 Univ Ave
Monroe, LA 71209-0460
(318) 342-1644

Northwestern State University of Louisiana
—Shreveport—

Full-Time Enrollments: 743   Evening Classes: Yes
Part-Time Enrollments: 211   Weekend Classes: No
Affiliation: Public   Distance Learning: Yes

NLN ACCREDITATION: Yes

BSN for non-RNs w/degree in other field: No

Articulation: Associate to Baccalaureate
                 Diploma to Baccalaureate
                 LPN to Baccalaureate
                 LPN to Associate

For Further Information Contact:

Dr Norann Planchock, Acting Director
Northwestern State University of Louisiana
1800 Line Ave
Shreveport, LA 71101
(318) 677-3100

Our Lady of Holy Cross College
—New Orleans—

Full-Time Enrollments: 101   Evening Classes: No
Part-Time Enrollments: 31   Weekend Classes: No
Affiliation: Religious Distance Learning: No

NLN ACCREDITATION: Yes

BSN for non-RNs w/degree in other field: No

Articulation: None

For Further Information Contact:

Dr Margaret T Shannon, Dean
Our Lady of Holy Cross College
4123 Woodland Dr
New Orleans, LA 70131
(504) 394-7744

Southeastern Louisiana University
—Hammond—

Full-Time Enrollments: 1071   Evening Classes: Yes
Part-Time Enrollments: 505   Weekend Classes: No
Affiliation: Public   Distance Learning: Yes

NLN ACCREDITATION: Yes

BSN for non-RNs w/degree in other field: No

Articulation: Associate to Baccalaureate
                 Diploma to Baccalaureate
                 LPN to Baccalaureate

For Further Information Contact:

Dr Ellienne T Tate, Dean
Southeastern Louisiana University
University Sta, Box 781
Hammond, LA 70402
(504) 549-3772

Southern University-Baton Rouge
—Baton Rouge—

Full-Time Enrollments: 514   Evening Classes: Yes
Part-Time Enrollments: 461   Weekend Classes: Yes
Affiliation: Public   Distance Learning: No

NLN ACCREDITATION: Yes

BSN for non-RNs w/degree in other field: No

Articulation: None

For Further Information Contact:

Dr Janet Rami, Dean
Southern University-Baton Rouge
Baton Rouge, LA 70813
(504) 771-2151

University of Southwestern Louisiana
—Lafayette—

Full-Time Enrollments: 1003   Evening Classes: Yes
Part-Time Enrollments: 179   Weekend Classes: No
Affiliation: Public   Distance Learning: No

NLN ACCREDITATION: Yes

BSN for non-RNs w/degree in other field: No

Articulation: Associate to Baccalaureate
                 LPN to Baccalaureate

For Further Information Contact:

Dr Evelyn Redding, Dean
University of Southwestern Louisiana
USL Sta, PO Box 42490
Lafayette, LA 70504
(318) 482-6808

William Carey College
—New Orleans—

Full-Time Enrollments: —   Evening Classes: —
Part-Time Enrollments: —   Weekend Classes: —
Affiliation: Religious Distance Learning: —

NLN ACCREDITATION: Yes

BSN for non-RNs w/degree in other field: No

Articulation: None

For Further Information Contact:

Dr Annette Barrar, Dean
William Carey College
2700 Napoleon Ave
New Orleans, LA 70115
(504) 865-1502

Maine

Husson College-Eastern Maine Medical Center
—Bangor—

Full-Time Enrollments:	166	Evening Classes:	Yes
Part-Time Enrollments:	52	Weekend Classes:	Yes
Affiliation:	Private	Distance Learning:	No

NLN ACCREDITATION: Yes

BSN for non-RNs w/degree in other field: No

Articulation: Associate to Baccalaureate
RN to MSN

For Further Information Contact:

Dr Elizabeth Burns, Dean
Husson College-Eastern Maine Medical Center
1 College Circle
Bangor, ME 04401
(207) 941-7000

Saint Joseph's College
—Standish—

Full-Time Enrollments:	149	Evening Classes:	No
Part-Time Enrollments:	1	Weekend Classes:	No
Affiliation:	Religious	Distance Learning:	Yes

NLN ACCREDITATION: Yes

BSN for non-RNs w/degree in other field: No

Articulation: Associate to Baccalaureate
Diploma to Baccalaureate
LPN to Baccalaureate

For Further Information Contact:

Dr Holley Gimpel, Chair
Saint Joseph's College
278 White Bridge Rd
Standish, ME 04084-5263
(207) 893-6766

University of Maine
—Orono—

Full-Time Enrollments:	460	Evening Classes:	—
Part-Time Enrollments:	14	Weekend Classes:	—
Affiliation:	Public	Distance Learning:	—

NLN ACCREDITATION: Yes

BSN for non-RNs w/degree in other field: No

Articulation: None

For Further Information Contact:

Dr Therese Shipps, Interim Director
University of Maine
5724 Dunn Hall
Orono, ME 04669
(207) 581-2600

University of Maine at Fort Kent
—Fort Kent—

Full-Time Enrollments:	67	Evening Classes:	Yes
Part-Time Enrollments:	10	Weekend Classes:	Yes
Affiliation:	Public	Distance Learning:	Yes

NLN ACCREDITATION: Yes

BSN for non-RNs w/degree in other field: No

Articulation: Associate to Baccalaureate

For Further Information Contact:

Mr Vincent Pelletier, Director
University of Maine at Fort Kent
25 Pleasant St
Fort Kent, ME 04743
(207) 834-3162

University of Southern Maine
—Portland—

Full-Time Enrollments:	108	Evening Classes:	Yes
Part-Time Enrollments:	63	Weekend Classes:	Yes
Affiliation:	Public	Distance Learning:	Yes

NLN ACCREDITATION: Yes

BSN for non-RNs w/degree in other field: No

Articulation: Associate to Baccalaureate
Diploma to Baccalaureate
RN to MSN

For Further Information Contact:

Dr Patricia Geary, Dean
University of Southern Maine
96 Falmouth St
Portland, ME 04103
(207) 780-4133

University of Southern Maine
—Portland—

Full-Time Enrollments:	29	Evening Classes:	Yes
Part-Time Enrollments:	1	Weekend Classes:	Yes
Affiliation:	Public	Distance Learning:	Yes

NLN ACCREDITATION: Yes

BSN for non-RNs w/degree in other field: No

Articulation: Associate to Baccalaureate
RN to MSN

For Further Information Contact:

Dr Patricia Geary, Dean
University of Southern Maine
96 Falmouth St
Portland, ME 04103
(207) 780-4133

Westbrook College\University of New England
—Portland—

Full-Time Enrollments:	54	Evening Classes:	Yes
Part-Time Enrollments:	—	Weekend Classes:	Yes
Affiliation:	Private	Distance Learning:	No

NLN ACCREDITATION: Yes

BSN for non-RNs w/degree in other field: No

Articulation: Associate to Baccalaureate

For Further Information Contact:

Dr Catherine Berardelli, Director
Westbrook College\University of New England
716 Stevens Ave
Portland, ME 04103
(207) 797-7261

Maryland

Columbia Union College
—Takoma Park—

Full-Time Enrollments:	73	Evening Classes:	Yes
Part-Time Enrollments:	2	Weekend Classes:	No
Affiliation:	Private	Distance Learning:	No

NLN ACCREDITATION: Yes

BSN for non-RNs w/degree in other field: Yes

Articulation: Associate to Baccalaureate
Diploma to Baccalaureate

For Further Information Contact:

Dr Shirley Wilson-Anderson, Chair
Columbia Union College
7600 Flower Ave
Takoma Park, MD 20912
(301) 891-4144

Coppin State College-Helene Fuld School of Nursing
—Baltimore—

Full-Time Enrollments:	149	Evening Classes:	Yes
Part-Time Enrollments:	1	Weekend Classes:	No
Affiliation:	Public	Distance Learning:	No

NLN ACCREDITATION: Yes

BSN for non-RNs w/degree in other field: No

Articulation: Associate to Baccalaureate
Diploma to Baccalaureate

For Further Information Contact:

Dr Doris Starks, Dean
Coppin State College-Helene Fuld School of Nursing
2500 W North Ave
Baltimore, MD 21216
(410) 383-5546

Johns Hopkins University
—Baltimore—

Full-Time Enrollments:	267	Evening Classes:	No
Part-Time Enrollments:	8	Weekend Classes:	No
Affiliation:	Private	Distance Learning:	No

NLN ACCREDITATION: Yes

BSN for non-RNs w/degree in other field: Yes

Articulation: None

For Further Information Contact:

Dr Sue Donaldson, Dean
Johns Hopkins University
1830 E Monument St #437
Baltimore, MD 21205-2100
(410) 955-7544

Salisbury State University
—Salisbury—

Full-Time Enrollments:	107	Evening Classes:	Yes
Part-Time Enrollments:	4	Weekend Classes:	No
Affiliation:	Public	Distance Learning:	No

NLN ACCREDITATION: Yes

BSN for non-RNs w/degree in other field: Yes

Articulation: Associate to Baccalaureate
Diploma to Baccalaureate

For Further Information Contact:

Dr Lisa Seldomridge, Chair
Salisbury State University
Salisbury, MD 21801
(410) 543-6402

Towson State University
—Towson—

Full-Time Enrollments:	155	Evening Classes:	Yes
Part-Time Enrollments:	16	Weekend Classes:	No
Affiliation:	Public	Distance Learning:	No

NLN ACCREDITATION: Yes

BSN for non-RNs w/degree in other field: No

Articulation: Associate to Baccalaureate
Diploma to Baccalaureate

For Further Information Contact:

Dr Cynthia E Kielinen, Chair
Towson State University
Towson, MD 21204
(410) 830-2067

University of Maryland
—Baltimore—

Full-Time Enrollments:	425	Evening Classes:	Yes
Part-Time Enrollments:	46	Weekend Classes:	No
Affiliation:	Public	Distance Learning:	Yes

NLN ACCREDITATION: Yes

BSN for non-RNs w/degree in other field: Yes

Articulation: Associate to Baccalaureate
Diploma to Baccalaureate
RN to MSN

For Further Information Contact:

Dr Barbara R Heller, Dean
University of Maryland
655 W Lombard St
Baltimore, MD 21201
(410) 706-6741

Villa Julie College/Union Memorial Hospital
—Stevenson—

Full-Time Enrollments:	173	Evening Classes:	Yes
Part-Time Enrollments:	153	Weekend Classes:	Yes
Affiliation:	Private	Distance Learning:	No

NLN ACCREDITATION: Yes

BSN for non-RNs w/degree in other field: No

Articulation: None

For Further Information Contact:

Dr Judith Feustle, Chair
Villa Julie College/Union Memorial Hospital
Greenspring Valley Rd
Stevenson, MD 21153
(410) 554-2055

Massachusetts

American International College
—Springfield—

Full-Time Enrollments:	178	Evening Classes:	No
Part-Time Enrollments:	—	Weekend Classes:	No
Affiliation:	Private	Distance Learning:	No

NLN ACCREDITATION: Yes

BSN for non-RNs w/degree in other field: No

Articulation: Associate to Baccalaureate

For Further Information Contact:

Dr Anne R Glanovsky, Director
American International College
1000 State St
Springfield, MA 01109
(413) 747-6361

Boston College
—Chestnut Hill—

Full-Time Enrollments:	322	Evening Classes:	No
Part-Time Enrollments:	—	Weekend Classes:	No
Affiliation:	Religious	Distance Learning:	No

NLN ACCREDITATION: Yes

BSN for non-RNs w/degree in other field: Yes

Articulation: None

For Further Information Contact:

Dr Barbara Hazard Munro, Dean
Boston College
140 Commonwealth Ave
Chestnut Hill, MA 02167
(617) 552-4274

College of Our Lady of the Elms
—Chicopee—

Full-Time Enrollments:	160	Evening Classes:	Yes
Part-Time Enrollments:	42	Weekend Classes:	Yes
Affiliation:	Religious	Distance Learning:	No

NLN ACCREDITATION: Yes

BSN for non-RNs w/degree in other field: No

Articulation: Associate to Baccalaureate
Diploma to Baccalaureate

For Further Information Contact:

Dr Jeannine Muldoon, Director
College of Our Lady of the Elms
291 Springfield St
Chicopee, MA 01013
(413) 594-2761

Curry College
—Milton—

Full-Time Enrollments:	148	Evening Classes:	Yes
Part-Time Enrollments:	30	Weekend Classes:	No
Affiliation:	Private	Distance Learning:	No

NLN ACCREDITATION: Yes

BSN for non-RNs w/degree in other field: No

Articulation: Diploma to Baccalaureate

For Further Information Contact:

Dr Elizabeth Kudzma, Chair
Curry College
1071 Blue Hill Ave
Milton, MA 02186
(617) 333-0500

Fitchburg State College
—Fitchburg—

Full-Time Enrollments:	349	Evening Classes:	No
Part-Time Enrollments:	—	Weekend Classes:	No
Affiliation:	Public	Distance Learning:	No

NLN ACCREDITATION: Yes

BSN for non-RNs w/degree in other field: No

Articulation: Associate to Baccalaureate

For Further Information Contact:

Dr Sophia Harrell, Chair
Fitchburg State College
160 Pearl St
Fitchburg, MA 01420
(508) 665-3221

Massachusetts General Hospital Institute of Health Professions
—Boston—

Full-Time Enrollments:	—	Evening Classes:	—
Part-Time Enrollments:	—	Weekend Classes:	—
Affiliation:	Private	Distance Learning:	—

NLN ACCREDITATION: Yes

BSN for non-RNs w/degree in other field: —

Articulation: —

For Further Information Contact:

Dr Arlene Lowenstein, Director
Massachusetts General Hospital Institute of Health Professions
101 Merrimac St
Boston, MA 02114-4719
(617) 726-3163

Northeastern University
—Boston—

Full-Time Enrollments:	558	Evening Classes:	Yes
Part-Time Enrollments:	—	Weekend Classes:	No
Affiliation:	Private	Distance Learning:	No

NLN ACCREDITATION: Yes

BSN for non-RNs w/degree in other field: No

Articulation: None

For Further Information Contact:

Dr Eileen Zungolo, Dean
Northeastern University
360 Huntington Ave
Boston, MA 02115
(617) 373-3102

Regis College
—Weston—

Full-Time Enrollments:	40	Evening Classes:	Yes
Part-Time Enrollments:	5	Weekend Classes:	—
Affiliation:	Religious	Distance Learning:	—

NLN ACCREDITATION: Yes

BSN for non-RNs w/degree in other field: No

Articulation: Associate to Baccalaureate
Diploma to Baccalaureate

For Further Information Contact:

Dr Amy Anderson, Chair
Regis College
235 Wells
Weston, MA 02193
(617) 768-7090

Salem State College-South Campus
—Salem—

Full-Time Enrollments:	380	Evening Classes:	—
Part-Time Enrollments:	95	Weekend Classes:	—
Affiliation:	Public	Distance Learning:	—

NLN ACCREDITATION: Yes

BSN for non-RNs w/degree in other field: No

Articulation: None

For Further Information Contact:

Dr Joanne Evans, Chair
Salem State College-South Campus
352 Lafayette
Salem, MA 01970
(508) 741-6649

Simmons College
—Boston—

Full-Time Enrollments:	—	Evening Classes:	—
Part-Time Enrollments:	—	Weekend Classes:	—
Affiliation:	Private	Distance Learning:	—

NLN ACCREDITATION: Yes

BSN for non-RNs w/degree in other field: —

Articulation: None

For Further Information Contact:

Dr Penelope Glynn, Chair
Simmons College
300 The Fenway
Boston, MA 02115
(617) 521-2531

University Massachusetts/Dartmouth
—North Dartmouth—

Full-Time Enrollments:	233	Evening Classes:	—
Part-Time Enrollments:	43	Weekend Classes:	—
Affiliation:	Public	Distance Learning:	—

NLN ACCREDITATION: Yes

BSN for non-RNs w/degree in other field: No

Articulation: Associate to Baccalaureate

For Further Information Contact:

Dr Elisabeth Pennington, Dean
University Massachusetts/Dartmouth
Old Westport Rd
North Dartmouth, MA 02747
(508) 999-8586

University of Massachusetts
—Amherst—

Full-Time Enrollments:	177	Evening Classes:	No
Part-Time Enrollments:	—	Weekend Classes:	No
Affiliation:	Public	Distance Learning:	Yes

NLN ACCREDITATION: Yes

BSN for non-RNs w/degree in other field: Yes

Articulation: Associate to Baccalaureate
Diploma to Baccalaureate

For Further Information Contact:

Dr Melanie C Dreher, Dean
University of Massachusetts
Arnold House Rm 317
Amherst, MA 01003
(413) 545-2703

University of Massachusetts
—Amherst—

Full-Time Enrollments:	29	Evening Classes:	No
Part-Time Enrollments:	—	Weekend Classes:	No
Affiliation:	Public	Distance Learning:	Yes

NLN ACCREDITATION: Yes

BSN for non-RNs w/degree in other field: No

Articulation: LPN to Baccalaureate
LPN to Associate

For Further Information Contact:

Dr Melanie C Dreher, Dean
University of Massachusetts
Arnold House Rm 317
Amherst, MA 01003
(413) 545-2703

University of Massachusetts, Lowell
—Lowell—

Full-Time Enrollments:	203	Evening Classes:	No
Part-Time Enrollments:	—	Weekend Classes:	No
Affiliation:	Public	Distance Learning:	Yes

NLN ACCREDITATION: Yes

BSN for non-RNs w/degree in other field: No

Articulation: Associate to Baccalaureate

For Further Information Contact:

Dr May Futrell, Chair
University of Massachusetts, Lowell
One Univ Ave
Lowell, MA 01854
(508) 934-4467

University of Massachusetts-Boston College of Nursing
—Boston—

Full-Time Enrollments:	301	Evening Classes:	Yes
Part-Time Enrollments:	164	Weekend Classes:	No
Affiliation:	Public	Distance Learning:	No

NLN ACCREDITATION: Yes

BSN for non-RNs w/degree in other field: No

Articulation: Associate to Baccalaureate

For Further Information Contact:

Dr Brenda S Cherry, Dean
University of Massachusetts-Boston College of Nursing
100 Morrissey Blvd
Boston, MA 02125-3393
(617) 287-7500

Worcester State University-Department of Nursing
—Worcester—

Full-Time Enrollments:	98	Evening Classes:	No
Part-Time Enrollments:	—	Weekend Classes:	No
Affiliation:	Public	Distance Learning:	No

NLN ACCREDITATION: Yes

BSN for non-RNs w/degree in other field: No

Articulation: Associate to Baccalaureate
Diploma to Baccalaureate

For Further Information Contact:

Dr Anne Brown, Chair
Worcester State University-Department of Nursing
486 Chandler St
Worcester, MA 01602
(508) 793-8129

Michigan

Andrews University
—Berrien Springs—

Full-Time Enrollments:	100	Evening Classes:	Yes
Part-Time Enrollments:	56	Weekend Classes:	No
Affiliation:	Religious	Distance Learning:	Yes

NLN ACCREDITATION: Yes

BSN for non-RNs w/degree in other field: Yes

Articulation: None

For Further Information Contact:

Dr Patricia Scott, Chair
Andrews University
Berrien Springs, MI 49104
(616) 471-3311

Eastern Michigan University
—Ypsilanti—

Full-Time Enrollments:	218	Evening Classes:	—
Part-Time Enrollments:	—	Weekend Classes:	—
Affiliation:	Public	Distance Learning:	—

NLN ACCREDITATION: Yes

BSN for non-RNs w/degree in other field: No

Articulation: None

For Further Information Contact:

Dr Regina Williams, Dept Head
Eastern Michigan University
228 King Hall
Ypsilanti, MI 48197
(313) 487-2310

Grand Valley State University
—Allendale—

Full-Time Enrollments:	209	Evening Classes:	No
Part-Time Enrollments:	7	Weekend Classes:	No
Affiliation:	Public	Distance Learning:	Yes

NLN ACCREDITATION: Yes

BSN for non-RNs w/degree in other field: Yes

Articulation: Associate to Baccalaureate
Diploma to Baccalaureate

For Further Information Contact:

Dr Mary Horan, Dean
Grand Valley State University
167 Lake Michigan Hall
Allendale, MI 49401
(616) 895-3558

Hope-Calvin Department of Nursing
—Grand Rapids—

Full-Time Enrollments:	137	Evening Classes:	No
Part-Time Enrollments:	1	Weekend Classes:	No
Affiliation:	Religious	Distance Learning:	No

NLN ACCREDITATION: Yes

BSN for non-RNs w/degree in other field: No

Articulation: None

For Further Information Contact:

Dr Marjorie Viehl, Chair
Hope-Calvin Department of Nursing
3201 Burton SE c/o Calvin Coll
Grand Rapids, MI 49546-4388
(616) 957-7076

Lake Superior State University
—Sault Ste Marie—

Full-Time Enrollments:	187	Evening Classes:	Yes
Part-Time Enrollments:	24	Weekend Classes:	Yes
Affiliation:	Public	Distance Learning:	Yes

NLN ACCREDITATION: Yes

BSN for non-RNs w/degree in other field: No

Articulation: Associate to Baccalaureate
Diploma to Baccalaureate

For Further Information Contact:

Dr Mae E Markstrom, Dean
Lake Superior State University
1000 College Dr
Sault Ste Marie, MI 49783
(906) 635-2599

Madonna University-College of Nursing & Health
—Livonia—

Full-Time Enrollments:	260	Evening Classes:	Yes
Part-Time Enrollments:	240	Weekend Classes:	Yes
Affiliation:	Religious	Distance Learning:	No

NLN ACCREDITATION: Yes

BSN for non-RNs w/degree in other field: No

Articulation: Associate to Baccalaureate

For Further Information Contact:

Dr Mary Wawrzynski, Dean
Madonna University-College of Nursing & Health
36600 Schoolcraft Rd
Livonia, MI 48150
(313) 432-5465

Michigan State University
—East Lansing—

Full-Time Enrollments:	151	Evening Classes:	No
Part-Time Enrollments:	123	Weekend Classes:	No
Affiliation:	Public	Distance Learning:	No

NLN ACCREDITATION: Yes

BSN for non-RNs w/degree in other field: No

Articulation: None

For Further Information Contact:

Dr Marilyn Rothert, Dean
Michigan State University
A230 Life Sciences Bldg
East Lansing, MI 48824-1317
(517) 353-4827

Northern Michigan University
—Marquette—

Full-Time Enrollments:	129	Evening Classes:	Yes
Part-Time Enrollments:	61	Weekend Classes:	Yes
Affiliation:	Public	Distance Learning:	Yes

NLN ACCREDITATION: Yes

BSN for non-RNs w/degree in other field: No

Articulation: Associate to Baccalaureate

For Further Information Contact:

Dr Betty Hill, Dean
Northern Michigan University
202 Magers Hall
Marquette, MI 49855
(906) 227-2830

Oakland University
—Rochester—

Full-Time Enrollments:	165	Evening Classes:	Yes
Part-Time Enrollments:	166	Weekend Classes:	No
Affiliation:	Public	Distance Learning:	Yes

NLN ACCREDITATION: Yes

BSN for non-RNs w/degree in other field: No

Articulation: Associate to Baccalaureate
Diploma to Baccalaureate

For Further Information Contact:

Dr Justine Speer, Dean
Oakland University
428 O'Dowd Hall
Rochester, MI 48309
(313) 370-4081

Saginaw Valley State University
—University Center—

Full-Time Enrollments:	120	Evening Classes:	No
Part-Time Enrollments:	—	Weekend Classes:	No
Affiliation:	Public	Distance Learning:	Yes

NLN ACCREDITATION: Yes

BSN for non-RNs w/degree in other field: No

Articulation: Associate to Baccalaureate

For Further Information Contact:

Dr Crystal M Lange, Dean
Saginaw Valley State University
7400 Bay Road
University Center, MI 48603
(517) 790-4145

University of Detroit-Mercy
—Detroit—

Full-Time Enrollments:	185	Evening Classes:	—
Part-Time Enrollments:	290	Weekend Classes:	—
Affiliation:	Private	Distance Learning:	—

NLN ACCREDITATION: Yes

BSN for non-RNs w/degree in other field: Yes

Articulation: None

For Further Information Contact:

Dr Marie L Friedemann, Associate Dean
University of Detroit-Mercy
8200 W Outer Dr
Detroit, MI 48219-3599
(313) 993-6132

University of Michigan
—Ann Arbor—

Full-Time Enrollments:	433	Evening Classes:	No
Part-Time Enrollments:	25	Weekend Classes:	No
Affiliation:	Public	Distance Learning:	Yes

NLN ACCREDITATION: Yes

BSN for non-RNs w/degree in other field: Yes

Articulation: Associate to Baccalaureate

For Further Information Contact:

Dr Ada S Hinshaw, Dean
University of Michigan
Rm 400 N Ingalls Bldg Rm1320
Ann Arbor, MI 48109-0482
(313) 764-7185

University of Michigan
—Flint—

Full-Time Enrollments: 165
Part-Time Enrollments: —
Affiliation: Public

Evening Classes: Yes
Weekend Classes: No
Distance Learning: No

NLN ACCREDITATION: Yes

BSN for non-RNs w/degree in other field: No

Articulation: None

For Further Information Contact:

Dr Ellen Woodman, Director
University of Michigan
303 E Kearsley St
Flint, MI 48502-2186
(810) 762-3420

Wayne State University
—Detroit—

Full-Time Enrollments: 262
Part-Time Enrollments: 80
Affiliation: Public

Evening Classes: Yes
Weekend Classes: Yes
Distance Learning: No

NLN ACCREDITATION: Yes

BSN for non-RNs w/degree in other field: Yes

Articulation: Associate to Baccalaureate
Diploma to Baccalaureate
RN to MSN

For Further Information Contact:

Dr Marjorie Isenberg, Associate Dean
Wayne State University
5557 Cass Avenue
Detroit, MI 48202
(313) 577-4070

Western Michigan University
—Kalamazoo—

Full-Time Enrollments: 42
Part-Time Enrollments: 2
Affiliation: Public

Evening Classes: Yes
Weekend Classes: No
Distance Learning: —

NLN ACCREDITATION: No

BSN for non-RNs w/degree in other field: No

Articulation: Diploma to Baccalaureate
LPN to Baccalaureate

For Further Information Contact:

Dr Bernadine M Lacey, Director
Western Michigan University
School of Nursing
Kalamazoo, MI 49008-5184
(616) 387-2887

Minnesota

Bethel College Nursing Department
—St Paul—

Full-Time Enrollments: —
Part-Time Enrollments: —
Affiliation: Religious

Evening Classes: —
Weekend Classes: —
Distance Learning: —

NLN ACCREDITATION: Yes

BSN for non-RNs w/degree in other field: —

Articulation: None

For Further Information Contact:

Dr Sagrid E Edman, Chair
Bethel College Nursing Department
3900 Bethel Dr
St Paul, MN 55112-6999
(612) 638-6368

College of St Benedict/St John's University
—St Joseph—

Full-Time Enrollments: 87
Part-Time Enrollments: 11
Affiliation: Religious

Evening Classes: No
Weekend Classes: No
Distance Learning: No

NLN ACCREDITATION: Yes

BSN for non-RNs w/degree in other field: No

Articulation: None

For Further Information Contact:

Dr Joann Wessman, Chair
College of St Benedict/St John's University
37 South College Ave
St Joseph, MN 56374-2099
(612) 363-5404

College of St Catherine-Department of Nursing
—St Paul—

Full-Time Enrollments: 175
Part-Time Enrollments: —
Affiliation: Religious

Evening Classes: Yes
Weekend Classes: Yes
Distance Learning: No

NLN ACCREDITATION: Yes

BSN for non-RNs w/degree in other field: No

Articulation: None

For Further Information Contact:

Ms Alice Swan, Chair
College of St Catherine-Department of Nursing
2004 Randolph Ave
St Paul, MN 55105
(612) 690-6583

College of St Scholastica
—Duluth—

Full-Time Enrollments:	102	Evening Classes:	No
Part-Time Enrollments:	3	Weekend Classes:	No
Affiliation:	Private	Distance Learning:	No

NLN ACCREDITATION: Yes

BSN for non-RNs w/degree in other field: No

Articulation: None

For Further Information Contact:

Dr Cecelia Taylor, Chair
College of St Scholastica
1200 Kenwood Ave
Duluth, MN 55811-4199
(218) 723-6025

Mankato State University-School of Nursing
—Mankato—

Full-Time Enrollments:	195	Evening Classes:	Yes
Part-Time Enrollments:	12	Weekend Classes:	Yes
Affiliation:	Public	Distance Learning:	Yes

NLN ACCREDITATION: Yes

BSN for non-RNs w/degree in other field: No

Articulation: LPN to Baccalaureate

For Further Information Contact:

Dr Mary Huntley, Interim Assoc Dean
Mankato State University-School of Nursing
MSU Box 27-PO Box 8400
Mankato, MN 56002-8400
(507) 389-6022

Minnesota Intercollegiate Nursing Consortium
—Northfield—

Full-Time Enrollments:	72	Evening Classes:	No
Part-Time Enrollments:	—	Weekend Classes:	No
Affiliation:	Religious	Distance Learning:	No

NLN ACCREDITATION: Yes

BSN for non-RNs w/degree in other field: No

Articulation: None

For Further Information Contact:

Dr Rita Glazebrook, Director
Minnesota Intercollegiate Nursing Consortium
1520 St Olaf Ave
Northfield, MN 55057-1098
(507) 646-3265

Tri College University-Concordia College
—Moorhead—

Full-Time Enrollments:	—	Evening Classes:	—
Part-Time Enrollments:	—	Weekend Classes:	—
Affiliation:	Public	Distance Learning:	—

NLN ACCREDITATION: Yes

BSN for non-RNs w/degree in other field: No

Articulation: None

For Further Information Contact:

Dr Lois F Nelson, Chair
Tri College University-Concordia College
901 S 8th St
Moorhead, MN 56562
(218) 299-3879

University of Minnesota
—Minneapolis—

Full-Time Enrollments:	98	Evening Classes:	No
Part-Time Enrollments:	98	Weekend Classes:	No
Affiliation:	Public	Distance Learning:	No

NLN ACCREDITATION: Yes

BSN for non-RNs w/degree in other field: No

Articulation: RN to MSN

For Further Information Contact:

Dr Sandra Edwardson, Dean
University of Minnesota
308 Harvard St SE 5-140
Minneapolis, MN 55455-0342
(612) 624-5959

Winona State University
—Winona—

Full-Time Enrollments:	203	Evening Classes:	No
Part-Time Enrollments:	5	Weekend Classes:	No
Affiliation:	Public	Distance Learning:	Yes

NLN ACCREDITATION: Yes

BSN for non-RNs w/degree in other field: No

Articulation: Associate to Baccalaureate
                  Diploma to Baccalaureate

For Further Information Contact:

Dr Timothy Gaspar, Dean
Winona State University
PO Box 5838 301 Stark Hall
Winona, MN 55987-5838
(507) 457-5122

Mississippi

Alcorn State University
—Natchez—

Full-Time Enrollments:	55	Evening Classes:	No
Part-Time Enrollments:	7	Weekend Classes:	No
Affiliation:	Public	Distance Learning:	No

NLN ACCREDITATION: Yes

BSN for non-RNs w/degree in other field: No

Articulation: None

For Further Information Contact:

Dr Joyce McManus, Chair
Alcorn State University
PO Box 18399
Natchez, MS 39122
(601) 442-3901

Delta State University
—Cleveland—

Full-Time Enrollments:	56	Evening Classes:	Yes
Part-Time Enrollments:	—	Weekend Classes:	Yes
Affiliation:	Public	Distance Learning:	Yes

NLN ACCREDITATION: Yes

BSN for non-RNs w/degree in other field: No

Articulation: Associate to Baccalaureate

For Further Information Contact:

Dr Barbara Powell, Dean
Delta State University
PO Box 3343
Cleveland, MS 38733
(601) 846-4268

Mississippi College
—Clinton—

Full-Time Enrollments:	112	Evening Classes:	Yes
Part-Time Enrollments:	9	Weekend Classes:	Yes
Affiliation:	Religious	Distance Learning:	—

NLN ACCREDITATION: Yes

BSN for non-RNs w/degree in other field: No

Articulation: None

For Further Information Contact:

Dr Mary J Padgett, Dean
Mississippi College
Box 4225
Clinton, MS 39058
(601) 925-3278

Mississippi University for Women
—Columbus—

Full-Time Enrollments:	93	Evening Classes:	Yes
Part-Time Enrollments:	—	Weekend Classes:	No
Affiliation:	Public	Distance Learning:	Yes

NLN ACCREDITATION: Yes

BSN for non-RNs w/degree in other field: No

Articulation: Associate to Baccalaureate

For Further Information Contact:

Dr Linda Cox, Director
Mississippi University for Women
Taylor Hall, PO Box W910
Columbus, MS 39701
(601) 329-7299

University of Mississippi Medical Center
—Jackson—

Full-Time Enrollments:	192	Evening Classes:	Yes
Part-Time Enrollments:	5	Weekend Classes:	Yes
Affiliation:	Public	Distance Learning:	No

NLN ACCREDITATION: Yes

BSN for non-RNs w/degree in other field: No

Articulation: RN to MSN

For Further Information Contact:

Dr Anne Peirce, Dean
University of Mississippi Medical Center
2500 N State St
Jackson, MS 39206-4505
(601) 984-6200

University of Southern Mississippi
—Hattiesburg—

Full-Time Enrollments:	279	Evening Classes:	No
Part-Time Enrollments:	—	Weekend Classes:	No
Affiliation:	Public	Distance Learning:	Yes

NLN ACCREDITATION: Yes

BSN for non-RNs w/degree in other field: No

Articulation: None

For Further Information Contact:

Dr Gerry Cadenhead, Interim Director
University of Southern Mississippi
PO Box 5095
Hattiesburg, MS 39406-5695
(601) 266-5639

William Carey College
—Gulfport—

Full-Time Enrollments:	202	Evening Classes:	No
Part-Time Enrollments:	10	Weekend Classes:	No
Affiliation:	Religious	Distance Learning:	No

NLN ACCREDITATION: Yes

BSN for non-RNs w/degree in other field: No

Articulation: None

For Further Information Contact:

Dr Annette Barrar, Dean
William Carey College
1856 Beach Dr
Gulfport, MS 39507
(601) 867-9201

Missouri

Avila College
—Kansas City—

Full-Time Enrollments:	61	Evening Classes:	Yes
Part-Time Enrollments:	2	Weekend Classes:	Yes
Affiliation:	Religious	Distance Learning:	No

NLN ACCREDITATION: Yes

BSN for non-RNs w/degree in other field: No

Articulation: None

For Further Information Contact:

Dr Susan Fetsch, Chair
Avila College
11901 Wornall Rd
Kansas City, MO 64145-1698
(816) 942-8400

Central Methodist College
—Fayette—

Full-Time Enrollments:	32	Evening Classes:	Yes
Part-Time Enrollments:	—	Weekend Classes:	—
Affiliation:	Religious	Distance Learning:	Yes

NLN ACCREDITATION: No

BSN for non-RNs w/degree in other field: No

Articulation: None

For Further Information Contact:

Dr Shirley Peterson, Chair
Central Methodist College
411 Central Methodist Sq
Fayette, MO 65248
(816) 248-3391 Ext 363

Central Missouri State University
—Warrensburg—

Full-Time Enrollments:	120	Evening Classes:	—
Part-Time Enrollments:	—	Weekend Classes:	—
Affiliation:	Public	Distance Learning:	—

NLN ACCREDITATION: Yes

BSN for non-RNs w/degree in other field: No

Articulation: None

For Further Information Contact:

Dr Elaine Frank-Ragan, Chair
Central Missouri State University
Dept of Nsg, SHC-106
Warrensburg, MO 64093
(816) 543-4775

Deaconess College of Nursing
—St Louis—

Full-Time Enrollments:	212	Evening Classes:	No
Part-Time Enrollments:	65	Weekend Classes:	No
Affiliation:	Private	Distance Learning:	No

NLN ACCREDITATION: Yes

BSN for non-RNs w/degree in other field: No

Articulation: Associate to Baccalaureate
Diploma to Baccalaureate

For Further Information Contact:

Dr Janet Barrett, Director
Deaconess College of Nursing
6150 Oakland Ave
St Louis, MO 63139-3297
(314) 768-3042

Graceland College
—Independence—

Full-Time Enrollments:	66	Evening Classes:	Yes
Part-Time Enrollments:	7	Weekend Classes:	No
Affiliation:	Religious	Distance Learning:	Yes

NLN ACCREDITATION: Yes

BSN for non-RNs w/degree in other field: No

Articulation: Associate to Baccalaureate
Diploma to Baccalaureate

For Further Information Contact:

Dr Sharon Kirkpatrick, Vice President
Graceland College
221 W Lexington Suite 110
Independence, MO 64050-3720
(816) 833-0524

Maryville University of St Louis
—St Louis—

Full-Time Enrollments:	52	Evening Classes:	Yes
Part-Time Enrollments:	123	Weekend Classes:	Yes
Affiliation:	Private	Distance Learning:	—

NLN ACCREDITATION: Yes

BSN for non-RNs w/degree in other field: No

Articulation: Associate to Baccalaureate

For Further Information Contact:

Dr Mary Margaret Mooney, Director
Maryville University of St Louis
13550 Conway Rd
St Louis, MO 63141-7299
(314) 529-9435

Missouri Southern State College
—Joplin—

Full-Time Enrollments:	44	Evening Classes:	—
Part-Time Enrollments:	—	Weekend Classes:	—
Affiliation:	Public	Distance Learning:	—

NLN ACCREDITATION: Yes

BSN for non-RNs w/degree in other field: No

Articulation: None

For Further Information Contact:

Dr Barbara Box, Director
Missouri Southern State College
3950 East Newman Rd
Joplin, MO 64801-1595
(417) 625-9322

Missouri Western State College
—St Joseph—

Full-Time Enrollments:	182	Evening Classes:	No
Part-Time Enrollments:	—	Weekend Classes:	No
Affiliation:	Public	Distance Learning:	No

NLN ACCREDITATION: Yes

BSN for non-RNs w/degree in other field: No

Articulation: Associate to Baccalaureate
RN to MSN

For Further Information Contact:

Dr Jeanne M Daffron, Chair
Missouri Western State College
4525 Downs Dr Suite ET 203
St Joseph, MO 64507
(816) 271-4404

Research College of Nursing
—Kansas City—

Full-Time Enrollments:	219	Evening Classes:	—
Part-Time Enrollments:	17	Weekend Classes:	—
Affiliation:	Private	Distance Learning:	—

NLN ACCREDITATION: Yes

BSN for non-RNs w/degree in other field: Yes

Articulation: None

For Further Information Contact:

Dr Nancy DeBasio, Dean
Research College of Nursing
2316 E Meyer Blvd
Kansas City, MO 64132
(816) 276-4700

Southeast Missouri State University
—Cape Girardeau—

Full-Time Enrollments:	136	Evening Classes:	Yes
Part-Time Enrollments:	—	Weekend Classes:	Yes
Affiliation:	Public	Distance Learning:	No

NLN ACCREDITATION: Yes

BSN for non-RNs w/degree in other field: No

Articulation: Associate to Baccalaureate
Diploma to Baccalaureate

For Further Information Contact:

Dr A Louise Hart, Chair
Southeast Missouri State University
One University Plaza
Cape Girardeau, MO 63701
(573) 651-2585

St Louis University School of Nursing
—St Louis—

Full-Time Enrollments:	311	Evening Classes:	Yes
Part-Time Enrollments:	25	Weekend Classes:	No
Affiliation:	Religious	Distance Learning:	No

NLN ACCREDITATION: Yes

BSN for non-RNs w/degree in other field: Yes

Articulation: Associate to Baccalaureate
Diploma to Baccalaureate
RN to MSN

For Further Information Contact:

Dr Judith Lewis, Director
St Louis University School of Nursing
3525 Caroline St
St Louis, MO 63104-1099
(314) 577-8900

St Luke's College of Nursing
—Kansas City—

Full-Time Enrollments:	82	Evening Classes:	—
Part-Time Enrollments:	24	Weekend Classes:	Yes
Affiliation:	Religious	Distance Learning:	—

NLN ACCREDITATION: Yes

BSN for non-RNs w/degree in other field: No

Articulation: Associate to Baccalaureate
Diploma to Baccalaureate

For Further Information Contact:

Dr Helen Jepson, Dean
St Luke's College of Nursing
4426 Wornall Rd
Kansas City, MO 64111
(816) 932-2239

Truman State University
—Kirksville—

Full-Time Enrollments:	194	Evening Classes:	—
Part-Time Enrollments:	—	Weekend Classes:	—
Affiliation:	Public	Distance Learning:	—

NLN ACCREDITATION: Yes

BSN for non-RNs w/degree in other field: No

Articulation: None

For Further Information Contact:

Dr Constance Ayers, Director
Truman State University
Barnett Hall 223
Kirksville, MO 63501
(816) 785-4557

University of Missouri-Columbia
—Columbia—

Full-Time Enrollments:	205	Evening Classes:	No
Part-Time Enrollments:	10	Weekend Classes:	Yes
Affiliation:	Public	Distance Learning:	Yes

NLN ACCREDITATION: Yes

BSN for non-RNs w/degree in other field: No

Articulation: None

For Further Information Contact:

Dr Toni J Sullivan, Dean
University of Missouri-Columbia
Nursing Bldg S410
Columbia, MO 65211
(573) 882-0278

University of Missouri-St Louis
—St Louis—

Full-Time Enrollments:	352	Evening Classes:	Yes
Part-Time Enrollments:	102	Weekend Classes:	No
Affiliation:	Public	Distance Learning:	Yes

NLN ACCREDITATION: Yes

BSN for non-RNs w/degree in other field: No

Articulation: Associate to Baccalaureate
Diploma to Baccalaureate

For Further Information Contact:

Dr Shirley Martin, Dean
University of Missouri-St Louis
8001 Natural Bridge
St Louis, MO 63121-4499
(314) 516-6067

William Jewell College
—Liberty—

Full-Time Enrollments:	115	Evening Classes:	No
Part-Time Enrollments:	—	Weekend Classes:	No
Affiliation:	Religious	Distance Learning:	No

NLN ACCREDITATION: Yes

BSN for non-RNs w/degree in other field: Yes

Articulation: None

For Further Information Contact:

Dr Joanne Kersten, Acting Chair
William Jewell College
500 College Hill
Liberty, MO 64068
(816) 781-7700

Montana

Carroll College
—Helena—

Full-Time Enrollments:	—	Evening Classes:	—
Part-Time Enrollments:	—	Weekend Classes:	—
Affiliation:	Private	Distance Learning:	—

NLN ACCREDITATION: Yes

BSN for non-RNs w/degree in other field: —

Articulation: None

For Further Information Contact:

Dr Maureen Quinn, Chair
Carroll College
1601 Benton Ave
Helena, MT 59625
(406) 447-5497

Montana State University
—Bozeman—

Full-Time Enrollments:	476	Evening Classes:	No
Part-Time Enrollments:	50	Weekend Classes:	No
Affiliation:	Public	Distance Learning:	No

NLN ACCREDITATION: Yes

BSN for non-RNs w/degree in other field: Yes

Articulation: Associate to Baccalaureate
Diploma to Baccalaureate

For Further Information Contact:

Dr Lea Acord, Dean
Montana State University
Bozeman, MT 59717
(406) 994-3783

Nebraska

Clarkson College-Department of Nursing
—Omaha—

Full-Time Enrollments:	151	Evening Classes:	—
Part-Time Enrollments:	92	Weekend Classes:	—
Affiliation:	Religious	Distance Learning:	—

NLN ACCREDITATION: Yes

BSN for non-RNs w/degree in other field: No

Articulation: None

For Further Information Contact:

Dr Charles Beauchamp, Dean
Clarkson College-Department of Nursing
101 S 42nd St
Omaha, NE 68131
(402) 552-3480

Creighton University (2 Branches)
—Omaha—

Full-Time Enrollments:	247	Evening Classes:	Yes
Part-Time Enrollments:	12	Weekend Classes:	No
Affiliation:	Religious	Distance Learning:	No

NLN ACCREDITATION: Yes

BSN for non-RNs w/degree in other field: No

Articulation: Associate to Baccalaureate
Diploma to Baccalaureate

For Further Information Contact:

Dr E Kitchen, Dean
Creighton University (2 Branches)
2500 California St
Omaha, NE 68178
(402) 280-2006

Midland Lutheran College
—Fremont—

Full-Time Enrollments:	64	Evening Classes:	Yes
Part-Time Enrollments:	—	Weekend Classes:	No
Affiliation:	Religious	Distance Learning:	Yes

NLN ACCREDITATION: Yes

BSN for non-RNs w/degree in other field: No

Articulation: None

For Further Information Contact:

Dr Nancy Harms, Chair
Midland Lutheran College
900 North Clarkson
Fremont, NE 68025
(402) 721-5480

Nebraska Methodist College of Nursing
—Omaha—

Full-Time Enrollments:	—	Evening Classes:	—
Part-Time Enrollments:	—	Weekend Classes:	—
Affiliation:	Private	Distance Learning:	—

NLN ACCREDITATION: Yes

BSN for non-RNs w/degree in other field: —

Articulation: None

For Further Information Contact:

Ms Nancy Mockelstrom, Chair
Nebraska Methodist College of Nursing
8501 West Dodge Rd
Omaha, NE 68114
(402) 390-4981

Union College in Lincoln
—Lincoln—

Full-Time Enrollments:	77	Evening Classes:	No
Part-Time Enrollments:	8	Weekend Classes:	No
Affiliation:	Religious	Distance Learning:	No

NLN ACCREDITATION: Yes

BSN for non-RNs w/degree in other field: Yes

Articulation: LPN to Baccalaureate

For Further Information Contact:

Dr Marilyn McArthur, Chair
Union College in Lincoln
3800 S 48th St
Lincoln, NE 68506
(402) 486-2524

University of Nebraska College of Nursing
(4 Branches)
—Omaha—

Full-Time Enrollments:	541	Evening Classes:	No
Part-Time Enrollments:	19	Weekend Classes:	No
Affiliation:	Public	Distance Learning:	Yes

NLN ACCREDITATION: Yes

BSN for non-RNs w/degree in other field: No

Articulation: None

For Further Information Contact:

Dr Ada Lindsey, Dean
University of Nebraska College of Nursing (4 Brchs)
600 South 42nd St
Omaha, NE 68198-5330
(402) 559-4109

Nevada

University of Nevada
—Las Vegas—

Full-Time Enrollments:	186	Evening Classes:	No
Part-Time Enrollments:	2	Weekend Classes:	No
Affiliation:	Public	Distance Learning:	Yes

NLN ACCREDITATION: Yes

BSN for non-RNs w/degree in other field: No

Articulation: Associate to Baccalaureate

For Further Information Contact:

Dr Rosemary Witt, Chair
University of Nevada
4505 Maryland Parkway
Las Vegas, NV 89154
(702) 895-3360

University of Nevada-Orvis School of Nursing
—Reno—

Full-Time Enrollments:	102	Evening Classes:	No
Part-Time Enrollments:	—	Weekend Classes:	No
Affiliation:	Public	Distance Learning:	Yes

NLN ACCREDITATION: Yes

BSN for non-RNs w/degree in other field: No

Articulation: Associate to Baccalaureate
Diploma to Baccalaureate

For Further Information Contact:

Dr Julie Johnson, Director
University of Nevada-Orvis School of Nursing
Reno, NV 89507-0052
(702) 784-6841

New Hampshire

Colby-Sawyer College
—New London—

Full-Time Enrollments:	17	Evening Classes:	No
Part-Time Enrollments:	3	Weekend Classes:	No
Affiliation:	Private	Distance Learning:	No

NLN ACCREDITATION: Yes

BSN for non-RNs w/degree in other field: No

Articulation: None

For Further Information Contact:

Ms Mary Colvin, Chair
Colby-Sawyer College
100 Main
New London, NH 03257
(603) 526-3000

Saint Anselm College
—Manchester—

Full-Time Enrollments:	272	Evening Classes:	Yes
Part-Time Enrollments:	2	Weekend Classes:	No
Affiliation:	Religious	Distance Learning:	No

NLN ACCREDITATION: Yes

BSN for non-RNs w/degree in other field: No

Articulation: None

For Further Information Contact:

Dr Joanne Farley, Director
Saint Anselm College
100 Saint Anselm Dr #1745
Manchester, NH 03102-1310
(603) 641-7084

University of New Hampshire-Nursing
Department
—Durham—

Full-Time Enrollments:	206	Evening Classes:	Yes
Part-Time Enrollments:	—	Weekend Classes:	No
Affiliation:	Public	Distance Learning:	Yes

NLN ACCREDITATION: Yes

BSN for non-RNs w/degree in other field: No

Articulation: Associate to Baccalaureate

For Further Information Contact:

Mrs Ann Kelley, Chair
University of New Hampshire-Nursing Department
Hewitt Hall
Durham, NH 03824
(603) 862-0450

New Jersey

Bloomfield College
—Bloomfield—

Full-Time Enrollments: 82   Evening Classes: Yes
Part-Time Enrollments: 7   Weekend Classes: Yes
Affiliation: Private   Distance Learning: No

NLN ACCREDITATION: Yes

BSN for non-RNs w/degree in other field: No

Articulation: Associate to Baccalaureate

For Further Information Contact:

Dr Carolyn Tuella, Chair
Bloomfield College
467 Franklin Ave
Bloomfield, NJ 07003
(201) 748-9000

Fairleigh Dickinson University
—Teaneck—

Full-Time Enrollments: 123   Evening Classes: Yes
Part-Time Enrollments: 77   Weekend Classes: No
Affiliation: Private   Distance Learning: Yes

NLN ACCREDITATION: Yes

BSN for non-RNs w/degree in other field: Yes

Articulation: None

For Further Information Contact:

Dr Caroline Jordet, Director
Fairleigh Dickinson University
1000 River Rd
Teaneck, NJ 07666
(201) 692-2888

Felician College
—Lodi—

Full-Time Enrollments: —   Evening Classes: —
Part-Time Enrollments: —   Weekend Classes: —
Affiliation: Private   Distance Learning: —

NLN ACCREDITATION: No

BSN for non-RNs w/degree in other field: —

Articulation: None

For Further Information Contact:

Dr Rona Levin, Director
Felician College
262 South Main St
Lodi, NJ 07644
(201) 778-1190

Rutgers-The State University of New Jersey
—Newark—

Full-Time Enrollments: 337   Evening Classes: Yes
Part-Time Enrollments: 19   Weekend Classes: No
Affiliation: Public   Distance Learning: Yes

NLN ACCREDITATION: Yes

BSN for non-RNs w/degree in other field: Yes

Articulation: None

For Further Information Contact:

Dr Hurdis Griffith, Dean
Rutgers-The State University of New Jersey
180 University Ave
Newark, NJ 07102
(201) 648-5142

Rutgers-The State University-Camden Campus
—Camden—

Full-Time Enrollments: 72   Evening Classes: No
Part-Time Enrollments: —   Weekend Classes: No
Affiliation: Public   Distance Learning: No

NLN ACCREDITATION: Yes

BSN for non-RNs w/degree in other field: No

Articulation: Associate to Baccalaureate
Diploma to Baccalaureate

For Further Information Contact:

Dr Mary Greipp, Chair
Rutgers-The State University-Camden Campus
311 N 5th St
Camden, NJ 08102
(609) 225-6226

Seton Hall University
—South Orange—

Full-Time Enrollments: 226   Evening Classes: Yes
Part-Time Enrollments: 48   Weekend Classes: —
Affiliation: Religious   Distance Learning: Yes

NLN ACCREDITATION: Yes

BSN for non-RNs w/degree in other field: Yes

Articulation: None

For Further Information Contact:

Dr Barbara A Beeker, Dean
Seton Hall University
S Orange Ave
South Orange, NJ 07079
(201) 761-9015

Trenton State College School of Nursing
—Trenton—

Full-Time Enrollments:	150	Evening Classes:	Yes
Part-Time Enrollments:	8	Weekend Classes:	No
Affiliation:	Public	Distance Learning:	No

NLN ACCREDITATION: Yes

BSN for non-RNs w/degree in other field:　　No

Articulation:　　Associate to Baccalaureate

For Further Information Contact:

Dr Laurie Sherwen, Dean
Trenton State College School of Nursing
Hillwood Lakes CN4700
Trenton, NJ 08650
(609) 771-2848

University of Medicine & Dentistry in New Jersey-Ramapo College
—Mahwah—

Full-Time Enrollments:	33	Evening Classes:	—
Part-Time Enrollments:	—	Weekend Classes:	—
Affiliation:	Public	Distance Learning:	—

NLN ACCREDITATION: Yes

BSN for non-RNs w/degree in other field:　　No

Articulation:　　None

For Further Information Contact:

Dr Katherine Burke, Coordinator
University of Medicine & Dentistry in New Jersey-Ramapo College
505 Ramapo Rd
Mahwah, NJ 07430-1680
(201) 529-7749

William Paterson College
—Wayne—

Full-Time Enrollments:	247	Evening Classes:	Yes
Part-Time Enrollments:	43	Weekend Classes:	No
Affiliation:	Public	Distance Learning:	No

NLN ACCREDITATION: Yes

BSN for non-RNs w/degree in other field:　　Yes

Articulation:　　Associate to Baccalaureate

For Further Information Contact:

Dr Sandra DeYoung, Chair
William Paterson College
300 Pompton Rd
Wayne, NJ 07470
(201) 595-2286

New Mexico

New Mexico State University
—Las Cruces—

Full-Time Enrollments:	122	Evening Classes:	Yes
Part-Time Enrollments:	—	Weekend Classes:	No
Affiliation:	Public	Distance Learning:	No

NLN ACCREDITATION: Yes

BSN for non-RNs w/degree in other field:　　No

Articulation:　　Associate to Baccalaureate

For Further Information Contact:

Dr Judith Karshmer, Dept Head
New Mexico State University
PO Box 30001 Dept 3185
Las Cruces, NM 88003-8001
(505) 646-3812

University of New Mexico-College of Nursing
—Albuquerque—

Full-Time Enrollments:	234	Evening Classes:	Yes
Part-Time Enrollments:	76	Weekend Classes:	No
Affiliation:	Public	Distance Learning:	Yes

NLN ACCREDITATION: Yes

BSN for non-RNs w/degree in other field:　　No

Articulation:　　Associate to Baccalaureate
　　　　　　　　Diploma to Baccalaureate
　　　　　　　　RN to MSN

For Further Information Contact:

Dr Donea Shane, Interim Dean
University of New Mexico-College of Nursing
Albuquerque, NM 87131-1061
(505) 277-4221

New York

Adelphi University-School of Nursing
—Garden City—

Full-Time Enrollments:	236	Evening Classes:	No
Part-Time Enrollments:	38	Weekend Classes:	No
Affiliation:	Private	Distance Learning:	No

NLN ACCREDITATION: Yes

BSN for non-RNs w/degree in other field:　　No

Articulation:　　None

For Further Information Contact:

Dr Caryle Wolahan, Dean
Adelphi University-School of Nursing
Box 516
Garden City, NY 11530
(516) 877-3000

Binghamton University
—Binghamton—

Full-Time Enrollments: 251
Part-Time Enrollments: 16
Affiliation: Public

Evening Classes: No
Weekend Classes: No
Distance Learning: Yes

NLN ACCREDITATION: Yes

BSN for non-RNs w/degree in other field: Yes

Articulation: Associate to Baccalaureate

For Further Information Contact:

Dr Mary S Collins, Dean
Binghamton University
Decker Sch of Nsg PO Box 6000
Binghamton, NY 13902-6000
(607) 777-2311

College of New Rochelle
—New Rochelle—

Full-Time Enrollments: 168
Part-Time Enrollments: 117
Affiliation: Private

Evening Classes: Yes
Weekend Classes: Yes
Distance Learning: No

NLN ACCREDITATION: Yes

BSN for non-RNs w/degree in other field: Yes

Articulation: Associate to Baccalaureate

For Further Information Contact:

Dr Connie Vance, Dean
College of New Rochelle
29 Castle Pl
New Rochelle, NY 10805
(914) 654-5244

City College School of Nursing of CUNY
—New York—

Full-Time Enrollments: 99
Part-Time Enrollments: —
Affiliation: Public

Evening Classes: —
Weekend Classes: —
Distance Learning: —

NLN ACCREDITATION: Yes

BSN for non-RNs w/degree in other field: No

Articulation: None

For Further Information Contact:

Dr Reuphenia James, Chair
City College School of Nursing of CUNY
138th & Convent Ave
New York, NY 10031
(212) 650-7178

Columbia University
—New York—

Full-Time Enrollments: —
Part-Time Enrollments: —
Affiliation: Private

Evening Classes: —
Weekend Classes: —
Distance Learning: —

NLN ACCREDITATION: Yes

BSN for non-RNs w/degree in other field: —

Articulation: None

For Further Information Contact:

Dr Mary O Mundinger, Dean
Columbia University
630 W 168th St
New York, NY 10032
(212) 305-5756

College of Mt St Vincent
—Riverdale—

Full-Time Enrollments: 230
Part-Time Enrollments: 80
Affiliation: Private

Evening Classes: —
Weekend Classes: —
Distance Learning: —

NLN ACCREDITATION: Yes

BSN for non-RNs w/degree in other field: Yes

Articulation: None

For Further Information Contact:

Dr Barbara Cohen, Director
College of Mt St Vincent
6301 Riverdale Ave
Riverdale, NY 10471-1093
(718) 405-3353

D'Youville College
—Buffalo—

Full-Time Enrollments: 138
Part-Time Enrollments: 32
Affiliation: Private

Evening Classes: Yes
Weekend Classes: Yes
Distance Learning: No

NLN ACCREDITATION: Yes

BSN for non-RNs w/degree in other field: No

Articulation: Associate to Baccalaureate

For Further Information Contact:

Dr Carol Batra, Dept Head
D'Youville College
585 Prospect Ave
Buffalo, NY 14213
(716) 881-7613

Dominican College of Blauvelt
—Orangeburg—

Full-Time Enrollments:	141	Evening Classes:	Yes
Part-Time Enrollments:	72	Weekend Classes:	Yes
Affiliation:	Private	Distance Learning:	No

NLN ACCREDITATION: Yes

BSN for non-RNs w/degree in other field: Yes

Articulation: Associate to Baccalaureate
Diploma to Baccalaureate
LPN to Baccalaureate

For Further Information Contact:

Dr Maureen Creegan, Director
Dominican College of Blauvelt
10 Western Highway
Orangeburg, NY 10962
(914) 359-7800

Elmira College
—Elmira—

Full-Time Enrollments:	67	Evening Classes:	Yes
Part-Time Enrollments:	22	Weekend Classes:	No
Affiliation:	Private	Distance Learning:	No

NLN ACCREDITATION: Yes

BSN for non-RNs w/degree in other field: No

Articulation: Associate to Baccalaureate
Diploma to Baccalaureate

For Further Information Contact:

Dr Anita Ogden, Director
Elmira College
Elmira, NY 14901
(607) 735-1890

Hartwick College
—Oneonta—

Full-Time Enrollments:	111	Evening Classes:	Yes
Part-Time Enrollments:	3	Weekend Classes:	—
Affiliation:	Private	Distance Learning:	—

NLN ACCREDITATION: Yes

BSN for non-RNs w/degree in other field: No

Articulation: Associate to Baccalaureate
Diploma to Baccalaureate

For Further Information Contact:

Dr Dianne C Miner, Chair
Hartwick College
Dept of Nsg
Oneonta, NY 13820
(607) 431-4780

Hunter College-Bellevue School of Nursing
—New York—

Full-Time Enrollments:	125	Evening Classes:	No
Part-Time Enrollments:	3	Weekend Classes:	No
Affiliation:	Public	Distance Learning:	No

NLN ACCREDITATION: Yes

BSN for non-RNs w/degree in other field: No

Articulation: Associate to Baccalaureate

For Further Information Contact:

Dr Evelynn C Gioiella, Dean
Hunter College-Bellevue School of Nursing
425 E 25 St
New York, NY 10010
(212) 481-7557

Keuka College
—Keuka Park—

Full-Time Enrollments:	53	Evening Classes:	No
Part-Time Enrollments:	2	Weekend Classes:	—
Affiliation:	Private	Distance Learning:	—

NLN ACCREDITATION: Yes

BSN for non-RNs w/degree in other field: No

Articulation: Associate to Baccalaureate

For Further Information Contact:

Dr Margaret England, Chair
Keuka College
Keuka Park, NY 14478-0098
(315) 536-5273

Lehman College of CUNY
—Bronx—

Full-Time Enrollments:	—	Evening Classes:	—
Part-Time Enrollments:	—	Weekend Classes:	—
Affiliation:	Public	Distance Learning:	—

NLN ACCREDITATION: Yes

BSN for non-RNs w/degree in other field: —

Articulation: None

For Further Information Contact:

Dr Ngogi Nkongho, Chair
Lehman College of CUNY
250 Bedford Park Blvd, W
Bronx, NY 10468-1589
(718) 960-8794

BACCALAUREATE DEGREE

Long Island University
—Brooklyn—

Full-Time Enrollments:	469	Evening Classes:	Yes
Part-Time Enrollments:	112	Weekend Classes:	Yes
Affiliation:	Private	Distance Learning:	—

NLN ACCREDITATION: Yes

BSN for non-RNs w/degree in other field: No

Articulation: None

For Further Information Contact:

Dr Esther Siegel, Dean
Long Island University
1 Univ Plaza
Brooklyn, NY 11201
(718) 488-1059

Molloy College
—Rockville Centre—

Full-Time Enrollments:	524	Evening Classes:	Yes
Part-Time Enrollments:	157	Weekend Classes:	Yes
Affiliation:	Private	Distance Learning:	—

NLN ACCREDITATION: Yes

BSN for non-RNs w/degree in other field: Yes

Articulation: Associate to Baccalaureate

For Further Information Contact:

Dr Gloria Gelfand, Chair
Molloy College
Rockville Centre, NY 11570
(516) 256-2220

Mt Saint Mary College
—Newburgh—

Full-Time Enrollments:	156	Evening Classes:	Yes
Part-Time Enrollments:	30	Weekend Classes:	Yes
Affiliation:	Private	Distance Learning:	—

NLN ACCREDITATION: Yes

BSN for non-RNs w/degree in other field: No

Articulation: None

For Further Information Contact:

Dr Linda Scheetz, Chair
Mt Saint Mary College
330 Powell Ave
Newburgh, NY 12550
(914) 561-0800

New York Institute of Technology
—Old Westbury—

Full-Time Enrollments:	10	Evening Classes:	Yes
Part-Time Enrollments:	7	Weekend Classes:	Yes
Affiliation:	Private	Distance Learning:	Yes

NLN ACCREDITATION: No

BSN for non-RNs w/degree in other field: No

Articulation: None

For Further Information Contact:

Dr Dolores Shapiro, Chair
New York Institute of Technology
PO Box 170
Old Westbury, NY 11568
(516) 686-7844

New York University
—New York—

Full-Time Enrollments:	400	Evening Classes:	Yes
Part-Time Enrollments:	48	Weekend Classes:	Yes
Affiliation:	Private	Distance Learning:	—

NLN ACCREDITATION: Yes

BSN for non-RNs w/degree in other field: Yes

Articulation: Associate to Baccalaureate

For Further Information Contact:

Dr Diane O McGivern, Dept Head
New York University
50 West 4th St
New York, NY 10012-1165
(212) 998-5300

Niagara University
—Niagara Univ—

Full-Time Enrollments:	157	Evening Classes:	Yes
Part-Time Enrollments:	31	Weekend Classes:	No
Affiliation:	Private	Distance Learning:	Yes

NLN ACCREDITATION: Yes

BSN for non-RNs w/degree in other field: No

Articulation: Associate to Baccalaureate
Diploma to Baccalaureate

For Further Information Contact:

Dr Dolores Bower, Dean
Niagara University
Niagara Univ, NY 14109-2203
(716) 286-8310

Pace University
—Pleasantville—

Full-Time Enrollments:	298	Evening Classes:	Yes
Part-Time Enrollments:	50	Weekend Classes:	No
Affiliation:	Private	Distance Learning:	No

NLN ACCREDITATION: Yes

BSN for non-RNs w/degree in other field: Yes

Articulation: Associate to Baccalaureate

For Further Information Contact:

Dr Martha Greenberg, Chair
Pace University
861 Bedford Rd
Pleasantville, NY 10570
(914) 773-3373

Regents College-University of the State of New York
—Albany—

Full-Time Enrollments:	—	Evening Classes:	No
Part-Time Enrollments:	734	Weekend Classes:	No
Affiliation:	Private	Distance Learning:	Yes

NLN ACCREDITATION: Yes

BSN for non-RNs w/degree in other field: No

Articulation: Associate to Baccalaureate
LPN to Associate

For Further Information Contact:

Dr Mary Beth Hanner, Dean
Regents College-University of the State of New York
7 Columbia Cir
Albany, NY 12203-5159
(518) 464-8500

Roberts Wesleyan College
—Rochester—

Full-Time Enrollments:	92	Evening Classes:	Yes
Part-Time Enrollments:	1	Weekend Classes:	No
Affiliation:	Religious	Distance Learning:	No

NLN ACCREDITATION: Yes

BSN for non-RNs w/degree in other field: No

Articulation: Associate to Baccalaureate

For Further Information Contact:

Dr Carol B Kenyon, Chair
Roberts Wesleyan College
2301 Westside Dr
Rochester, NY 14624
(716) 594-6330

Russell Sage College
—Troy—

Full-Time Enrollments:	148	Evening Classes:	Yes
Part-Time Enrollments:	11	Weekend Classes:	Yes
Affiliation:	Private	Distance Learning:	No

NLN ACCREDITATION: Yes

BSN for non-RNs w/degree in other field: No

Articulation: Associate to Baccalaureate

For Further Information Contact:

Dr Linnea Jatulis, Chair
Russell Sage College
Troy, NY 12180
(518) 270-2231

St John Fisher College
—Rochester—

Full-Time Enrollments:	159	Evening Classes:	Yes
Part-Time Enrollments:	19	Weekend Classes:	No
Affiliation:	Religious	Distance Learning:	No

NLN ACCREDITATION: Yes

BSN for non-RNs w/degree in other field: No

Articulation: Associate to Baccalaureate

For Further Information Contact:

Dr Kathleen Powers, Chair
St John Fisher College
3690 East Avenue
Rochester, NY 14618
(716) 385-8241

SUNY at Brockport
—Brockport—

Full-Time Enrollments:	148	Evening Classes:	No
Part-Time Enrollments:	—	Weekend Classes:	No
Affiliation:	Public	Distance Learning:	No

NLN ACCREDITATION: Yes

BSN for non-RNs w/degree in other field: No

Articulation: Associate to Baccalaureate

For Further Information Contact:

Dr Kathryn M Wood, Chair
SUNY at Brockport
Brockport, NY 14420
(716) 395-2355

SUNY at Buffalo
—Buffalo—

Full-Time Enrollments:	138	Evening Classes:	Yes
Part-Time Enrollments:	13	Weekend Classes:	No
Affiliation:	Public	Distance Learning:	Yes

NLN ACCREDITATION: Yes

BSN for non-RNs w/degree in other field: No

Articulation: Associate to Baccalaureate
Diploma to Baccalaureate

For Further Information Contact:

Dr Mecca S Cranley, Dean
SUNY at Buffalo
1010 Kimball Tower
Buffalo, NY 14214
(716) 829-2533

SUNY at Stony Brook
—Stony Brook—

Full-Time Enrollments:	70	Evening Classes:	No
Part-Time Enrollments:	2	Weekend Classes:	No
Affiliation:	Public	Distance Learning:	No

NLN ACCREDITATION: Yes

BSN for non-RNs w/degree in other field: Yes

Articulation: None

For Further Information Contact:

Dr Lenora McClean, Dean
SUNY at Stony Brook
Stony Brook, NY 11794-8240
(516) 444-3260

SUNY-College at Plattsburgh
—Plattsburgh—

Full-Time Enrollments:	240	Evening Classes:	Yes
Part-Time Enrollments:	5	Weekend Classes:	No
Affiliation:	Public	Distance Learning:	Yes

NLN ACCREDITATION: Yes

BSN for non-RNs w/degree in other field: Yes

Articulation: Associate to Baccalaureate
Diploma to Baccalaureate

For Further Information Contact:

Dr Crawford Beebe, Chair
SUNY-College at Plattsburgh
Dept of Nursing
Plattsburgh, NY 12901
(518) 564-3124

SUNY-Health Science Center
—Brooklyn—

Full-Time Enrollments:	71	Evening Classes:	Yes
Part-Time Enrollments:	11	Weekend Classes:	No
Affiliation:	Public	Distance Learning:	Yes

NLN ACCREDITATION: Yes

BSN for non-RNs w/degree in other field: No

Articulation: Associate to Baccalaureate

For Further Information Contact:

Dr Mary Ella Graham, Dean
SUNY-Health Science Center
450 Clarkson Ave Box 22
Brooklyn, NY 11203
(718) 270-7672

Syracuse University
—Syracuse—

Full-Time Enrollments:	415	Evening Classes:	—
Part-Time Enrollments:	6	Weekend Classes:	—
Affiliation:	Private	Distance Learning:	—

NLN ACCREDITATION: Yes

BSN for non-RNs w/degree in other field: No

Articulation: None

For Further Information Contact:

Dr Grace H Chickadonz, Dean
Syracuse University
426 Ostrom Ave
Syracuse, NY 13210
(315) 443-2141

University of Rochester
—Rochester—

Full-Time Enrollments:	158	Evening Classes:	No
Part-Time Enrollments:	13	Weekend Classes:	No
Affiliation:	Private	Distance Learning:	No

NLN ACCREDITATION: Yes

BSN for non-RNs w/degree in other field: No

Articulation: Associate to Baccalaureate

For Further Information Contact:

Ms Rita D'Aoust, Coordinator
University of Rochester
601 Elmwood Ave Box 703
Rochester, NY 14642
(716) 275-8831

Utica College-Syracuse University
—Utica—

Full-Time Enrollments:	71	Evening Classes:	Yes
Part-Time Enrollments:	7	Weekend Classes:	No
Affiliation:	Private	Distance Learning:	Yes

NLN ACCREDITATION: Yes

BSN for non-RNs w/degree in other field: Yes

Articulation: Associate to Baccalaureate

For Further Information Contact:

Dr Mary K Maroney, Director
Utica College-Syracuse University
1600 Burrstone Rd
Utica, NY 13502
(315) 792-3059

Wagner College
—Staten Island—

Full-Time Enrollments:	139	Evening Classes:	Yes
Part-Time Enrollments:	43	Weekend Classes:	No
Affiliation:	Private	Distance Learning:	No

NLN ACCREDITATION: Yes

BSN for non-RNs w/degree in other field: Yes

Articulation: None

For Further Information Contact:

Mrs Julia Barchitta, Dept Head
Wagner College
631 Howard Ave
Staten Island, NY 10301
(718) 390-3436

North Carolina

Barton College
—Wilson—

Full-Time Enrollments:	79	Evening Classes:	—
Part-Time Enrollments:	—	Weekend Classes:	Yes
Affiliation:	Religious	Distance Learning:	No

NLN ACCREDITATION: Yes

BSN for non-RNs w/degree in other field: Yes

Articulation: None

For Further Information Contact:

Dr Evelyn Pruden, Dean
Barton College
College Station
Wilson, NC 27893
(919) 399-6401

East Carolina University
—Greenville—

Full-Time Enrollments:	341	Evening Classes:	No
Part-Time Enrollments:	62	Weekend Classes:	No
Affiliation:	Public	Distance Learning:	No

NLN ACCREDITATION: Yes

BSN for non-RNs w/degree in other field: No

Articulation: Associate to Baccalaureate
Diploma to Baccalaureate

For Further Information Contact:

Dr Phyllis N Horns, Dean
East Carolina University
5th Street
Greenville, NC 27858-4353
(919) 328-6099

Lenoir Rhyne College
—Hickory—

Full-Time Enrollments:	136	Evening Classes:	Yes
Part-Time Enrollments:	5	Weekend Classes:	No
Affiliation:	Religious	Distance Learning:	No

NLN ACCREDITATION: Yes

BSN for non-RNs w/degree in other field: No

Articulation: Associate to Baccalaureate

For Further Information Contact:

Dr Linda Reece, Chair
Lenoir Rhyne College
PO Box 7292
Hickory, NC 28603
(704) 328-7282

North Carolina Agricultural & Technical State University
—Greensboro—

Full-Time Enrollments:	132	Evening Classes:	Yes
Part-Time Enrollments:	21	Weekend Classes:	No
Affiliation:	Public	Distance Learning:	No

NLN ACCREDITATION: Yes

BSN for non-RNs w/degree in other field: No

Articulation: LPN to Baccalaureate

For Further Information Contact:

Dr Janice Brewingston, Interim Dean
North Carolina Agricultural & Technical State University
Greensboro, NC 27411
(910) 334-7751

North Carolina Central University
—Durham—

Full-Time Enrollments:	110	Evening Classes:	No
Part-Time Enrollments:	4	Weekend Classes:	No
Affiliation:	Public	Distance Learning:	No

NLN ACCREDITATION: Yes

BSN for non-RNs w/degree in other field: No

Articulation: Associate to Baccalaureate

For Further Information Contact:

Dr Kaye McDonald, Chair
North Carolina Central University
PO Box 19798
Durham, NC 27707
(919) 560-6322

Queens College
—Charlotte—

Full-Time Enrollments:	30	Evening Classes:	Yes
Part-Time Enrollments:	17	Weekend Classes:	Yes
Affiliation:	Religious	Distance Learning:	No

NLN ACCREDITATION: Yes

BSN for non-RNs w/degree in other field: No

Articulation: Diploma to Baccalaureate

For Further Information Contact:

Dr Joan McGill, Chair
Queens College
1900 Selwyn Ave
Charlotte, NC 28274
(704) 337-2276

University of North Carolina at Chapel Hill
—Chapel Hill—

Full-Time Enrollments:	259	Evening Classes:	Yes
Part-Time Enrollments:	14	Weekend Classes:	No
Affiliation:	Public	Distance Learning:	No

NLN ACCREDITATION: Yes

BSN for non-RNs w/degree in other field: No

Articulation: Associate to Baccalaureate

For Further Information Contact:

Dr Cynthia M Freund, Dean
University of North Carolina at Chapel Hill
Carrington Hall-CB #7460
Chapel Hill, NC 27599-7460
(919) 966-4260

University of North Carolina at Charlotte
—Charlotte—

Full-Time Enrollments:	170	Evening Classes:	Yes
Part-Time Enrollments:	33	Weekend Classes:	Yes
Affiliation:	Public	Distance Learning:	Yes

NLN ACCREDITATION: Yes

BSN for non-RNs w/degree in other field: No

Articulation: Associate to Baccalaureate

For Further Information Contact:

Dr Sue Marquis Bishop, Dean
University of North Carolina at Charlotte
Charlotte, NC 28223
(704) 547-4650

University of North Carolina at Greensboro
—Greensboro—

Full-Time Enrollments:	180	Evening Classes:	Yes
Part-Time Enrollments:	4	Weekend Classes:	No
Affiliation:	Public	Distance Learning:	Yes

NLN ACCREDITATION: Yes

BSN for non-RNs w/degree in other field: Yes

Articulation: Associate to Baccalaureate

For Further Information Contact:

Dr Lynne Pearcey, Dean
University of North Carolina at Greensboro
School of Nursing
Greensboro, NC 27412-5001
(910) 334-5010

University of North Carolina at Wilmington
—Wilmington—

Full-Time Enrollments:	131	Evening Classes:	Yes
Part-Time Enrollments:	7	Weekend Classes:	Yes
Affiliation:	Public	Distance Learning:	Yes

NLN ACCREDITATION: Yes

BSN for non-RNs w/degree in other field: No

Articulation: Associate to Baccalaureate

For Further Information Contaot:

Dr Virginia Adams, Dean
University of North Carolina at Wilmington
601 South College Rd
Wilmington, NC 28403
(910) 962-3784

Western Carolina University
—Cullowhee—

Full-Time Enrollments:	87	Evening Classes:	Yes
Part-Time Enrollments:	—	Weekend Classes:	No
Affiliation:	Public	Distance Learning:	No

NLN ACCREDITATION: Yes

BSN for non-RNs w/degree in other field: No

Articulation: Associate to Baccalaureate

For Further Information Contact:

Dr Sharon Jacques, Dept Head
Western Carolina University
207 Moore Hall
Cullowhee, NC 28723
(704) 227-7467

Winston-Salem State University
—Winston-Salem—

Full-Time Enrollments:	188	Evening Classes:	Yes
Part-Time Enrollments:	—	Weekend Classes:	Yes
Affiliation:	Public	Distance Learning:	No

NLN ACCREDITATION: Yes

BSN for non-RNs w/degree in other field: No

Articulation: Associate to Baccalaureate
Diploma to Baccalaureate
LPN to Baccalaureate

For Further Information Contact:

Dr Bettie Glenn, Chair
Winston-Salem State University
PO Box 13326
Winston-Salem, NC 27110
(910) 750-2660

North Dakota

Dickinson State University
—Dickinson—

Full-Time Enrollments:	—	Evening Classes:	—
Part-Time Enrollments:	—	Weekend Classes:	—
Affiliation:	Public	Distance Learning:	—

NLN ACCREDITATION: Yes

BSN for non-RNs w/degree in other field: —

Articulation: None

For Further Information Contact:

Dr Sandra Affeldt, Chair
Dickinson State University
291 Campus Dr
Dickinson, ND 58601
(701) 227-2172

Jamestown College
—Jamestown—

Full-Time Enrollments:	63	Evening Classes:	No
Part-Time Enrollments:	—	Weekend Classes:	No
Affiliation:	Private	Distance Learning:	No

NLN ACCREDITATION: Yes

BSN for non-RNs w/degree in other field: No

Articulation: LPN to Baccalaureate

For Further Information Contact:

Dr Geneal Hall, Chair
Jamestown College
6010 College Lane
Jamestown, ND 58405
(701) 252-3467

Medcenter One College of Nursing
—Bismarck—

Full-Time Enrollments:	66	Evening Classes:	No
Part-Time Enrollments:	3	Weekend Classes:	No
Affiliation:	Private	Distance Learning:	No

NLN ACCREDITATION: Yes

BSN for non-RNs w/degree in other field: No

Articulation: None

For Further Information Contact:

Dr Karen Kristensen, Provost
Medcenter One College of Nursing
512 North 7th St
Bismarck, ND 58501
(701) 323-6270

Minot State University
—Minot—

Full-Time Enrollments:	76	Evening Classes:	—
Part-Time Enrollments:	13	Weekend Classes:	—
Affiliation:	Public	Distance Learning:	Yes

NLN ACCREDITATION: Yes

BSN for non-RNs w/degree in other field: No

Articulation: None

For Further Information Contact:

Dr V C Fabricius, Dean
Minot State University
500 University Ave,W
Minot, ND 58707
(701) 858-3101

Tri College University-North Dakota State University
—Fargo—

Full-Time Enrollments:	100	Evening Classes:	Yes
Part-Time Enrollments:	3	Weekend Classes:	No
Affiliation:	Public	Distance Learning:	No

NLN ACCREDITATION: Yes

BSN for non-RNs w/degree in other field:　No

Articulation:　LPN to Baccalaureate

For Further Information Contact:

Dr Lois F Nelson, Chair
Tri College University-North Dakota State University
PO Box 5630
Fargo, ND 58105
(218) 299-3879

University of Mary
—Bismarck—

Full-Time Enrollments:	117	Evening Classes:	Yes
Part-Time Enrollments:	—	Weekend Classes:	No
Affiliation:	Religious	Distance Learning:	Yes

NLN ACCREDITATION: Yes

BSN for non-RNs w/degree in other field:　No

Articulation:　Associate to Baccalaureate
　　　　　Diploma to Baccalaureate
　　　　　LPN to Baccalaureate

For Further Information Contact:

Dr Betty Rambur, Chair
University of Mary
7500 Univ Dr
Bismarck, ND 58504
(701) 255-7500

University of North Dakota
—Grand Forks—

Full-Time Enrollments:	232	Evening Classes:	Yes
Part-Time Enrollments:	34	Weekend Classes:	Yes
Affiliation:	Public	Distance Learning:	No

NLN ACCREDITATION: Yes

BSN for non-RNs w/degree in other field:　No

Articulation:　Associate to Baccalaureate
　　　　　LPN to Baccalaureate

For Further Information Contact:

Dr Elizabeth Nichols, Dean
University of North Dakota
Box 9025 Univ Station
Grand Forks, ND 58202
(701) 777-4173

Ohio

Bowling Green State University c/o Medical College of Ohio
—Toledo—

Full-Time Enrollments:	108	Evening Classes:	Yes
Part-Time Enrollments:	4	Weekend Classes:	Yes
Affiliation:	Public	Distance Learning:	Yes

NLN ACCREDITATION: Yes

BSN for non-RNs w/degree in other field:　No

Articulation:　Associate to Baccalaureate

For Further Information Contact:

Dr Joyce Shoemaker, Dean
Bowling Green State University c/o Medical College of Ohio
PO Box 10008
Toledo, OH 43699-0008
(419) 381-5800

Capital University
—Columbus—

Full-Time Enrollments:	283	Evening Classes:	Yes
Part-Time Enrollments:	9	Weekend Classes:	Yes
Affiliation:	Religious	Distance Learning:	No

NLN ACCREDITATION: Yes

BSN for non-RNs w/degree in other field:　No

Articulation:　None

For Further Information Contact:

Dr Doris S Edwards, Dean
Capital University
2199 E Main St
Columbus, OH 43209-2394
(614) 236-6703

Case Western Reserve University-F P Bolton
—Cleveland—

Full-Time Enrollments:	230	Evening Classes:	Yes
Part-Time Enrollments:	2	Weekend Classes:	Yes
Affiliation:	Private	Distance Learning:	Yes

NLN ACCREDITATION: Yes

BSN for non-RNs w/degree in other field:　No

Articulation:　None

For Further Information Contact:

Dr Joyce Fitzpatrick, Dean
Case Western Reserve University-F P Bolton
10900 Euclid Ave
Cleveland, OH 44106-4904
(216) 368-2540

Cedarville College School of Nursing
—Cedarville—

Full-Time Enrollments:	273	Evening Classes:	Yes
Part-Time Enrollments:	—	Weekend Classes:	No
Affiliation:	Religious	Distance Learning:	No

NLN ACCREDITATION: Yes

BSN for non-RNs w/degree in other field: No

Articulation: None

For Further Information Contact:

Dr Irene B Alyn, Chair
Cedarville College School of Nursing
Box 601
Cedarville, OH 45314-0601
(937) 766-7715

Cleveland State University
—Cleveland—

Full-Time Enrollments:	160	Evening Classes:	No
Part-Time Enrollments:	17	Weekend Classes:	No
Affiliation:	Public	Distance Learning:	No

NLN ACCREDITATION: Yes

BSN for non-RNs w/degree in other field: No

Articulation: Associate to Baccalaureate
Diploma to Baccalaureate

For Further Information Contact:

Dr Lois Owen, Chair
Cleveland State University
1860 E 22nd
Cleveland, OH 44115-2407
(216) 687-3598

College of Mt St Joseph
—Cincinnati—

Full-Time Enrollments:	130	Evening Classes:	Yes
Part-Time Enrollments:	23	Weekend Classes:	Yes
Affiliation:	Religious	Distance Learning:	No

NLN ACCREDITATION: Yes

BSN for non-RNs w/degree in other field: No

Articulation: Associate to Baccalaureate
Diploma to Baccalaureate

For Further Information Contact:

Dr Ignatius Perkins, Chair
College of Mt St Joseph
5701 Delhi Rd
Cincinnati, OH 45233-1670
(513) 244-4511

Franciscan University of Steubenville BSN Program
—Steubenville—

Full-Time Enrollments:	84	Evening Classes:	Yes
Part-Time Enrollments:	—	Weekend Classes:	—
Affiliation:	Religious	Distance Learning:	—

NLN ACCREDITATION: Yes

BSN for non-RNs w/degree in other field: No

Articulation: Associate to Baccalaureate
Diploma to Baccalaureate
LPN to Baccalaureate

For Further Information Contact:

Ms Carolyn S Miller, Chair
Franciscan University of Steubenville BSN Program
University Blvd
Steubenville, OH 43952-6701
(614) 283-6324

Kent State University
—Kent—

Full-Time Enrollments:	647	Evening Classes:	Yes
Part-Time Enrollments:	123	Weekend Classes:	Yes
Affiliation:	Public	Distance Learning:	—

NLN ACCREDITATION: Yes

BSN for non-RNs w/degree in other field: Yes

Articulation: None

For Further Information Contact:

Dr Davina Gosnell, Dean
Kent State University
113 Henderson Hall Box 5190
Kent, OH 44242-0001
(330) 672-7930

Lourdes College
—Sylvania—

Full-Time Enrollments:	63	Evening Classes:	Yes
Part-Time Enrollments:	25	Weekend Classes:	Yes
Affiliation:	Religious	Distance Learning:	No

NLN ACCREDITATION: Yes

BSN for non-RNs w/degree in other field: No

Articulation: Associate to Baccalaureate
Diploma to Baccalaureate

For Further Information Contact:

Ms Rebecca Zechman, Director
Lourdes College
6832 Convent Blvd
Sylvania, OH 43560-2898
(419) 885-3211

Malone College-Department of Nursing Education
—Canton—

Full-Time Enrollments:	134	Evening Classes:	Yes
Part-Time Enrollments:	8	Weekend Classes:	No
Affiliation:	Religious	Distance Learning:	No

NLN ACCREDITATION: Yes

BSN for non-RNs w/degree in other field:　No

Articulation:　None

For Further Information Contact:

Dr Loretta Reinhart, Chair
Malone College-Department of Nursing Education
515 25th St NW
Canton, OH 44709-3897
(330) 471-8166

Mt Carmel College of Nursing
—Columbus—

Full-Time Enrollments:	304	Evening Classes:	No
Part-Time Enrollments:	44	Weekend Classes:	No
Affiliation:	Religious	Distance Learning:	No

NLN ACCREDITATION: Yes

BSN for non-RNs w/degree in other field:　No

Articulation:　None

For Further Information Contact:

Dr Ann E Schiele, President
Mt Carmel College of Nursing
127 S Davis Ave
Columbus, OH 43222-1504
(614) 234-5032

Ohio State University College of Nursing
—Columbus—

Full-Time Enrollments:	370	Evening Classes:	Yes
Part-Time Enrollments:	81	Weekend Classes:	No
Affiliation:	Public	Distance Learning:	No

NLN ACCREDITATION: Yes

BSN for non-RNs w/degree in other field:　No

Articulation:　None

For Further Information Contact:

Dr Carole A Anderson, Dean
Ohio State University College of Nursing
1585 Neil Ave
Columbus, OH 43210-1289
(614) 292-8900

Otterbein College BSN Program
—Westerville—

Full-Time Enrollments:	113	Evening Classes:	—
Part-Time Enrollments:	92	Weekend Classes:	—
Affiliation:	Private	Distance Learning:	—

NLN ACCREDITATION: Yes

BSN for non-RNs w/degree in other field:　No

Articulation:　None

For Further Information Contact:

Dr Judy Strayer, Chair
Otterbein College BSN Program
155 W Main St
Westerville, OH 43081
(614) 890-3000

University of Akron College of Nursing
—Akron—

Full-Time Enrollments:	536	Evening Classes:	Yes
Part-Time Enrollments:	—	Weekend Classes:	No
Affiliation:	Public	Distance Learning:	No

NLN ACCREDITATION: Yes

BSN for non-RNs w/degree in other field:　No

Articulation:　Associate to Baccalaureate
Diploma to Baccalaureate
LPN to Baccalaureate

For Further Information Contact:

Dr J Dunham-Taylor, Interim Dean
University of Akron College of Nursing
209 Carroll St
Akron, OH 44325-3701
(216) 972-7552

University of Cincinnati-College of Nursing & Health
—Cincinnati—

Full-Time Enrollments:	343	Evening Classes:	No
Part-Time Enrollments:	29	Weekend Classes:	No
Affiliation:	Public	Distance Learning:	Yes

NLN ACCREDITATION: Yes

BSN for non-RNs w/degree in other field:　Yes

Articulation:　Associate to Baccalaureate
Diploma to Baccalaureate

For Further Information Contact:

Dr Andrea R Lindell, Dean
University of Cincinnati-College of Nursing & Health
3110 Vine St
Cincinnati, OH 44221
(513) 558-5070

University of Toledo-Medical College of Ohio
—Toledo—

Full-Time Enrollments:	113	Evening Classes:	Yes
Part-Time Enrollments:	5	Weekend Classes:	Yes
Affiliation:	Public	Distance Learning:	Yes

NLN ACCREDITATION: Yes

BSN for non-RNs w/degree in other field: No

Articulation: Associate to Baccalaureate

For Further Information Contact:

Dr Joyce Shoemaker, Dean
University of Toledo-Medical College of Ohio
PO Box 10008
Toledo, OH 43699-0008
(419) 381-5800

Ursuline College
—Pepper Pike—

Full-Time Enrollments:	234	Evening Classes:	Yes
Part-Time Enrollments:	91	Weekend Classes:	Yes
Affiliation:	Private	Distance Learning:	No

NLN ACCREDITATION: Yes

BSN for non-RNs w/degree in other field: Yes

Articulation: Associate to Baccalaureate
Diploma to Baccalaureate

For Further Information Contact:

Dr Carole F Cashion, Dean
Ursuline College
2550 Lander Rd
Pepper Pike, OH 44124-4398
(216) 449-4200

Wright State University-Miami Valley College of Nursing
—Dayton—

Full-Time Enrollments:	283	Evening Classes:	No
Part-Time Enrollments:	103	Weekend Classes:	No
Affiliation:	Public	Distance Learning:	Yes

NLN ACCREDITATION: Yes

BSN for non-RNs w/degree in other field: No

Articulation: Associate to Baccalaureate

For Further Information Contact:

Dr Jane C Swart, Dean
Wright State University-Miami Valley College of Nursing
3640 Colonel Glenn Hwy
Dayton, OH 45435
(937) 775-3133

Xavier University
—Cincinnati—

Full-Time Enrollments:	58	Evening Classes:	Yes
Part-Time Enrollments:	2	Weekend Classes:	—
Affiliation:	Religious	Distance Learning:	—

NLN ACCREDITATION: Yes

BSN for non-RNs w/degree in other field: No

Articulation: None

For Further Information Contact:

Dr Evelyn Lutz, Interim Chair
Xavier University
3800 Victory Parkway
Cincinnati, OH 45207
(513) 745-3815

Youngstown State University
—Youngstown—

Full-Time Enrollments:	148	Evening Classes:	—
Part-Time Enrollments:	2	Weekend Classes:	No
Affiliation:	Public	Distance Learning:	No

NLN ACCREDITATION: Yes

BSN for non-RNs w/degree in other field: No

Articulation: Associate to Baccalaureate
Diploma to Baccalaureate

For Further Information Contact:

Dr Patricia McCarthy, Chair
Youngstown State University
410 Wick Ave
Youngstown, OH 44555-0002
(330) 742-3293

Oklahoma

East Central University
—Ada—

Full-Time Enrollments:	130	Evening Classes:	Yes
Part-Time Enrollments:	6	Weekend Classes:	—
Affiliation:	Public	Distance Learning:	Yes

NLN ACCREDITATION: Yes

BSN for non-RNs w/degree in other field: No

Articulation: Associate to Baccalaureate

For Further Information Contact:

Dr E Schmelling, Chair
East Central University
1000 E 14th
Ada, OK 74820
(405) 332-8000

Langston University
—Langston—

Full-Time Enrollments:	105	**Evening Classes:**	—
Part-Time Enrollments:	2	**Weekend Classes:**	—
Affiliation:	Public	**Distance Learning:**	—

NLN ACCREDITATION: Yes

BSN for non-RNs w/degree in other field: No

Articulation: None

For Further Information Contact:

Dr C Kornegay, Director
Langston University
3rd Fl Univ Women Bldg
Langston, OK 73050
(405) 466-3411

Northwestern Oklahoma State University
—Alva—

Full-Time Enrollments:	57	**Evening Classes:**	Yes
Part-Time Enrollments:	1	**Weekend Classes:**	No
Affiliation:	Public	**Distance Learning:**	Yes

NLN ACCREDITATION: Yes

BSN for non-RNs w/degree in other field: No

Articulation: Associate to Baccalaureate

For Further Information Contact:

Mrs Doris Ferguson, Dean
Northwestern Oklahoma State University
Alva, OK 73717
(405) 327-1700

Oklahoma Baptist University
—Shawnee—

Full-Time Enrollments:	63	**Evening Classes:**	Yes
Part-Time Enrollments:	2	**Weekend Classes:**	No
Affiliation:	Religious	**Distance Learning:**	No

NLN ACCREDITATION: Yes

BSN for non-RNs w/degree in other field: No

Articulation: None

For Further Information Contact:

Dr Claudine F Dickey, Dean
Oklahoma Baptist University
500 W Univ PO Box 61805
Shawnee, OK 74801
(405) 878-2081

Oklahoma City University School of Nursing
—Oklahoma City—

Full-Time Enrollments:	52	**Evening Classes:**	No
Part-Time Enrollments:	16	**Weekend Classes:**	No
Affiliation:	Religious	**Distance Learning:**	No

NLN ACCREDITATION: Yes

BSN for non-RNs w/degree in other field: No

Articulation: Associate to Baccalaureate

For Further Information Contact:

Dr Andrea West, Interim Dean
Oklahoma City University School of Nursing
2501 N Blackwelder Box 96B
Oklahoma City, OK 73106-1498
(405) 272-7203

Oral Roberts University
—Tulsa—

Full-Time Enrollments:	44	**Evening Classes:**	Yes
Part-Time Enrollments:	5	**Weekend Classes:**	No
Affiliation:	Religious	**Distance Learning:**	No

NLN ACCREDITATION: Yes

BSN for non-RNs w/degree in other field: No

Articulation: None

For Further Information Contact:

Dr Kenda Jezek, Dean
Oral Roberts University
7777 S Lewis Ave
Tulsa, OK 74171
(918) 495-6198

Southern Nazarene University
—Bethany—

Full-Time Enrollments:	85	**Evening Classes:**	—
Part-Time Enrollments:	4	**Weekend Classes:**	—
Affiliation:	Religious	**Distance Learning:**	—

NLN ACCREDITATION: Yes

BSN for non-RNs w/degree in other field: No

Articulation: None

For Further Information Contact:

Dr Donna Eckhart, Chair
Southern Nazarene University
6729 NW 39th Expressway
Bethany, OK 73008
(405) 491-6365

Southwestern Oklahoma State University
—Weatherford—

Full-Time Enrollments:	66	Evening Classes:	No
Part-Time Enrollments:	—	Weekend Classes:	Yes
Affiliation:	Public	Distance Learning:	No

NLN ACCREDITATION: Yes

BSN for non-RNs w/degree in other field: No

Articulation: Associate to Baccalaureate

For Further Information Contact:

Dr Patricia Meyer, Chair
Southwestern Oklahoma State University
100 Campus Dr
Weatherford, OK 73096-3098
(405) 774-3261

University of Central Oklahoma
—Edmond—

Full-Time Enrollments:	175	Evening Classes:	No
Part-Time Enrollments:	1	Weekend Classes:	No
Affiliation:	Public	Distance Learning:	—

NLN ACCREDITATION: Yes

BSN for non-RNs w/degree in other field: No

Articulation: Associate to Baccalaureate

For Further Information Contact:

Dr Patricia LaGrow, Chair
University of Central Oklahoma
100 N Univ Dr
Edmond, OK 73060
(405) 341-2980

University of Oklahoma-Health Science Center
—Oklahoma City—

Full-Time Enrollments:	192	Evening Classes:	Yes
Part-Time Enrollments:	24	Weekend Classes:	Yes
Affiliation:	Public	Distance Learning:	Yes

NLN ACCREDITATION: Yes

BSN for non-RNs w/degree in other field: No

Articulation: Associate to Baccalaureate

For Further Information Contact:

Dr Patricia Forni, Dean
University of Oklahoma-Health Science Center
PO Box 26901
Oklahoma City, OK 73190
(405) 271-2125

University of Tulsa
—Tulsa—

Full-Time Enrollments:	99	Evening Classes:	—
Part-Time Enrollments:	4	Weekend Classes:	—
Affiliation:	Private	Distance Learning:	—

NLN ACCREDITATION: Yes

BSN for non-RNs w/degree in other field: No

Articulation: None

For Further Information Contact:

Dr Susan Gaston, Director
University of Tulsa
600 S College
Tulsa, OK 74104
(918) 631-3116

Oregon

Linfield College-Good Samaritan
—Portland—

Full-Time Enrollments:	—	Evening Classes:	—
Part-Time Enrollments:	—	Weekend Classes:	—
Affiliation:	Religious	Distance Learning:	—

NLN ACCREDITATION: Yes

BSN for non-RNs w/degree in other field: —

Articulation: None

For Further Information Contact:

Dr Pamela Harris, Dean
Linfield College-Good Samaritan
2255 N W Northrup R304
Portland, OR 97210
(503) 229-7651

Oregon Health Sciences University School of Nursing
—Portland—

Full-Time Enrollments:	323	Evening Classes:	Yes
Part-Time Enrollments:	9	Weekend Classes:	Yes
Affiliation:	Public	Distance Learning:	Yes

NLN ACCREDITATION: Yes

BSN for non-RNs w/degree in other field: No

Articulation: Associate to Baccalaureate

For Further Information Contact:

Dr Kathleen Potempa, Dean
Oregon Health Sciences University School of Nursing
3181 SW Sam Jackson Park Rd
Portland, OR 97201
(503) 494-7791

University of Portland
—Portland—

Full-Time Enrollments:	121	Evening Classes:	Yes
Part-Time Enrollments:	3	Weekend Classes:	No
Affiliation:	Religious	Distance Learning:	Yes

NLN ACCREDITATION: Yes

BSN for non-RNs w/degree in other field: No

Articulation: None

For Further Information Contact:

Dr Susan R Moscato, Interim Dean
University of Portland
5000 N Willamette Blvd
Portland, OR 97203
(503) 283-7211

Pennsylvania

Allentown College of St Francis De Sales
—Center Valley—

Full-Time Enrollments:	116	Evening Classes:	Yes
Part-Time Enrollments:	12	Weekend Classes:	Yes
Affiliation:	Private	Distance Learning:	Yes

NLN ACCREDITATION: Yes

BSN for non-RNs w/degree in other field: No

Articulation: Associate to Baccalaureate

For Further Information Contact:

Dr Karen Moore Schaefer, Chair
Allentown College of St Francis De Sales
2755 Station Ave
Center Valley, PA 18034-9568
(610) 282-1100

Bloomsburg University
—Bloomsburg—

Full-Time Enrollments:	224	Evening Classes:	Yes
Part-Time Enrollments:	8	Weekend Classes:	No
Affiliation:	Public	Distance Learning:	No

NLN ACCREDITATION: Yes

BSN for non-RNs w/degree in other field: Yes

Articulation: Associate to Baccalaureate
Diploma to Baccalaureate

For Further Information Contact:

Dr Christine Alichnie, Chair
Bloomsburg University
3109 McCormick Center
Bloomsburg, PA 17815
(717) 389-4423

Carlow College
—Pittsburgh—

Full-Time Enrollments:	249	Evening Classes:	Yes
Part-Time Enrollments:	—	Weekend Classes:	Yes
Affiliation:	Religious	Distance Learning:	Yes

NLN ACCREDITATION: Yes

BSN for non-RNs w/degree in other field: No

Articulation: Associate to Baccalaureate
Diploma to Baccalaureate
RN to MSN

For Further Information Contact:

Dr Lorraine Rodrigues-Fisher, Chair
Carlow College
3333 5th Ave
Pittsburgh, PA 15213
(412) 578-6116

Cedar Crest College
—Allentown—

Full-Time Enrollments:	99	Evening Classes:	Yes
Part-Time Enrollments:	60	Weekend Classes:	No
Affiliation:	Private	Distance Learning:	No

NLN ACCREDITATION: Yes

BSN for non-RNs w/degree in other field: No

Articulation: Associate to Baccalaureate
Diploma to Baccalaureate

For Further Information Contact:

Dr Eloise R Lee, Chair
Cedar Crest College
100 College Dr
Allentown, PA 18104-6196
(610) 437-4471

College Misericordia
—Dallas—

Full-Time Enrollments:	104	Evening Classes:	Yes
Part-Time Enrollments:	3	Weekend Classes:	Yes
Affiliation:	Private	Distance Learning:	Yes

NLN ACCREDITATION: Yes

BSN for non-RNs w/degree in other field: No

Articulation: Associate to Baccalaureate

For Further Information Contact:

Dr Helen Streubert, Chair
College Misericordia
301 Lake Street
Dallas, PA 18612
(717) 675-2181

Duquesne University
—Pittsburgh—

Full-Time Enrollments:	261	Evening Classes:	Yes
Part-Time Enrollments:	14	Weekend Classes:	No
Affiliation:	Religious	Distance Learning:	—

NLN ACCREDITATION: Yes

BSN for non-RNs w/degree in other field: Yes

Articulation: Associate to Baccalaureate

For Further Information Contact:

Dr Mary de Chesnay, Dean
Duquesne University
600 Forbes Ave
Pittsburgh, PA 15282
(412) 396-6550

East Stroudsburg University
—East Stroudsburg—

Full-Time Enrollments:	72	Evening Classes:	No
Part-Time Enrollments:	2	Weekend Classes:	No
Affiliation:	Public	Distance Learning:	No

NLN ACCREDITATION: Yes

BSN for non-RNs w/degree in other field: No

Articulation: Associate to Baccalaureate
Diploma to Baccalaureate

For Further Information Contact:

Dr Mark Kilker, Chair
East Stroudsburg University
200 Prospect St
East Stroudsburg, PA 18301
(717) 422-3474

Edinboro University of Pennsylvania
—Edinboro—

Full-Time Enrollments:	216	Evening Classes:	Yes
Part-Time Enrollments:	—	Weekend Classes:	No
Affiliation:	Public	Distance Learning:	No

NLN ACCREDITATION: Yes

BSN for non-RNs w/degree in other field: No

Articulation: Associate to Baccalaureate
Diploma to Baccalaureate
LPN to Baccalaureate

For Further Information Contact:

Dr Mary L Keller, Chair
Edinboro University of Pennsylvania
Centennial Hall
Edinboro, PA 16444
(814) 732-2424

Gannon University-Department of Nursing
—Erie—

Full-Time Enrollments:	141	Evening Classes:	No
Part-Time Enrollments:	—	Weekend Classes:	No
Affiliation:	Religious	Distance Learning:	No

NLN ACCREDITATION: Yes

BSN for non-RNs w/degree in other field: No

Articulation: Associate to Baccalaureate
Diploma to Baccalaureate
RN to MSN

For Further Information Contact:

Dr Beverly Bartlett, Interim Chair
Gannon University-Department of Nursing
University Square
Erie, PA 16541
(814) 838-5520

Holy Family College
—Philadelphia—

Full-Time Enrollments:	331	Evening Classes:	Yes
Part-Time Enrollments:	163	Weekend Classes:	Yes
Affiliation:	Religious	Distance Learning:	No

NLN ACCREDITATION: Yes

BSN for non-RNs w/degree in other field: No

Articulation: Associate to Baccalaureate

For Further Information Contact:

Dr Jane Cardea, Head
Holy Family College
Grant & Frankford Ave
Philadelphia, PA 19114-2094
(215) 637-7700

Indiana University of Pennsylvania
—Indiana—

Full-Time Enrollments:	315	Evening Classes:	Yes
Part-Time Enrollments:	—	Weekend Classes:	No
Affiliation:	Public	Distance Learning:	No

NLN ACCREDITATION: Yes

BSN for non-RNs w/degree in other field: No

Articulation: None

For Further Information Contact:

Mrs Jodell Kuzneski, Chair
Indiana University of Pennsylvania
210 Johnson Hall
Indiana, PA 15705
(412) 357-2557

La Salle University
—Philadelphia—

Full-Time Enrollments:	136	Evening Classes:	Yes
Part-Time Enrollments:	15	Weekend Classes:	Yes
Affiliation:	Religious	Distance Learning:	No

NLN ACCREDITATION: Yes

BSN for non-RNs w/degree in other field: Yes

Articulation: Associate to Baccalaureate
Diploma to Baccalaureate

For Further Information Contact:

Dr C Flynn Capers, Interim Dean
La Salle University
1900 West Olney Ave
Philadelphia, PA 19141
(215) 951-4130

Lycoming College
—Williamsport—

Full-Time Enrollments:	116	Evening Classes:	Yes
Part-Time Enrollments:	—	Weekend Classes:	No
Affiliation:	Religious	Distance Learning:	No

NLN ACCREDITATION: Yes

BSN for non-RNs w/degree in other field: Yes

Articulation: None

For Further Information Contact:

Dr Doris Parrish, Chair
Lycoming College
700 College Pl
Williamsport, PA 17701
(717) 321-4250

Mansfield University
—Mansfield—

Full-Time Enrollments:	137	Evening Classes:	No
Part-Time Enrollments:	1	Weekend Classes:	No
Affiliation:	Public	Distance Learning:	No

NLN ACCREDITATION: Yes

BSN for non-RNs w/degree in other field: No

Articulation: None

For Further Information Contact:

Mrs Janeen Bartlett Sheehe, Chair
Mansfield University
Robert Packer Dept of Nsg
Mansfield, PA 16933
(717) 662-4522

Marywood College
—Scranton—

Full-Time Enrollments:	66	Evening Classes:	No
Part-Time Enrollments:	18	Weekend Classes:	No
Affiliation:	Religious	Distance Learning:	Yes

NLN ACCREDITATION: Yes

BSN for non-RNs w/degree in other field: No

Articulation: Associate to Baccalaureate
Diploma to Baccalaureate

For Further Information Contact:

Dr Mary Alice Golden, Chair
Marywood College
2300 Adams Ave
Scranton, PA 18509
(717) 348-6275

Messiah College
—Grantham—

Full-Time Enrollments:	236	Evening Classes:	—
Part-Time Enrollments:	—	Weekend Classes:	—
Affiliation:	Religious	Distance Learning:	—

NLN ACCREDITATION: Yes

BSN for non-RNs w/degree in other field: Yes

Articulation: None

For Further Information Contact:

Dr Sandra Jamison, Chair
Messiah College
Dept of Nursing
Grantham, PA 17027
(717) 691-6029

Neumann College
—Aston—

Full-Time Enrollments:	102	Evening Classes:	Yes
Part-Time Enrollments:	82	Weekend Classes:	Yes
Affiliation:	Religious	Distance Learning:	—

NLN ACCREDITATION: Yes

BSN for non-RNs w/degree in other field: No

Articulation: Associate to Baccalaureate

For Further Information Contact:

Dr Jill B Derstine, Chair
Neumann College
1 Neumann Dr
Aston, PA 19014-1297
(215) 558-5560

Pennsylvania State University
—University Park—

Full-Time Enrollments:	268	Evening Classes:	Yes
Part-Time Enrollments:	7	Weekend Classes:	No
Affiliation:	Public	Distance Learning:	Yes

NLN ACCREDITATION: Yes

BSN for non-RNs w/degree in other field:　No

Articulation:　Associate to Baccalaureate
　　　　　　　Diploma to Baccalaureate

For Further Information Contact:

Dr Sarah Hall Gueldner, Director
Pennsylvania State University
201 Hlth Human Development E
University Park, PA 16802
(814) 863-0245

St Francis College
—Loretto—

Full-Time Enrollments:	—	Evening Classes:	—
Part-Time Enrollments:	—	Weekend Classes:	—
Affiliation:	Religious	Distance Learning:	—

NLN ACCREDITATION: Yes

BSN for non-RNs w/degree in other field:　—

Articulation:　—

For Further Information Contact:

Dr Jean M Samii, Chair
St Francis College
800 E Lancaster Ave
Loretto, PA 15940
(814) 472-3027

Temple University-College of Allied Health Professions
—Philadelphia—

Full-Time Enrollments:	142	Evening Classes:	No
Part-Time Enrollments:	10	Weekend Classes:	No
Affiliation:	Public	Distance Learning:	No

NLN ACCREDITATION: Yes

BSN for non-RNs w/degree in other field:　No

Articulation:　None

For Further Information Contact:

Dr Catherine Bevil, Chair
Temple University-College of Allied Health Professions
3307 N Broad St
Philadelphia, PA 19140
(215) 707-4687

Thiel College
—Greenville—

Full-Time Enrollments:	59	Evening Classes:	No
Part-Time Enrollments:	2	Weekend Classes:	No
Affiliation:	Religious	Distance Learning:	No

NLN ACCREDITATION: Yes

BSN for non-RNs w/degree in other field:　No

Articulation:　None

For Further Information Contact:

Dr Evelyn Ramming, Director
Thiel College
75 College Ave
Greenville, PA 16125
(412) 589-2053

Thomas Jefferson University-College of Health Professions
—Philadelphia—

Full-Time Enrollments:	190	Evening Classes:	—
Part-Time Enrollments:	71	Weekend Classes:	—
Affiliation:	Private	Distance Learning:	—

NLN ACCREDITATION: Yes

BSN for non-RNs w/degree in other field:　Yes

Articulation:　None

For Further Information Contact:

Dr Pamela Watson, Chair
Thomas Jefferson University-College of Health Professions
130 S 9th St Suite 1200
Philadelphia, PA 19107
(215) 928-7939

University of Pennsylvania
—Philadelphia—

Full-Time Enrollments:	420	Evening Classes:	Yes
Part-Time Enrollments:	36	Weekend Classes:	No
Affiliation:	Private	Distance Learning:	Yes

NLN ACCREDITATION: Yes

BSN for non-RNs w/degree in other field:　No

Articulation:　None

For Further Information Contact:

Dr Norma Lang, Dean
University of Pennsylvania
420 Guardian Dr
Philadelphia, PA 19104-6096
(215) 898-8442

University of Pittsburgh-Community System of Higher Education
—Pittsburgh—

Full-Time Enrollments:	326	Evening Classes:	Yes
Part-Time Enrollments:	27	Weekend Classes:	No
Affiliation:	Public	Distance Learning:	No

NLN ACCREDITATION: Yes

BSN for non-RNs w/degree in other field: Yes

Articulation: Associate to Baccalaureate
Diploma to Baccalaureate
RN to MSN

For Further Information Contact:

Dr Ellen Beam Rudy, Dean
University of Pittsburgh-Community System of Higher Education
3500 Victoria St
Pittsburgh, PA 15261
(412) 624-2400

University of Scranton
—Scranton—

Full-Time Enrollments:	154	Evening Classes:	Yes
Part-Time Enrollments:	3	Weekend Classes:	No
Affiliation:	Religious	Distance Learning:	Yes

NLN ACCREDITATION: Yes

BSN for non-RNs w/degree in other field: No

Articulation: None

For Further Information Contact:

Dr Patricia Harrington, Chair
University of Scranton
107 A O'Hara Hall
Scranton, PA 18510-4595
(717) 941-7673

Villanova University-Department of Nursing
—Villanova—

Full-Time Enrollments:	393	Evening Classes:	Yes
Part-Time Enrollments:	1	Weekend Classes:	—
Affiliation:	Religious	Distance Learning:	—

NLN ACCREDITATION: Yes

BSN for non-RNs w/degree in other field: No

Articulation: Associate to Baccalaureate

For Further Information Contact:

Dr M Louise Fitzpatrick, Dean
Villanova University-Department of Nursing
800 Lancaster Ave
Villanova, PA 19085-1690
(610) 519-4900

Waynesburg College-Department of Nursing
—Waynesburg—

Full-Time Enrollments:	180	Evening Classes:	Yes
Part-Time Enrollments:	6	Weekend Classes:	No
Affiliation:	Religious	Distance Learning:	No

NLN ACCREDITATION: Yes

BSN for non-RNs w/degree in other field: No

Articulation: None

For Further Information Contact:

Dr Joan Clites, Director
Waynesburg College-Department of Nursing
51 West College St
Waynesburg, PA 15370
(412) 852-3356

West Chester University
—West Chester—

Full-Time Enrollments:	168	Evening Classes:	Yes
Part-Time Enrollments:	13	Weekend Classes:	No
Affiliation:	Public	Distance Learning:	No

NLN ACCREDITATION: Yes

BSN for non-RNs w/degree in other field: No

Articulation: None

For Further Information Contact:

Ms Ann Coghlan Stowe, Chair
West Chester University
Box 1041 S Church St
West Chester, PA 19383
(610) 436-2331

Widener University-School of Nursing
—Chester—

Full-Time Enrollments:	294	Evening Classes:	Yes
Part-Time Enrollments:	94	Weekend Classes:	Yes
Affiliation:	Private	Distance Learning:	No

NLN ACCREDITATION: Yes

BSN for non-RNs w/degree in other field: No

Articulation: Associate to Baccalaureate

For Further Information Contact:

Dr Marge Barbiere, Dean
Widener University-School of Nursing
One University Place
Chester, PA 19013-5792
(610) 499-4213

Wilkes University, Department of Nursing
—Wilkes-Barre—

Full-Time Enrollments:	82	Evening Classes:	Yes
Part-Time Enrollments:	48	Weekend Classes:	Yes
Affiliation:	Private	Distance Learning:	Yes

NLN ACCREDITATION: Yes

BSN for non-RNs w/degree in other field: No

Articulation: Associate to Baccalaureate
Diploma to Baccalaureate

For Further Information Contact:

Dr Ann M Kolanowski, Chair
Wilkes University, Department of Nursing
109 S Franklin St
Wilkes-Barre, PA 18766
(717) 824-4651

York College of Pennsylvania
—York—

Full-Time Enrollments:	297	Evening Classes:	Yes
Part-Time Enrollments:	99	Weekend Classes:	No
Affiliation:	Private	Distance Learning:	Yes

NLN ACCREDITATION: Yes

BSN for non-RNs w/degree in other field: No

Articulation: Associate to Baccalaureate

For Further Information Contact:

Dr Joan Reider, Chair
York College of Pennsylvania
Country Club Rd
York, PA 17405-7199
(717) 846-7788

Puerto Rico

Antillian Adventist University
—Mayaguez—

Full-Time Enrollments:	—	Evening Classes:	—
Part-Time Enrollments:	—	Weekend Classes:	—
Affiliation:	Religious	Distance Learning:	—

NLN ACCREDITATION: No

BSN for non-RNs w/degree in other field: —

Articulation: —

For Further Information Contact:

Prof Alicia Bruno, Director
Antillian Adventist University
PO Box 118
Mayaguez, PR 00681
(787) 834-9595

Caribbean University
—Bayamon—

Full-Time Enrollments:	10	Evening Classes:	Yes
Part-Time Enrollments:	15	Weekend Classes:	Yes
Affiliation:	Public	Distance Learning:	—

NLN ACCREDITATION: No

BSN for non-RNs w/degree in other field: No

Articulation: Associate to Baccalaureate

For Further Information Contact:

Ms Saria Cruz, Director
Caribbean University
Box 493
Bayamon, PR 00960-6093
(787) 780-0070

Columbia College
—Caguas—

Full-Time Enrollments:	—	Evening Classes:	—
Part-Time Enrollments:	—	Weekend Classes:	—
Affiliation:	Private	Distance Learning:	—

NLN ACCREDITATION: No

BSN for non-RNs w/degree in other field: —

Articulation: None

For Further Information Contact:

Mr Hector Colon Del Valle, Coordinator
Columbia College
PO Box 8517
Caguas, PR 00726-8517
(787) 743-4041

Instituto De Educacion Universal
—San Juan—

Full-Time Enrollments:	—	Evening Classes:	—
Part-Time Enrollments:	—	Weekend Classes:	—
Affiliation:	Private	Distance Learning:	—

NLN ACCREDITATION: No

BSN for non-RNs w/degree in other field: —

Articulation: None

For Further Information Contact:

Dr Miguel Ortiz, Director
Instituto De Educacion Universal
PO Box 195432
San Juan, PR 00919-5432
(787) 766-2915

Interamerican University
—Aguadilla—

Full-Time Enrollments: — Evening Classes: —
Part-Time Enrollments: — Weekend Classes: —
Affiliation: Private Distance Learning: —

NLN ACCREDITATION: No

BSN for non-RNs w/degree in other field: —

Articulation: None

For Further Information Contact:

Mrs Ana Delgado Hernandez, Coordinator
Interamerican University
Box 925
Aguadilla, PR 00605
(787) 891-0925 Ext 205

Interamerican University of Puerto Rico
—Arecibo—

Full-Time Enrollments: — Evening Classes: —
Part-Time Enrollments: — Weekend Classes: —
Affiliation: Private Distance Learning: —

NLN ACCREDITATION: No

BSN for non-RNs w/degree in other field: —

Articulation: None

For Further Information Contact:

Mrs Delia Brenes, Director
Interamerican University of Puerto Rico
PO Box 4050
Arecibo, PR 00613
(787) 878-5475

Interamerican University of Puerto Rico
—Guayama—

Full-Time Enrollments: 59 Evening Classes: Yes
Part-Time Enrollments: — Weekend Classes: No
Affiliation: Private Distance Learning: No

NLN ACCREDITATION: No

BSN for non-RNs w/degree in other field: No

Articulation: Associate to Baccalaureate

For Further Information Contact:

Dr Angela DeJesus Alicea, Director
Interamerican University of Puerto Rico
Box 1559
Guayama, PR 00785
(787) 864-2222

Interamerican University of Puerto Rico
—San German—

Full-Time Enrollments: — Evening Classes: —
Part-Time Enrollments: — Weekend Classes: —
Affiliation: Private Distance Learning: —

NLN ACCREDITATION: No

BSN for non-RNs w/degree in other field: —

Articulation: None

For Further Information Contact:

Mrs Maritza Ortiz, Director
Interamerican University of Puerto Rico
Box 5106
San German, PR 00683
(787) 264-1912

Interamerican University of Puerto Rico
—San Juan—

Full-Time Enrollments: 298 Evening Classes: Yes
Part-Time Enrollments: 4 Weekend Classes: No
Affiliation: Private Distance Learning: No

NLN ACCREDITATION: Yes

BSN for non-RNs w/degree in other field: No

Articulation: Associate to Baccalaureate

For Further Information Contact:

Dr Gloria E Ortiz, Director
Interamerican University of Puerto Rico
PO Box 191293
San Juan, PR 00919-1293
(787) 766-3066

Pontificia University Catolica de Puerto Rico
—Ponce—

Full-Time Enrollments: 520 Evening Classes: —
Part-Time Enrollments: 80 Weekend Classes: Yes
Affiliation: Religious Distance Learning: No

NLN ACCREDITATION: Yes

BSN for non-RNs w/degree in other field: No

Articulation: Associate to Baccalaureate

For Further Information Contact:

Dr Carmen Madera, Director
Pontificia University Catolica de Puerto Rico
2250 Ave Las Americas
Ponce, PR 00732
(787) 841-2000

Universidad Central De Bayamon
—Bayamon—

Full-Time Enrollments:	264	Evening Classes:	—
Part-Time Enrollments:	—	Weekend Classes:	—
Affiliation:	Religious	Distance Learning:	—

NLN ACCREDITATION: No

BSN for non-RNs w/degree in other field: No

Articulation: None

For Further Information Contact:

Prof Lydia Villamil, Director
Universidad Central De Bayamon
Box 1725
Bayamon, PR 00960-1725
(787) 786-3030

Universidad Metropolitana
—Rio Piedras—

Full-Time Enrollments:	171	Evening Classes:	Yes
Part-Time Enrollments:	7	Weekend Classes:	No
Affiliation:	Private	Distance Learning:	No

NLN ACCREDITATION: Yes

BSN for non-RNs w/degree in other field: No

Articulation: None

For Further Information Contact:

Mrs Carmen Bigas, Director
Universidad Metropolitana
Box 21150
Rio Piedras, PR 00928
(787) 766-1717

University of Puerto Rico at Mayaguez
—Mayaguez—

Full-Time Enrollments:	—	Evening Classes:	—
Part-Time Enrollments:	—	Weekend Classes:	—
Affiliation:	Public	Distance Learning:	—

NLN ACCREDITATION: Yes

BSN for non-RNs w/degree in other field: —

Articulation: None

For Further Information Contact:

Dr Hayden Rios, Director
University of Puerto Rico at Mayaguez
PO Box 5000
Mayaguez, PR 00681-5000
(787) 832-4040

University of Puerto Rico-Arecibo Technical College
—Arecibo—

Full-Time Enrollments:	—	Evening Classes:	—
Part-Time Enrollments:	—	Weekend Classes:	—
Affiliation:	Public	Distance Learning:	—

NLN ACCREDITATION: No

BSN for non-RNs w/degree in other field: —

Articulation: None

For Further Information Contact:

Mrs Migdalia Lopez Forty, Director
University of Puerto Rico-Arecibo Technical College
Box 4010
Arecibo, PR 00613-4010
(787) 878-2830

University of Puerto Rico-Humacao
—Humacao—

Full-Time Enrollments:	168	Evening Classes:	—
Part-Time Enrollments:	—	Weekend Classes:	—
Affiliation:	Public	Distance Learning:	—

NLN ACCREDITATION: Yes

BSN for non-RNs w/degree in other field: No

Articulation: None

For Further Information Contact:

Prof Alida Santana Troche, Director
University of Puerto Rico-Humacao
Station
Humacao, PR 00790
(787) 850-9493

University of Puerto Rico-Medical Science Campus
—San Juan—

Full-Time Enrollments:	184	Evening Classes:	Yes
Part-Time Enrollments:	—	Weekend Classes:	—
Affiliation:	Public	Distance Learning:	—

NLN ACCREDITATION: Yes

BSN for non-RNs w/degree in other field: No

Articulation: Associate to Baccalaureate

For Further Information Contact:

Mrs Irma R Ortiz, Director
University of Puerto Rico-Medical Science Campus
PO Box 365067
San Juan, PR 00936-5067
(787) 758-2525

University of Sacred Heart
—Santurce—

Full-Time Enrollments:	90	Evening Classes:	Yes
Part-Time Enrollments:	12	Weekend Classes:	Yes
Affiliation:	Religious	Distance Learning:	No

NLN ACCREDITATION: Yes

BSN for non-RNs w/degree in other field: No

Articulation: Associate to Baccalaureate
Diploma to Baccalaureate

For Further Information Contact:

Dr Amelia Yordan, Director
University of Sacred Heart
PO Box 12383, Loiza St
Santurce, PR 00914-2383
(787) 728-1515

Rhode Island

Rhode Island College
—Providence—

Full-Time Enrollments:	199	Evening Classes:	Yes
Part-Time Enrollments:	148	Weekend Classes:	No
Affiliation:	Public	Distance Learning:	No

NLN ACCREDITATION: Yes

BSN for non-RNs w/degree in other field: No

Articulation: Associate to Baccalaureate

For Further Information Contact:

Dr Patricia Thomas, Chair
Rhode Island College
600 Mount Pleasant Ave
Providence, RI 02908
(401) 456-8014

Salve Regina University
—Newport—

Full-Time Enrollments:	—	Evening Classes:	—
Part-Time Enrollments:	—	Weekend Classes:	—
Affiliation:	Religious	Distance Learning:	—

NLN ACCREDITATION: Yes

BSN for non-RNs w/degree in other field: —

Articulation: —

For Further Information Contact:

Dr Eileen Donnelly, Chair
Salve Regina University
100 Ochre Point Ave
Newport, RI 02840
(401) 847-6650

University of Rhode Island
—Kingston—

Full-Time Enrollments:	400	Evening Classes:	Yes
Part-Time Enrollments:	26	Weekend Classes:	No
Affiliation:	Public	Distance Learning:	No

NLN ACCREDITATION: Yes

BSN for non-RNs w/degree in other field: No

Articulation: None

For Further Information Contact:

Dr Dayle Joseph, Interim Dean
University of Rhode Island
White Hall
Kingston, RI 02881
(401) 874-2766

South Carolina

Bob Jones University
—Greenville—

Full-Time Enrollments:	—	Evening Classes:	—
Part-Time Enrollments:	—	Weekend Classes:	—
Affiliation:	Religious	Distance Learning:	—

NLN ACCREDITATION: No

BSN for non-RNs w/degree in other field: —

Articulation: —

For Further Information Contact:

Dr Kathleen Crispin, Chair
Bob Jones University
1700 Wade Hampton Blvd
Greenville, SC 29614
(864) 242-5100

Charleston Southern University School of Nursing
—Charleston—

Full-Time Enrollments:	23	Evening Classes:	No
Part-Time Enrollments:	—	Weekend Classes:	No
Affiliation:	Religious	Distance Learning:	No

NLN ACCREDITATION.

BSN for non-RNs w/degree in other field: No

Articulation: None

For Further Information Contact:

Miss Lonell Jones, Acting Dean
Charleston Southern University School of Nursing
PO Box 118087
Charleston, SC 29423-8087
(803) 863-7032

Clemson University
—Clemson—

Full-Time Enrollments:	378	Evening Classes:	Yes
Part-Time Enrollments:	29	Weekend Classes:	No
Affiliation:	Public	Distance Learning:	Yes

NLN ACCREDITATION: Yes

BSN for non-RNs w/degree in other field: No

Articulation: Associate to Baccalaureate
RN to MSN

For Further Information Contact:

Dr Barbara Logan, Director
Clemson University
Box 341703
Clemson, SC 29634-1703
(803) 656-0383

Lander University
—Greenwood—

Full-Time Enrollments:	121	Evening Classes:	Yes
Part-Time Enrollments:	27	Weekend Classes:	No
Affiliation:	Public	Distance Learning:	No

NLN ACCREDITATION: Yes

BSN for non-RNs w/degree in other field: No

Articulation: Associate to Baccalaureate

For Further Information Contact:

Dr Barbara Freese, Dean
Lander University
320 Stanley Ave
Greenwood, SC 29649
(864) 388-8337

Medical University of South Carolina
—Charleston—

Full-Time Enrollments:	166	Evening Classes:	Yes
Part-Time Enrollments:	32	Weekend Classes:	No
Affiliation:	Public	Distance Learning:	No

NLN ACCREDITATION: Yes

BSN for non-RNs w/degree in other field: No

Articulation: Associate to Baccalaureate
LPN to Baccalaureate
RN to MSN

For Further Information Contact:

Dr Jean D'Meza Leuner, Associate Dean
Medical University of South Carolina
171 Ashley Ave
Charleston, SC 29425
(803) 792-3815

South Carolina State University
—Orangeburg—

Full-Time Enrollments:	23	Evening Classes:	No
Part-Time Enrollments:	4	Weekend Classes:	Yes
Affiliation:	Public	Distance Learning:	No

NLN ACCREDITATION: Yes

BSN for non-RNs w/degree in other field: Yes

Articulation: Associate to Baccalaureate

For Further Information Contact:

Dr Sylvia Whiting, Chair
South Carolina State University
PO Box 7158
Orangeburg, SC 29117
(803) 536-8193

University of South Carolina
—Columbia—

Full-Time Enrollments:	472	Evening Classes:	Yes
Part-Time Enrollments:	75	Weekend Classes:	—
Affiliation:	Public	Distance Learning:	Yes

NLN ACCREDITATION: Yes

BSN for non-RNs w/degree in other field: No

Articulation: Associate to Baccalaureate

For Further Information Contact:

Dr Sue Young, Associate Dean
University of South Carolina
Williams Brice Bldg
Columbia, SC 29208
(803) 777-7113

University of South Carolina Spartanburg
—Spartanburg—

Full-Time Enrollments:	77	Evening Classes:	Yes
Part-Time Enrollments:	16	Weekend Classes:	No
Affiliation:	Public	Distance Learning:	No

NLN ACCREDITATION: Yes

BSN for non-RNs w/degree in other field: No

Articulation: Associate to Baccalaureate
Diploma to Baccalaureate
LPN to Baccalaureate

For Further Information Contact:

Dr Jim Ferrell, Chair
University of South Carolina Spartanburg
800 University Way
Spartanburg, SC 29303
(864) 503-5441

South Dakota

Augustana College
—Sioux Falls—

Full-Time Enrollments:	118	Evening Classes:	Yes
Part-Time Enrollments:	8	Weekend Classes:	No
Affiliation:	Religious	Distance Learning:	No

NLN ACCREDITATION: Yes

BSN for non-RNs w/degree in other field: No

Articulation: None

For Further Information Contact:

Dr Mary Brendtro, Chair
Augustana College
29 & South Summit
Sioux Falls, SD 57197
(605) 336-4724

Mount Marty College
—Yankton—

Full-Time Enrollments:	80	Evening Classes:	Yes
Part-Time Enrollments:	—	Weekend Classes:	No
Affiliation:	Religious	Distance Learning:	No

NLN ACCREDITATION: Yes

BSN for non-RNs w/degree in other field: No

Articulation: None

For Further Information Contact:

Sr Corinne Lemmer, Director
Mount Marty College
1100 W 8th St
Yankton, SD 57078
(605) 668-1594

Presentation College
—Aberdeen—

Full-Time Enrollments:	3	Evening Classes:	—
Part-Time Enrollments:	42	Weekend Classes:	—
Affiliation:	Religious	Distance Learning:	No

NLN ACCREDITATION: Yes

BSN for non-RNs w/degree in other field: No

Articulation: Associate to Baccalaureate
Diploma to Baccalaureate

For Further Information Contact:

Mr Thomas Stenvig, Chair
Presentation College
1500 North Main St
Aberdeen, SD 57401
(605) 229-8473

South Dakota State University
—Brookings—

Full-Time Enrollments:	312	Evening Classes:	No
Part-Time Enrollments:	—	Weekend Classes:	No
Affiliation:	Public	Distance Learning:	Yes

NLN ACCREDITATION: Yes

BSN for non-RNs w/degree in other field: No

Articulation: None

For Further Information Contact:

Dr Roberta Olson, Dean
South Dakota State University
Box 2275
Brookings, SD 57007-0098
(605) 688-5178

Tennessee

Austin Peay State University
—Clarksville—

Full-Time Enrollments:	149	Evening Classes:	No
Part-Time Enrollments:	—	Weekend Classes:	No
Affiliation:	Public	Distance Learning:	No

NLN ACCREDITATION: Yes

BSN for non-RNs w/degree in other field: No

Articulation: Associate to Baccalaureate
Diploma to Baccalaureate

For Further Information Contact:

Dr Wynella B Badgett, Dean
Austin Peay State University
Clarksville, TN 37040
(615) 648-7710

Baptist Memorial College
—Memphis—

Full-Time Enrollments:	100	Evening Classes:	Yes
Part-Time Enrollments:	—	Weekend Classes:	—
Affiliation:	Religious	Distance Learning:	—

NLN ACCREDITATION: No

BSN for non-RNs w/degree in other field: No

Articulation: Associate to Baccalaureate
Diploma to Baccalaureate

For Further Information Contact:

Mrs Anne Plumb, Interim Dean
Baptist Memorial College
1003 Monroe Ave
Memphis, TN 38104
(901) 227-5730

Belmont University
—Nashville—

Full-Time Enrollments: —   Evening Classes: —
Part-Time Enrollments: —   Weekend Classes: —
Affiliation: Religious   Distance Learning: —

NLN ACCREDITATION: Yes

BSN for non-RNs w/degree in other field: —

Articulation: None

For Further Information Contact:

Debra Wollaber, Interim Chair
Belmont University
1900 Belmont Blvd
Nashville, TN 37212
(615) 386-4117

Carson Newman College
—Jefferson City—

Full-Time Enrollments: 115   Evening Classes: Yes
Part-Time Enrollments: —   Weekend Classes: No
Affiliation: Religious   Distance Learning: No

NLN ACCREDITATION: Yes

BSN for non-RNs w/degree in other field: No

Articulation: Associate to Baccalaureate
Diploma to Baccalaureate

For Further Information Contact:

Dr Ann Harley, Dean
Carson Newman College
Div of Nursing
Jefferson City, TN 37760
(423) 471-3425

Cumberland University
—Lebanon—

Full-Time Enrollments: 68   Evening Classes: Yes
Part-Time Enrollments: 2   Weekend Classes: No
Affiliation: Private   Distance Learning: No

NLN ACCREDITATION: Yes

BSN for non-RNs w/degree in other field: Yes

Articulation: None

For Further Information Contact:

Mrs Linda Watlington, Chair
Cumberland University
South Greenwood St
Lebanon, TN 37087
(615) 443-8417

East Tennessee State University
—Johnson City—

Full-Time Enrollments: 287   Evening Classes: Yes
Part-Time Enrollments: 5   Weekend Classes: No
Affiliation: Public   Distance Learning: Yes

NLN ACCREDITATION: Yes

BSN for non-RNs w/degree in other field: No

Articulation: Associate to Baccalaureate
Diploma to Baccalaureate

For Further Information Contact:

Dr Joellen Edwards, Dean
East Tennessee State University
PO Box 70617
Johnson City, TN 37614-0617
(423) 439-7051

Middle Tennessee State University-Nursing Department
—Murfreesboro—

Full-Time Enrollments: 142   Evening Classes: Yes
Part-Time Enrollments: —   Weekend Classes: —
Affiliation: Public   Distance Learning: —

NLN ACCREDITATION: Yes

BSN for non-RNs w/degree in other field: No

Articulation: Associate to Baccalaureate

For Further Information Contact:

Dr Judith Wakim, Director
Middle Tennessee State University-Nursing Department
Box 81 E Main St
Murfreesboro, TN 37132
(615) 898-2437

Milligan College
—Milligan College—

Full-Time Enrollments: 109   Evening Classes: Yes
Part-Time Enrollments: —   Weekend Classes: No
Affiliation: Religious   Distance Learning: No

NLN ACCREDITATION: No

BSN for non-RNs w/degree in other field: No

Articulation: Associate to Baccalaureate
Diploma to Baccalaureate

For Further Information Contact:

Dr Elizabeth Smith, Chair
Milligan College
Box 500
Milligan College, TN 37682
(423) 461-8555

Tennessee State University-School of Nursing
—Nashville—

Full-Time Enrollments: 100   Evening Classes: Yes
Part-Time Enrollments: —   Weekend Classes: No
Affiliation: Public   Distance Learning: No

NLN ACCREDITATION: Yes

BSN for non-RNs w/degree in other field: No

Articulation: Associate to Baccalaureate

For Further Information Contact:

Dr Yvonne Stringfield, Director
Tennessee State University-School of Nursing
3500 John A Merritt Blvd
Nashville, TN 37209
(615) 320-3016

Tennessee Technological University
—Cookeville—

Full-Time Enrollments: 83   Evening Classes: No
Part-Time Enrollments: —   Weekend Classes: No
Affiliation: Public   Distance Learning: No

NLN ACCREDITATION: Yes

BSN for non-RNs w/degree in other field: No

Articulation: None

For Further Information Contact:

Dr Barbara Reynolds, Dean
Tennessee Technological University
Box 5001
Cookeville, TN 38505
(615) 372-3213

The University of Memphis
—Memphis—

Full-Time Enrollments: 148   Evening Classes: Yes
Part-Time Enrollments: 70   Weekend Classes: No
Affiliation: Public   Distance Learning: Yes

NLN ACCREDITATION: Yes

BSN for non-RNs w/degree in other field: No

Articulation: None

For Further Information Contact:

Dr Toni Bargagliotti, Dean
The University of Memphis
Memphis, TN 38152
(901) 678-2020

Union University
—Jackson—

Full-Time Enrollments: 109   Evening Classes: Yes
Part-Time Enrollments: —   Weekend Classes: Yes
Affiliation: Religious   Distance Learning: No

NLN ACCREDITATION: Yes

BSN for non-RNs w/degree in other field: No

Articulation: None

For Further Information Contact:

Dr Carla Sanderson, Dean
Union University
Jackson, TN 38305-9901
(901) 661-1818

University of Tennessee College of Nursing
—Memphis—

Full-Time Enrollments: 55   Evening Classes: No
Part-Time Enrollments: —   Weekend Classes: No
Affiliation: Public   Distance Learning: Yes

NLN ACCREDITATION: Yes

BSN for non-RNs w/degree in other field: Yes

Articulation: Associate to Baccalaureate

For Further Information Contact:

Dr Michael A Carter, Dean
University of Tennessee College of Nursing
877 Madison Ave
Memphis, TN 38163
(901) 448-6128

University of Tennessee at Chattanooga
—Chattanooga—

Full-Time Enrollments: 330   Evening Classes: Yes
Part-Time Enrollments: —   Weekend Classes: No
Affiliation: Public   Distance Learning: No

NLN ACCREDITATION: Yes

BSN for non-RNs w/degree in other field: No

Articulation: Associate to Baccalaureate
RN to MSN

For Further Information Contact:

Dr Pamela Holder, Director
University of Tennessee at Chattanooga
615 McCallie Ave
Chattanooga, TN 37403-8598
(423) 755-4750

University of Tennessee at Knoxville
—Knoxville—

Full-Time Enrollments:	46	Evening Classes:	No
Part-Time Enrollments:	10	Weekend Classes:	No
Affiliation:	Public	Distance Learning:	No

NLN ACCREDITATION: Yes

BSN for non-RNs w/degree in other field: No

Articulation: Associate to Baccalaureate

For Further Information Contact:

Dr Joan Creasia, Dean
University of Tennessee at Knoxville
1200 Volunteer Blvd
Knoxville, TN 37996-4180
(423) 974-7584

University of Tennessee at Knoxville
—Knoxville—

Full-Time Enrollments:	194	Evening Classes:	Yes
Part-Time Enrollments:	10	Weekend Classes:	No
Affiliation:	Public	Distance Learning:	No

NLN ACCREDITATION: Yes

BSN for non-RNs w/degree in other field: No

Articulation: Associate to Baccalaureate

For Further Information Contact:

Dr Joan Creasia, Dean
University of Tennessee at Knoxville
1200 Volunteer Blvd
Knoxville, TN 37996-4110
(423) 974-7584

University of Tennessee at Martin
—Martin—

Full-Time Enrollments:	96	Evening Classes:	Yes
Part-Time Enrollments:	10	Weekend Classes:	No
Affiliation:	Public	Distance Learning:	Yes

NLN ACCREDITATION: Yes

BSN for non-RNs w/degree in other field: No

Articulation: Associate to Baccalaureate
                 Diploma to Baccalaureate

For Further Information Contact:

Dr V Strickland Seng, Chair
University of Tennessee at Martin
Dept of Nsg
Martin, TN 38238
(901) 587-7131

Vanderbilt University
—Nashville—

Full-Time Enrollments:	—	Evening Classes:	—
Part-Time Enrollments:	—	Weekend Classes:	—
Affiliation:	Private	Distance Learning:	—

NLN ACCREDITATION: Yes

BSN for non-RNs w/degree in other field: —

Articulation: —

For Further Information Contact:

Dr Colleen Conway-Welch, Dean
Vanderbilt University
21st Ave, S
Nashville, TN 37240
(615) 322-3804

Texas

Abilene Inter Collegiate School
—Abilene—

Full-Time Enrollments:	92	Evening Classes:	No
Part-Time Enrollments:	—	Weekend Classes:	No
Affiliation:	Religious	Distance Learning:	No

NLN ACCREDITATION: Yes

BSN for non-RNs w/degree in other field: No

Articulation: Associate to Baccalaureate
                 Diploma to Baccalaureate

For Further Information Contact:

Dr Corine N Bonnet, Dean
Abilene Inter Collegiate School
2149 Hickory
Abilene, TX 79601
(915) 672-2441

Baylor University School of Nursing
—Dallas—

Full-Time Enrollments:	207	Evening Classes:	Yes
Part-Time Enrollments:	36	Weekend Classes:	No
Affiliation:	Religious	Distance Learning:	No

NLN ACCREDITATION: Yes

BSN for non-RNs w/degree in other field: No

Articulation: None

For Further Information Contact:

Dr Phyllis S Karns, Dean
Baylor University School of Nursing
3700 Worth St
Dallas, TX 75246
(214) 820-3361

East Texas Baptist University
—Marshall—

Full-Time Enrollments:	41	Evening Classes:	No
Part-Time Enrollments:	3	Weekend Classes:	No
Affiliation:	Religious	Distance Learning:	No

NLN ACCREDITATION: Yes

BSN for non-RNs w/degree in other field:　No

Articulation:　None

For Further Information Contact:

Dr Ella Herriage, Director
East Texas Baptist University
1209 North Grove
Marshall, TX 75670
(903) 935-7963

Houston Baptist University
—Houston—

Full-Time Enrollments:	86	Evening Classes:	No
Part-Time Enrollments:	—	Weekend Classes:	No
Affiliation:	Religious	Distance Learning:	No

NLN ACCREDITATION: Yes

BSN for non-RNs w/degree in other field:　No

Articulation:　Associate to Baccalaureate

For Further Information Contact:

Dr Nancy C Yuill, Dean
Houston Baptist University
7502 Fondren Rd
Houston, TX 77074-3298
(713) 995-3300

Lamar University
—Beaumont—

Full-Time Enrollments:	146	Evening Classes:	No
Part-Time Enrollments:	—	Weekend Classes:	No
Affiliation:	Public	Distance Learning:	No

NLN ACCREDITATION: Yes

BSN for non-RNs w/degree in other field:　No

Articulation:　Associate to Baccalaureate

For Further Information Contact:

Dr Alexia Green, Chair
Lamar University
PO Box 10081
Beaumont, TX 77710
(409) 880-8817

Midwestern State University
—Wichita Falls—

Full-Time Enrollments:	251	Evening Classes:	Yes
Part-Time Enrollments:	—	Weekend Classes:	No
Affiliation:	Public	Distance Learning:	No

NLN ACCREDITATION: Yes

BSN for non-RNs w/degree in other field:　No

Articulation:　Associate to Baccalaureate

For Further Information Contact:

Dr Susan Sportsman, Director
Midwestern State University
3410 Taft Blvd
Wichita Falls, TX 76308
(817) 689-4597

Prairie View A & M University College of Nursing
—Houston—

Full-Time Enrollments:	226	Evening Classes:	Yes
Part-Time Enrollments:	50	Weekend Classes:	Yes
Affiliation:	Public	Distance Learning:	Yes

NLN ACCREDITATION: Yes

BSN for non-RNs w/degree in other field:　No

Articulation:　None

For Further Information Contact:

Dr Dollie Brathwaite, Dean
Prairie View A & M University College of Nursing
6436 Fannin
Houston, TX 77030
(713) 797-7007

Stephen F Austin State University
—Nacogdoches—

Full-Time Enrollments:	81	Evening Classes:	—
Part-Time Enrollments:	1	Weekend Classes:	—
Affiliation:	Public	Distance Learning:	—

NLN ACCREDITATION: Yes

BSN for non-RNs w/degree in other field:　No

Articulation:　None

For Further Information Contact:

Dr Glenda Walker, Director
Stephen F Austin State University
PO Box 6156
Nacogdoches, TX 75962
(409) 468-3604

Tarelton State University
—Stephenville—

Full-Time Enrollments:	64	Evening Classes:	—
Part-Time Enrollments:	17	Weekend Classes:	—
Affiliation:	Public	Distance Learning:	—

NLN ACCREDITATION: No

BSN for non-RNs w/degree in other field: No

Articulation: None

For Further Information Contact:

Dr Elaine Evans, Director
Tarelton State University
Box T-500
Stephenville, TX 76402
(817) 968-9139

Texas A&M University-Corpus Christi
—Corpus Christi—

Full-Time Enrollments:	66	Evening Classes:	Yes
Part-Time Enrollments:	21	Weekend Classes:	No
Affiliation:	Public	Distance Learning:	Yes

NLN ACCREDITATION: Yes

BSN for non-RNs w/degree in other field: No

Articulation: Associate to Baccalaureate
Diploma to Baccalaureate
RN to MSN

For Further Information Contact:

Dr Rebecca P Jones, Director
Texas A&M University-Corpus Christi
6300 Ocean Dr
Corpus Christi, TX 78412
(512) 994-2648

Texas Christian University-Harris College of Nursing
—Fort Worth—

Full-Time Enrollments:	329	Evening Classes:	No
Part-Time Enrollments:	19	Weekend Classes:	No
Affiliation:	Private	Distance Learning:	No

NLN ACCREDITATION: Yes

BSN for non-RNs w/degree in other field: Yes

Articulation: None

For Further Information Contact:

Dr Kathleen Bond, Dean
Texas Christian University-Harris College of Nursing
2800 Bowie
Fort Worth, TX 76129
(817) 921-7652

Texas Technical University Health Sciences Center
—Lubbock—

Full-Time Enrollments:	199	Evening Classes:	Yes
Part-Time Enrollments:	124	Weekend Classes:	Yes
Affiliation:	Public	Distance Learning:	Yes

NLN ACCREDITATION: Yes

BSN for non-RNs w/degree in other field: No

Articulation: Associate to Baccalaureate

For Further Information Contact:

Dr Patricia Yoder Wise, Dean
Texas Technical University Health Sciences Center
3601 4th St
Lubbock, TX 79430
(806) 743-2737

Texas Woman's University
—Denton—

Full-Time Enrollments:	261	Evening Classes:	Yes
Part-Time Enrollments:	361	Weekend Classes:	No
Affiliation:	Public	Distance Learning:	No

NLN ACCREDITATION: Yes

BSN for non-RNs w/degree in other field: No

Articulation: None

For Further Information Contact:

Dr Carolyn Gunning, Dean
Texas Woman's University
TWU Station, Box 425498
Denton, TX 76204-5498
(817) 898-2401

University of Mary Hardin-Baylor School of Nursing
—Belton—

Full-Time Enrollments:	118	Evening Classes:	Yes
Part-Time Enrollments:	3	Weekend Classes:	No
Affiliation:	Religious	Distance Learning:	No

NLN ACCREDITATION: Yes

BSN for non-RNs w/degree in other field: No

Articulation: None

For Further Information Contact:

Dr Nancy Schoenrock, Dean
University of Mary Hardin-Baylor School of Nursing
UMH-B Station Box 8015
Belton, TX 76513
(817) 939-4662

University of Texas Health Science Center
—Houston—

Full-Time Enrollments:	126	Evening Classes:	—
Part-Time Enrollments:	9	Weekend Classes:	—
Affiliation:	Public	Distance Learning:	—

NLN ACCREDITATION: Yes

BSN for non-RNs w/degree in other field: No

Articulation: None

For Further Information Contact:

Dr Patricia L Starck, Dean
University of Texas Health Science Center
1100 Holcombe Blvd
Houston, TX 77030
(713) 500-4472

University of Texas at Tyler
—Tyler—

Full-Time Enrollments:	204	Evening Classes:	Yes
Part-Time Enrollments:	43	Weekend Classes:	No
Affiliation:	Public	Distance Learning:	Yes

NLN ACCREDITATION: Yes

BSN for non-RNs w/degree in other field: No

Articulation: Associate to Baccalaureate
LPN to Baccalaureate

For Further Information Contact:

Dr Linda Klotz, Director
University of Texas at Tyler
3900 Univ Blvd
Tyler, TX 75799
(903) 566-7320

University of Texas-Arlington
—Arlington—

Full-Time Enrollments:	289	Evening Classes:	No
Part-Time Enrollments:	40	Weekend Classes:	Yes
Affiliation:	Public	Distance Learning:	Yes

NLN ACCREDITATION: Yes

BSN for non-RNs w/degree in other field: No

Articulation: Associate to Baccalaureate

For Further Information Contact:

Dr Elizabeth Poster, Dean
University of Texas-Arlington
Box 19407
Arlington, TX 76019
(817) 272-2776

University of Texas-Austin
—Austin—

Full-Time Enrollments:	200	Evening Classes:	No
Part-Time Enrollments:	5	Weekend Classes:	No
Affiliation:	Public	Distance Learning:	No

NLN ACCREDITATION: Yes

BSN for non-RNs w/degree in other field: No

Articulation: None

For Further Information Contact:

Dr Dolores Sands, Dean
University of Texas-Austin
1700 Red River
Austin, TX 78701-1499
(512) 471-7311

University of Texas-El Paso
—El Paso—

Full-Time Enrollments:	225	Evening Classes:	No
Part-Time Enrollments:	64	Weekend Classes:	No
Affiliation:	Public	Distance Learning:	No

NLN ACCREDITATION: Yes

BSN for non-RNs w/degree in other field: No

Articulation: Associate to Baccalaureate
Diploma to Baccalaureate
RN to MSN

For Further Information Contact:

Dr Helen Castillo, Chair
University of Texas-El Paso
1101 N Campbell
El Paso, TX 79902
(915) 747-5880

University of Texas-Galveston
—Galveston—

Full-Time Enrollments:	165	Evening Classes:	Yes
Part-Time Enrollments:	41	Weekend Classes:	—
Affiliation:	Public	Distance Learning:	Yes

NLN ACCREDITATION: Yes

BSN for non-RNs w/degree in other field: No

Articulation: None

For Further Information Contact:

Dr Jeanette Hartsorn, Associate Dean
University of Texas-Galveston
301 University Blvd
Galveston, TX 77555
(409) 772-1181

University of Texas-Health Science Center
—San Antonio—

Full-Time Enrollments:	337	Evening Classes:	Yes
Part-Time Enrollments:	79	Weekend Classes:	Yes
Affiliation:	Public	Distance Learning:	Yes

NLN ACCREDITATION: Yes

BSN for non-RNs w/degree in other field: No

Articulation: Associate to Baccalaureate
Diploma to Baccalaureate

For Further Information Contact:

Dr Patty L Hawken, Dean
University of Texas-Health Science Center
7703 Floyd Curl
San Antonio, TX 78284-7942
(210) 567-5800

University of Texas-Pan American
—Edinburg—

Full-Time Enrollments:	94	Evening Classes:	Yes
Part-Time Enrollments:	—	Weekend Classes:	Yes
Affiliation:	Public	Distance Learning:	—

NLN ACCREDITATION: Yes

BSN for non-RNs w/degree in other field: No

Articulation: None

For Further Information Contact:

Dr Carolina Huerta, Chair
University of Texas-Pan American
1201 West University Dr
Edinburg, TX 78539
(210) 381-3491

University of the Incarnate Word
—San Antonio—

Full-Time Enrollments:	231	Evening Classes:	Yes
Part-Time Enrollments:	—	Weekend Classes:	—
Affiliation:	Religious	Distance Learning:	—

NLN ACCREDITATION: Yes

BSN for non-RNs w/degree in other field: No

Articulation: None

For Further Information Contact:

Dr Brenda Jackson, Director
University of the Incarnate Word
4301 Broadway
San Antonio, TX 78209
(210) 829-6029

West Texas A&M University
—Canyon—

Full-Time Enrollments:	146	Evening Classes:	No
Part-Time Enrollments:	13	Weekend Classes:	No
Affiliation:	Public	Distance Learning:	No

NLN ACCREDITATION: Yes

BSN for non-RNs w/degree in other field: No

Articulation: Associate to Baccalaureate
LPN to Baccalaureate

For Further Information Contact:

Dr Mary J Walsh, Div Head
West Texas A&M University
Box 969
Canyon, TX 79016
(806) 656-2630

Utah

Brigham Young University
—Provo—

Full-Time Enrollments:	207	Evening Classes:	No
Part-Time Enrollments:	—	Weekend Classes:	No
Affiliation:	Religious	Distance Learning:	No

NLN ACCREDITATION: Yes

BSN for non-RNs w/degree in other field: No

Articulation: Associate to Baccalaureate
LPN to Baccalaureate

For Further Information Contact:

Dr Sandra Rogers, Dean
Brigham Young University
Provo, UT 84602
(801) 378-6547

University of Utah
—Salt Lake City—

Full-Time Enrollments:	226	Evening Classes:	—
Part-Time Enrollments:	22	Weekend Classes:	—
Affiliation:	Public	Distance Learning:	Yes

NLN ACCREDITATION: Yes

BSN for non-RNs w/degree in other field: No

Articulation: Associate to Baccalaureate
RN to MSN

For Further Information Contact:

Dr Linda K Amos, Dean
University of Utah
25 S Medical Dr
Salt Lake City, UT 84112
(801) 581-8794

Westminster College-St Mark's
—Salt Lake City—

Full-Time Enrollments:	—	Evening Classes:	—
Part-Time Enrollments:	—	Weekend Classes:	—
Affiliation:	Private	Distance Learning:	—

NLN ACCREDITATION: Yes

BSN for non-RNs w/degree in other field: —

Articulation: None

For Further Information Contact:

Dr Imogene Rigdon, Dean
Westminster College-St Mark's
1840 S 13th St, E
Salt Lake City, UT 84105
(801) 488-4233

Vermont

University of Vermont-School of Nursing
—Burlington—

Full-Time Enrollments:	223	Evening Classes:	Yes
Part-Time Enrollments:	20	Weekend Classes:	No
Affiliation:	Public	Distance Learning:	No

NLN ACCREDITATION: Yes

BSN for non-RNs w/degree in other field: No

Articulation: None

For Further Information Contact:

Dr Marie McGrath, Interim Dean
University of Vermont-School of Nursing
216 Rowell Bldg
Burlington, VT 05405
(802) 656-3830

Virgin Islands

University of the Virgin Islands
—St Thomas—

Full-Time Enrollments:	45	Evening Classes:	No
Part-Time Enrollments:	27	Weekend Classes:	No
Affiliation:	Public	Distance Learning:	Yes

NLN ACCREDITATION: Yes

BSN for non-RNs w/degree in other field: No

Articulation: Associate to Baccalaureate

For Further Information Contact:

Dr Edith Ramsay-Johnson, Chair
University of the Virgin Islands
#2 John Brewers Bay
St Thomas, VI 00801
(809) 776-9200

Virginia

Christopher Newport University
—Newport News—

Full-Time Enrollments:	38	Evening Classes:	—
Part-Time Enrollments:	—	Weekend Classes:	—
Affiliation:	Public	Distance Learning:	—

NLN ACCREDITATION: Yes

BSN for non-RNs w/degree in other field: No

Articulation: None

For Further Information Contact:

Karin Polifko-Harris, Chair
Christopher Newport University
50 Shoe Lane
Newport News, VA 23606
(757) 594-7252

Eastern Mennonite University
—Harrisonburg—

Full-Time Enrollments:	113	Evening Classes:	No
Part-Time Enrollments:	3	Weekend Classes:	No
Affiliation:	Religious	Distance Learning:	No

NLN ACCREDITATION: Yes

BSN for non-RNs w/degree in other field: No

Articulation: None

For Further Information Contact:

Dr Marie Morris, Dept Head
Eastern Mennonite University
1200 Park Rd
Harrisonburg, VA 22801
(540) 432-4100

George Mason University
—Fairfax—

Full-Time Enrollments:	234	Evening Classes:	Yes
Part-Time Enrollments:	274	Weekend Classes:	No
Affiliation:	Public	Distance Learning:	No

NLN ACCREDITATION: Yes

BSN for non-RNs w/degree in other field: No

Articulation: Associate to Baccalaureate
Diploma to Baccalaureate
LPN to Baccalaureate

For Further Information Contact:

Dr Rita M Carty, Dean
George Mason University
4400 Univ Dr
Fairfax, VA 22030
(703) 993-1918

Hampton University
—Hampton—

Full-Time Enrollments:	250	Evening Classes:	Yes
Part-Time Enrollments:	30	Weekend Classes:	—
Affiliation:	Private	Distance Learning:	—

NLN ACCREDITATION: Yes

BSN for non-RNs w/degree in other field: No

Articulation: Associate to Baccalaureate

For Further Information Contact:

Dr Arlene Montgomery, Interim Dean
Hampton University
Hampton, VA 23668
(757) 727-5252

James Madison University
—Harrisonburg—

Full-Time Enrollments:	205	Evening Classes:	Yes
Part-Time Enrollments:	4	Weekend Classes:	No
Affiliation:	Public	Distance Learning:	No

NLN ACCREDITATION: Yes

BSN for non-RNs w/degree in other field: Yes

Articulation: Associate to Baccalaureate
Diploma to Baccalaureate

For Further Information Contact:

Dr Vida S Huber, Dept Head
James Madison University
Main St
Harrisonburg, VA 22807
(540) 568-6314

Liberty University
—Lynchburg—

Full-Time Enrollments:	145	Evening Classes:	Yes
Part-Time Enrollments:	3	Weekend Classes:	No
Affiliation:	Religious	Distance Learning:	No

NLN ACCREDITATION: Yes

BSN for non-RNs w/degree in other field: No

Articulation: None

For Further Information Contact:

Dr Deanna Britt, Chair
Liberty University
1971 University Blvd
Lynchburg, VA 24502
(804) 582-2519

Lynchburg College
—Lynchburg—

Full-Time Enrollments:	111	Evening Classes:	No
Part-Time Enrollments:	8	Weekend Classes:	No
Affiliation:	Religious	Distance Learning:	No

NLN ACCREDITATION: Yes

BSN for non-RNs w/degree in other field: No

Articulation: None

For Further Information Contact:

Dr Nancy Whitman, Chair
Lynchburg College
1501 Lakeside Dr
Lynchburg, VA 24501
(804) 544-8324

Norfolk State University
—Norfolk—

Full-Time Enrollments:	—	Evening Classes:	—
Part-Time Enrollments:	—	Weekend Classes:	—
Affiliation:	Public	Distance Learning:	—

NLN ACCREDITATION: Yes

BSN for non-RNs w/degree in other field: —

Articulation: None

For Further Information Contact:

Candace C Rogers, Acting Dept Head
Norfolk State University
2401 Corprew Ave
Norfolk, VA 23504
(804) 683-9014

Old Dominion University-School of Sciences
—Norfolk—

Full-Time Enrollments:	179	Evening Classes:	Yes
Part-Time Enrollments:	38	Weekend Classes:	Yes
Affiliation:	Public	Distance Learning:	Yes

NLN ACCREDITATION: Yes

BSN for non-RNs w/degree in other field: No

Articulation: None

For Further Information Contact:

Dr Brenda Nichols, Chair
Old Dominion University-School of Sciences
361 Technology Bldg
Norfolk, VA 23529
(757) 683-4299

Radford University School of Nursing
—Radford—

Full-Time Enrollments:	141	Evening Classes:	Yes
Part-Time Enrollments:	—	Weekend Classes:	Yes
Affiliation:	Public	Distance Learning:	Yes

NLN ACCREDITATION: Yes

BSN for non-RNs w/degree in other field: No

Articulation: Associate to Baccalaureate

For Further Information Contact:

Dr Hardy Boettcher, Chair
Radford University School of Nursing
PO Box 6964
Radford, VA 24142
(540) 831-5415

University of Virginia
—Charlottesville—

Full-Time Enrollments:	264	Evening Classes:	No
Part-Time Enrollments:	2	Weekend Classes:	No
Affiliation:	Public	Distance Learning:	No

NLN ACCREDITATION: Yes

BSN for non-RNs w/degree in other field: Yes

Articulation: None

For Further Information Contact:

Dr Doris Greiner, Associate Dean
University of Virginia
McLeod Hall
Charlottesville, VA 22903
(804) 924-2743

Virginia Commonwealth University-Medical College of Virginia
—Richmond—

Full-Time Enrollments:	149	Evening Classes:	Yes
Part-Time Enrollments:	30	Weekend Classes:	Yes
Affiliation:	Public	Distance Learning:	No

NLN ACCREDITATION: Yes

BSN for non-RNs w/degree in other field: No

Articulation: Associate to Baccalaureate

For Further Information Contact:

Dr Nancy Langston, Dean
Virginia Commonwealth University-Medical College of Virginia
1220 E Broad St Box 980567
Richmond, VA 23298-0567
(804) 828-5174

Washington

Intercollegiate Center for Nursing Education
—Spokane—

Full-Time Enrollments:	258	Evening Classes:	Yes
Part-Time Enrollments:	6	Weekend Classes:	No
Affiliation:	Public	Distance Learning:	Yes

NLN ACCREDITATION: Yes

BSN for non-RNs w/degree in other field: No

Articulation: None

For Further Information Contact:

Dr Thelma L Cleveland, Dean
Intercollegiate Center for Nursing Education
W 2917 Ft George Wright Dr
Spokane, WA 99204
(509) 324-7333

Pacific Lutheran University
—Tacoma—

Full-Time Enrollments:	261	Evening Classes:	Yes
Part-Time Enrollments:	1	Weekend Classes:	—
Affiliation:	Religious	Distance Learning:	—

NLN ACCREDITATION: Yes

BSN for non-RNs w/degree in other field: No

Articulation: None

For Further Information Contact:

Dr Dorothy Langan, Dean
Pacific Lutheran University
Tacoma, WA 98447
(206) 535-7674

Seattle Pacific University
—Seattle—

Full-Time Enrollments:	121	Evening Classes:	Yes
Part-Time Enrollments:	23	Weekend Classes:	Yes
Affiliation:	Religious	Distance Learning:	Yes

NLN ACCREDITATION: Yes

BSN for non-RNs w/degree in other field: No

Articulation: Associate to Baccalaureate
Diploma to Baccalaureate

For Further Information Contact:

Dr Annalee Oakes, Dean
Seattle Pacific University
3307 3rd Ave W at Nickerson
Seattle, WA 98119
(206) 281-2608

Seattle University
—Seattle—

Full-Time Enrollments:	240	Evening Classes:	Yes
Part-Time Enrollments:	37	Weekend Classes:	Yes
Affiliation:	Private	Distance Learning:	—

NLN ACCREDITATION: Yes

BSN for non-RNs w/degree in other field: No

Articulation: None

For Further Information Contact:

Dr Luth Tenorio, Dean
Seattle University
Broadway and Madison
Seattle, WA 98122-4460
(206) 296-5676

University of Washington
—Seattle—

Full-Time Enrollments:	123	Evening Classes:	Yes
Part-Time Enrollments:	4	Weekend Classes:	Yes
Affiliation:	Public	Distance Learning:	No

NLN ACCREDITATION: Yes

BSN for non-RNs w/degree in other field: No

Articulation: Associate to Baccalaureate

For Further Information Contact:

Dr Susan Woods, Associate Dean
University of Washington
School of Nsg Box 357260
Seattle, WA 98195-7260
(206) 543-4152

Walla Walla College School of Nursing
—Portland, OR—

Full-Time Enrollments:	105	Evening Classes:	No
Part-Time Enrollments:	12	Weekend Classes:	No
Affiliation:	Religious	Distance Learning:	No

NLN ACCREDITATION: Yes

BSN for non-RNs w/degree in other field: No

Articulation: None

For Further Information Contact:

Dr Lucille Krull, Dean
Walla Walla College School of Nursing
10345 SE Market
Portland, OR, WA 97216
(503) 251-6115

West Virginia

Alderson-Broaddus College
—Philippi—

Full-Time Enrollments:	95	Evening Classes:	No
Part-Time Enrollments:	—	Weekend Classes:	No
Affiliation:	Religious	Distance Learning:	No

NLN ACCREDITATION: Yes

BSN for non-RNs w/degree in other field: No

Articulation: Associate to Baccalaureate
Diploma to Baccalaureate
LPN to Baccalaureate

For Further Information Contact:

Dr M Sharon Boni, Chair
Alderson-Broaddus College
Philippi, WV 26416
(304) 457-1700

Marshall University
—Huntington—

Full-Time Enrollments:	190	Evening Classes:	Yes
Part-Time Enrollments:	22	Weekend Classes:	No
Affiliation:	Public	Distance Learning:	Yes

NLN ACCREDITATION: Yes

BSN for non-RNs w/degree in other field: No

Articulation: Associate to Baccalaureate
Diploma to Baccalaureate

For Further Information Contact:

Dr Lynne Welch, Dean
Marshall University
400 Hal Greer Blvd
Huntington, WV 25701
(304) 696-2616

Shepherd College
—Shepherdstown—

Full-Time Enrollments:	53	Evening Classes:	Yes
Part-Time Enrollments:	—	Weekend Classes:	—
Affiliation:	Public	Distance Learning:	—

NLN ACCREDITATION: Yes

BSN for non-RNs w/degree in other field: No

Articulation: None

For Further Information Contact:

Dr Charlotte Anderson, Chair
Shepherd College
Shepherdstown, WV 25443
(304) 876-2511

The College of West Virginia
—Beckley—

Full-Time Enrollments:	120	Evening Classes:	Yes
Part-Time Enrollments:	—	Weekend Classes:	Yes
Affiliation:	Private	Distance Learning:	Yes

NLN ACCREDITATION: Yes

BSN for non-RNs w/degree in other field: No

Articulation: None

For Further Information Contact:

Dr Patsy Haslam, Dean
The College of West Virginia
609 South Kanawha St
Beckley, WV 25801
(304) 253-7351

University of Charleston
—Charleston—

Full-Time Enrollments:	120	Evening Classes:	Yes
Part-Time Enrollments:	15	Weekend Classes:	No
Affiliation:	Private	Distance Learning:	No

NLN ACCREDITATION: Yes

BSN for non-RNs w/degree in other field: No

Articulation: None

For Further Information Contact:

Dr Sandra S Bowles, Dean
University of Charleston
2300 MacCorkle Ave SE
Charleston, WV 25304
(304) 357-4835

West Liberty State College
—West Liberty—

Full-Time Enrollments:	68	Evening Classes:	Yes
Part-Time Enrollments:	14	Weekend Classes:	—
Affiliation:	Public	Distance Learning:	—

NLN ACCREDITATION: Yes

BSN for non-RNs w/degree in other field: No

Articulation: None

For Further Information Contact:

Dr Donna A Lukich, Chair
West Liberty State College
West Liberty, WV 26074
(304) 336-8108

West Virginia University
—Morgantown—

Full-Time Enrollments:	250	Evening Classes:	No
Part-Time Enrollments:	25	Weekend Classes:	No
Affiliation:	Public	Distance Learning:	Yes

NLN ACCREDITATION: Yes

BSN for non-RNs w/degree in other field: No

Articulation: None

For Further Information Contact:

Dr E Jane Martin, Dean
West Virginia University
PO Box 9600
Morgantown, WV 26506-9600
(304) 293-4831

West Virginia Wesleyan College
—Buckhannon—

Full-Time Enrollments:	80	Evening Classes:	—
Part-Time Enrollments:	—	Weekend Classes:	—
Affiliation:	Religious	Distance Learning:	Yes

NLN ACCREDITATION: Yes

BSN for non-RNs w/degree in other field: No

Articulation: None

For Further Information Contact:

Dr Nancy Alfred, Chair
West Virginia Wesleyan College
59 College Ave Box 22
Buckhannon, WV 26201
(304) 473-8224

Wheeling Jesuit University
—Wheeling—

Full-Time Enrollments:	—	Evening Classes:	—
Part-Time Enrollments:	—	Weekend Classes:	—
Affiliation:	Religious	Distance Learning:	—

NLN ACCREDITATION: Yes

BSN for non-RNs w/degree in other field: —

Articulation: None

For Further Information Contact:

Dr Rose M Kutlenios, Chair
Wheeling Jesuit University
316 Washington Ave
Wheeling, WV 26003
(304) 243-2227

Wisconsin

Alverno College
—Milwaukee—

Full-Time Enrollments:	284	Evening Classes:	No
Part-Time Enrollments:	78	Weekend Classes:	Yes
Affiliation:	Religious	Distance Learning:	No

NLN ACCREDITATION: Yes

BSN for non-RNs w/degree in other field: No

Articulation: Associate to Baccalaureate
Diploma to Baccalaureate

For Further Information Contact:

Dr Jean Bartels, Chair
Alverno College
3401 S 39th St PO Box 343922
Milwaukee, WI 53234-3922
(414) 382-6271

Bellin College of Nursing
—Green Bay—

Full-Time Enrollments:	179	Evening Classes:	No
Part-Time Enrollments:	12	Weekend Classes:	No
Affiliation:	Private	Distance Learning:	No

NLN ACCREDITATION: Yes

BSN for non-RNs w/degree in other field: No

Articulation: None

For Further Information Contact:

Dr Kathleen Harr, Vice President
Bellin College of Nursing
725 S Webster Box 23400
Green Bay, WI 54305-3400
(414) 433-3794

Cardinal Stritch College
—Milwaukee—

Full-Time Enrollments:	—	Evening Classes:	—
Part-Time Enrollments:	—	Weekend Classes:	—
Affiliation:	Religious	Distance Learning:	—

NLN ACCREDITATION: Yes

BSN for non-RNs w/degree in other field: —

Articulation: —

For Further Information Contact:

Dr Zaiga G Kalnins, Chair
Cardinal Stritch College
6801 North Yates Rd
Milwaukee, WI 53217
(414) 352-5400

Columbia College of Nursing
—Milwaukee—

Full-Time Enrollments:	211	Evening Classes:	Yes
Part-Time Enrollments:	117	Weekend Classes:	No
Affiliation:	Private	Distance Learning:	No

NLN ACCREDITATION: Yes

BSN for non-RNs w/degree in other field: No

Articulation: None

For Further Information Contact:

Dr Marian Snyder, Dean
Columbia College of Nursing
2121 E Newport Ave
Milwaukee, WI 53211
(414) 961-4202

Concordia University Wisconsin
—Mequon—

Full-Time Enrollments:	77	Evening Classes:	Yes
Part-Time Enrollments:	8	Weekend Classes:	No
Affiliation:	Religious	Distance Learning:	Yes

NLN ACCREDITATION: Yes

BSN for non-RNs w/degree in other field: No

Articulation: Associate to Baccalaureate
LPN to Baccalaureate

For Further Information Contact:

Mrs Grace Peterson, Chair
Concordia University Wisconsin
12800 N Lake Shore Dr
Mequon, WI 53097
(414) 243-5700

Edgewood College
—Madison—

Full-Time Enrollments:	142	Evening Classes:	Yes
Part-Time Enrollments:	—	Weekend Classes:	Yes
Affiliation:	Religious	Distance Learning:	—

NLN ACCREDITATION: Yes

BSN for non-RNs w/degree in other field: No

Articulation: Associate to Baccalaureate

For Further Information Contact:

Dr Virginia Wirtz, Chair
Edgewood College
855 Woodrow St
Madison, WI 53711
(608) 257-4861

Marian College of Fond du Lac
—Fond du Lac—

Full-Time Enrollments: 222   Evening Classes: —
Part-Time Enrollments: 19   Weekend Classes: —
Affiliation: Religious   Distance Learning: —

    NLN ACCREDITATION: Yes

BSN for non-RNs w/degree in other field: No

Articulation: None

For Further Information Contact:

    Dr Elizabeth Parato, Chair
    Marian College of Fond du Lac
    45 S National Ave
    Fond du Lac, WI 54935
    (414) 923-8094

Marquette University-College of Nursing
—Milwaukee—

Full-Time Enrollments: 354   Evening Classes: Yes
Part-Time Enrollments: 13   Weekend Classes: Yes
Affiliation: Religious   Distance Learning: Yes

    NLN ACCREDITATION: Yes

BSN for non-RNs w/degree in other field: No

Articulation: Associate to Baccalaureate

For Further Information Contact:

    Dr Madeline Wake, Dean
    Marquette University-College of Nursing
    530 N 16 Box 1881
    Milwaukee, WI 53201-1881
    (414) 288-3812

Milwaukee School of Engineering-School of Nursing
—Milwaukee—

Full-Time Enrollments: 29   Evening Classes: —
Part-Time Enrollments: —   Weekend Classes: —
Affiliation: Private   Distance Learning: —

    NLN ACCREDITATION: No

BSN for non-RNs w/degree in other field: No

Articulation: None

For Further Information Contact:

    Dr Mary Louise Brown, Chair
    Milwaukee School of Engineering-School of Nursing
    1025 N Broadway PO Box 644
    Milwaukee, WI 53201-0644
    (414) 277-4516

University of Wisconsin-Eau Claire
—Eau Claire—

Full-Time Enrollments: 244   Evening Classes: —
Part-Time Enrollments: 53   Weekend Classes: —
Affiliation: Public   Distance Learning: —

    NLN ACCREDITATION: Yes

BSN for non-RNs w/degree in other field: No

Articulation: None

For Further Information Contact:

    Dr Marjorie Bottoms, Associate Dean
    University of Wisconsin-Eau Claire
    105 Garfield Ave Box 4004
    Eau Claire, WI 54702-4004
    (715) 836-5287

University of Wisconsin-Madison
—Madison—

Full-Time Enrollments: 231   Evening Classes: Yes
Part-Time Enrollments: 43   Weekend Classes: No
Affiliation: Public   Distance Learning: Yes

    NLN ACCREDITATION: Yes

BSN for non-RNs w/degree in other field: No

Articulation: Associate to Baccalaureate

For Further Information Contact:

    Dr Vivian Littlefield, Dean
    University of Wisconsin-Madison
    600 Highland Ave
    Madison, WI 53792-2455
    (608) 263-5155

University of Wisconsin-Milwaukee
—Milwaukee—

Full-Time Enrollments: 240   Evening Classes: Yes
Part-Time Enrollments: 94   Weekend Classes: —
Affiliation: Public   Distance Learning: Yes

    NLN ACCREDITATION: Yes

BSN for non-RNs w/degree in other field: Yes

Articulation: Associate to Baccalaureate

For Further Information Contact:

    Dr Sharon Hoffman, Dean
    University of Wisconsin-Milwaukee
    PO Box 413
    Milwaukee, WI 53201
    (414) 229-4189

University of Wisconsin-Oshkosh
—Oshkosh—

Full-Time Enrollments:	613	Evening Classes:	No
Part-Time Enrollments:	—	Weekend Classes:	No
Affiliation:	Public	Distance Learning:	Yes

NLN ACCREDITATION: Yes

BSN for non-RNs w/degree in other field: No

Articulation: None

For Further Information Contact:

Dr Merritt E Knox, Dean
University of Wisconsin-Oshkosh
800 Algoma Blvd
Oshkosh, WI 54901
(414) 424-1028

Viterbo College
—La Crosse—

Full-Time Enrollments:	343	Evening Classes:	Yes
Part-Time Enrollments:	24	Weekend Classes:	No
Affiliation:	Religious	Distance Learning:	Yes

NLN ACCREDITATION: Yes

BSN for non-RNs w/degree in other field: No

Articulation: Associate to Baccalaureate
Diploma to Baccalaureate

For Further Information Contact:

Dr Vivien Edwards, Dean
Viterbo College
815 S 9th St
La Crosse, WI 54601
(608) 796-3673

Wyoming

University of Wyoming School of Nursing
—Laramie—

Full-Time Enrollments:	94	Evening Classes:	No
Part-Time Enrollments:	1	Weekend Classes:	No
Affiliation:	Public	Distance Learning:	Yes

NLN ACCREDITATION: Yes

BSN for non-RNs w/degree in other field: No

Articulation: Associate to Baccalaureate
Diploma to Baccalaureate
RN to MSN

For Further Information Contact:

Dr Marcia Dale, Dean
University of Wyoming School of Nursing
PO Box 3065
Laramie, WY 82071-3065
(307) 766-4292

Section 3
Diploma Programs
by State

Arkansas

Baptist School of Nursing
—Little Rock—

Full-Time Enrollments:	394	Evening Classes:	No
Part-Time Enrollments:	—	Weekend Classes:	No
Affiliation:	Religious	Distance Learning:	No

NLN ACCREDITATION: Yes

Articulation: Diploma to Baccalaureate

For Further Information Contact:

Dr Shirlene Harris, Director
Baptist School of Nursing
11900 Colonel Glenn Rd
Little Rock, AR 72210-2820
(501) 202-7402

Jefferson School of Nursing
—Pine Bluff—

Full-Time Enrollments:	133	Evening Classes:	No
Part-Time Enrollments:	—	Weekend Classes:	No
Affiliation:	Private	Distance Learning:	No

NLN ACCREDITATION: Yes

Articulation: Diploma to Baccalaureate

For Further Information Contact:

Mrs Jessie M Clemmons, Director
Jefferson School of Nursing
1515 West 42nd Ave
Pine Bluff, AR 71603
(501) 541-7850

Connecticut

Bridgeport Hospital School of Nursing
—Bridgeport—

Full-Time Enrollments:	60	Evening Classes:	No
Part-Time Enrollments:	56	Weekend Classes:	No
Affiliation:	Private	Distance Learning:	No

NLN ACCREDITATION: Yes

Articulation: Diploma to Baccalaureate

For Further Information Contact:

Dr Karin Fiscella, Director
Bridgeport Hospital School of Nursing
200 Mill Hill Ave
Bridgeport, CT 06610
(203) 384-3485

St Francis Hospital School of Nursing
—Hartford—

Full-Time Enrollments:	54	Evening Classes:	No
Part-Time Enrollments:	—	Weekend Classes:	No
Affiliation:	Private	Distance Learning:	No

NLN ACCREDITATION: Yes

Articulation: Diploma to Baccalaureate

For Further Information Contact:

Dr Rosemary Hathaway, Director
St Francis Hospital School of Nursing
260 Ashley St
Hartford, CT 06105
(860) 714-6001

Delaware

Beebe School of Nursing
—Lewes—

Full-Time Enrollments:	66	Evening Classes:	No
Part-Time Enrollments:	—	Weekend Classes:	No
Affiliation:	Private	Distance Learning:	No

NLN ACCREDITATION: Yes

Articulation: Diploma to Baccalaureate

For Further Information Contact:

Mrs Constance E Bushey, Director
Beebe School of Nursing
424 Savannah Rd
Lewes, DE 19958
(302) 645-3251

Illinois

Graham Hospital School of Nursing
—Canton—

Full-Time Enrollments:	40	Evening Classes:	No
Part-Time Enrollments:	4	Weekend Classes:	No
Affiliation:	Private	Distance Learning:	No

NLN ACCREDITATION: Yes

Articulation: None

For Further Information Contact:

Ms Susan Livingston, Director
Graham Hospital School of Nursing
210 W Walnut St
Canton, IL 61520
(309) 647-5240

Methodist Medical Center School of Nursing
—Peoria—

Full-Time Enrollments:	162	Evening Classes:	No
Part-Time Enrollments:	12	Weekend Classes:	No
Affiliation:	Private	Distance Learning:	No

NLN ACCREDITATION: Yes

Articulation: Diploma to Baccalaureate

For Further Information Contact:

Dr Anne Gray, Director
Methodist Medical Center School of Nursing
221 NE Glen Oak Ave
Peoria, IL 61636
(309) 672-5514

Ravenswood Hospital Medical Center School of Nursing
—Chicago—

Full-Time Enrollments:	271	Evening Classes:	No
Part-Time Enrollments:	—	Weekend Classes:	No
Affiliation:	Private	Distance Learning:	No

NLN ACCREDITATION: Yes

Articulation: Diploma to Baccalaureate

For Further Information Contact:

Ms Phyllis Thomson, Director
Ravenswood Hospital Medical Center School of Nursing
2318 West Irving Pk Rd Bldg C
Chicago, IL 60618-3824
(312) 463-9191

St Francis Hospital School of Nursing
—Evanston—

Full-Time Enrollments:	23	Evening Classes:	No
Part-Time Enrollments:	4	Weekend Classes:	No
Affiliation:	Religious	Distance Learning:	No

NLN ACCREDITATION: Yes

Articulation: None

For Further Information Contact:

Ms Barbara Wejman, Director
St Francis Hospital School of Nursing
319 Ridge Ave
Evanston, IL 60202
(847) 316-6230

Indiana

St Elizabeth Hospital School of Nursing
—Lafayette—

Full-Time Enrollments:	137	Evening Classes:	No
Part-Time Enrollments:	17	Weekend Classes:	No
Affiliation:	Religious	Distance Learning:	No

NLN ACCREDITATION: Yes

Articulation: Diploma to Baccalaureate

For Further Information Contact:

Mr John R Jezierski, Director
St Elizabeth Hospital School of Nursing
1508 Tippecanoe St
Lafayette, IN 47904
(317) 423-6408

Iowa

Allen Memorial Hospital-School of Nursing
—Waterloo—

Full-Time Enrollments:	22	Evening Classes:	No
Part-Time Enrollments:	2	Weekend Classes:	No
Affiliation:	Private	Distance Learning:	No

NLN ACCREDITATION: Yes

Articulation: Diploma to Baccalaureate

For Further Information Contact:

Dr Jane Hasek, Chancellor
Allen Memorial Hospital-School of Nursing
1825 Logan Ave
Waterloo, IA 50703
(319) 235-3649

Iowa Methodist School of Nursing
—Des Moines—

Full-Time Enrollments:	100	Evening Classes:	No
Part-Time Enrollments:	40	Weekend Classes:	No
Affiliation:	Private	Distance Learning:	No

NLN ACCREDITATION: Yes

Articulation: Diploma to Baccalaureate

For Further Information Contact:

Mrs Pamela Bradley, Director
Iowa Methodist School of Nursing
1117 Pleasant St
Des Moines, IA 50309-1499
(515) 241-6901

Diploma Programs

Jennie Edmundson Memorial Hospital School of Nursing
—Council Bluffs—

Full-Time Enrollments:	—	Evening Classes:	—
Part-Time Enrollments:	—	Weekend Classes:	—
Affiliation:	Private	Distance Learning:	—

NLN ACCREDITATION: Yes

Articulation: None

For Further Information Contact:

Mrs Marjorie Matzen, Director
Jennie Edmundson Memorial Hospital School of Nursing
933 E Pierce St
Council Bluffs, IA 51501
(712) 328-6100

Mercy Hospital School of Nursing
—Des Moines—

Full-Time Enrollments:	112	Evening Classes:	No
Part-Time Enrollments:	—	Weekend Classes:	No
Affiliation:	Religious	Distance Learning:	No

NLN ACCREDITATION: Yes

Articulation: Diploma to Baccalaureate

For Further Information Contact:

Mrs Helen Roberts, Director
Mercy Hospital School of Nursing
928 6th Ave
Des Moines, IA 50309
(515) 247-3180

St Luke's School of Nursing and Allied Health
—Sioux City—

Full-Time Enrollments:	58	Evening Classes:	No
Part-Time Enrollments:	—	Weekend Classes:	No
Affiliation:	Private	Distance Learning:	No

NLN ACCREDITATION: Yes

Articulation: Diploma to Baccalaureate

For Further Information Contact:

Ms Regene Osborne, Director
St Luke's School of Nursing and Allied Health
2720 Stone Park Blvd
Sioux City, IA 51104-0263
(712) 279-3172

Louisiana

Baton Rouge General Medical Center
—Baton Rouge—

Full-Time Enrollments:	65	Evening Classes:	No
Part-Time Enrollments:	—	Weekend Classes:	No
Affiliation:	Private	Distance Learning:	No

NLN ACCREDITATION: Yes

Articulation: Diploma to Baccalaureate

For Further Information Contact:

Mrs Laura H Thigpen, Director
Baton Rouge General Medical Center
PO Box 2511
Baton Rouge, LA 70821
(504) 387-7623

Maryland

MacQueen Gibbs Willis School of Nursing, Memorial
—Easton—

Full-Time Enrollments:	46	Evening Classes:	—
Part-Time Enrollments:	—	Weekend Classes:	—
Affiliation:	Private	Distance Learning:	No

NLN ACCREDITATION: Yes

Articulation: Diploma to Baccalaureate

For Further Information Contact:

Ms Joan Coccaro, Director
MacQueen Gibbs Willis School of Nursing, Memorial
S Washington St
Easton, MD 21601
(410) 822-1000

Union Memorial Hospital School of Nursing
—Baltimore—

Full-Time Enrollments:	—	Evening Classes:	Yes
Part-Time Enrollments:	114	Weekend Classes:	Yes
Affiliation:	Private	Distance Learning:	No

NLN ACCREDITATION: Yes

Articulation: None

For Further Information Contact:

Dr Judith Feustle, Director
Union Memorial Hospital School of Nursing
201 E Univ Pkwy
Baltimore, MD 21218
(410) 554-2739

Massachusetts

Bay State Medical Center School of Nursing
—Springfield—

Full-Time Enrollments:	126	Evening Classes:	No
Part-Time Enrollments:	4	Weekend Classes:	No
Affiliation:	Private	Distance Learning:	No

NLN ACCREDITATION: Yes

Articulation: Diploma to Baccalaureate

For Further Information Contact:

Mrs Patricia A Miller, Director
Bay State Medical Center School of Nursing
759 Chestnut St
Springfield, MA 01199
(413) 784-3367

Brockton Hospital School of Nursing
—Brockton—

Full-Time Enrollments:	122	Evening Classes:	Yes
Part-Time Enrollments:	131	Weekend Classes:	Yes
Affiliation:	Private	Distance Learning:	No

NLN ACCREDITATION: Yes

Articulation: Diploma to Baccalaureate

For Further Information Contact:

Mrs Rula Harb, Director
Brockton Hospital School of Nursing
680 Centre St
Brockton, MA 02402
(508) 941-7044

Framingham Union Hospital School of Nursing
—Framingham—

Full-Time Enrollments:	28	Evening Classes:	No
Part-Time Enrollments:	23	Weekend Classes:	No
Affiliation:	Private	Distance Learning:	No

NLN ACCREDITATION: Yes

Articulation: Diploma to Baccalaureate

For Further Information Contact:

Mrs Joyce E Russell, Director
Framingham Union Hospital School of Nursing
85 Lincoln St
Framingham, MA 01701
(508) 383-1752

Lawrence Memorial Hospital School of Nursing
—Medford—

Full-Time Enrollments:	—	Evening Classes:	—
Part-Time Enrollments:	—	Weekend Classes:	—
Affiliation:	Private	Distance Learning:	—

NLN ACCREDITATION: Yes

Articulation: —

For Further Information Contact:

Mrs Marie B McCarthy, Vice President
Lawrence Memorial Hospital School of Nursing
170 Governors Ave
Medford, MA 02155
(617) 396-9250

New England Baptist Hospital School of Nursing
—Boston—

Full-Time Enrollments:	40	Evening Classes:	No
Part-Time Enrollments:	1	Weekend Classes:	No
Affiliation:	Private	Distance Learning:	No

NLN ACCREDITATION: Yes

Articulation: Diploma to Baccalaureate

For Further Information Contact:

Ms Elaine Kelter, Director
New England Baptist Hospital School of Nursing
220 Fisher Ave
Boston, MA 02120
(617) 739-5266

Somerville Hospital School of Nursing
—Somerville—

Full-Time Enrollments:	75	Evening Classes:	Yes
Part-Time Enrollments:	—	Weekend Classes:	Yes
Affiliation:	Private	Distance Learning:	No

NLN ACCREDITATION: Yes

Articulation: None

For Further Information Contact:

Mrs Princess Everton, Director
Somerville Hospital School of Nursing
125 Lowell St
Somerville, MA 02143
(617) 666-4400

St Elizabeth's Hospital School of Nursing
—Brighton—

Full-Time Enrollments:	119	Evening Classes:	No
Part-Time Enrollments:	5	Weekend Classes:	No
Affiliation:	Religious	Distance Learning:	No

NLN ACCREDITATION: Yes

Articulation: Diploma to Baccalaureate

For Further Information Contact:

Miss Helen C Fagan, Director
St Elizabeth's Hospital School of Nursing
159 Washington St
Brighton, MA 02135
(617) 789-2366

Michigan

Bronson Methodist Hospital School of Nursing
—Kalamazoo—

Full-Time Enrollments:	87	Evening Classes:	No
Part-Time Enrollments:	6	Weekend Classes:	No
Affiliation:	Private	Distance Learning:	No

NLN ACCREDITATION: Yes

Articulation: None

For Further Information Contact:

Ms Rosemarie Nedeau-Cayo, Director
Bronson Methodist Hospital School of Nursing
252 E Lovell St
Kalamazoo, MI 49007
(616) 341-7862

Henry Ford Hospital School of Nursing
—Detroit—

Full-Time Enrollments:	—	Evening Classes:	—
Part-Time Enrollments:	—	Weekend Classes:	—
Affiliation:	Private	Distance Learning:	—

NLN ACCREDITATION: Yes

Articulation: None

For Further Information Contact:

Dr Teresa Wehrwein, Director
Henry Ford Hospital School of Nursing
2921 W Grand Blvd
Detroit, MI 48202
(313) 972-1928

Missouri

Lutheran Medical Center School of Nursing
—St Louis—

Full-Time Enrollments:	61	Evening Classes:	No
Part-Time Enrollments:	24	Weekend Classes:	No
Affiliation:	Private	Distance Learning:	No

NLN ACCREDITATION: Yes

Articulation: Diploma to Baccalaureate

For Further Information Contact:

Mrs Jean Horrall, Director
Lutheran Medical Center School of Nursing
3547 S Jefferson Ave
St Louis, MO 63118-3999
(314) 577-5855

Missouri Baptist Hospital School of Nursing
—St Louis—

Full-Time Enrollments:	78	Evening Classes:	No
Part-Time Enrollments:	68	Weekend Classes:	No
Affiliation:	Private	Distance Learning:	No

NLN ACCREDITATION: Yes

Articulation: Diploma to Baccalaureate

For Further Information Contact:

Miss Pamela Dick, Director
Missouri Baptist Hospital School of Nursing
3015 N Ballas Rd
St Louis, MO 63131
(314) 569-5191

St John's School of Nursing
—Springfield—

Full-Time Enrollments:	99	Evening Classes:	No
Part-Time Enrollments:	—	Weekend Classes:	No
Affiliation:	Religious	Distance Learning:	No

NLN ACCREDITATION: Yes

Articulation: None

For Further Information Contact:

Miss Virginia Mayeux, Director
St John's School of Nursing
4431 S Fremont
Springfield, MO 65804-7307
(417) 885-2069

Nebraska

Bryan Memorial Hospital School of Nursing
—Lincoln—

Full-Time Enrollments:	127	Evening Classes:	No
Part-Time Enrollments:	—	Weekend Classes:	No
Affiliation:	Private	Distance Learning:	Yes

NLN ACCREDITATION: Yes

Articulation: Diploma to Baccalaureate

For Further Information Contact:

Mrs Phylis Hollamon, Director
Bryan Memorial Hospital School of Nursing
5000 Sumner St
Lincoln, NE 68506
(402) 483-3867

New Jersey

Ann May School of Nursing, Jersey Shore Medical Center
—Neptune—

Full-Time Enrollments:	56	Evening Classes:	No
Part-Time Enrollments:	—	Weekend Classes:	No
Affiliation:	Private	Distance Learning:	No

NLN ACCREDITATION: Yes

Articulation: None

For Further Information Contact:

Mrs Arlene Farmer, Director
Ann May School of Nursing, Jersey Shore Medical Center
1945 Corlies Ave
Neptune, NJ 07753
(908) 776-4200

Bayonne Hospital School of Nursing
—Bayonne—

Full-Time Enrollments:	52	Evening Classes:	No
Part-Time Enrollments:	7	Weekend Classes:	No
Affiliation:	Public	Distance Learning:	No

NLN ACCREDITATION: Yes

Articulation: Diploma to Baccalaureate

For Further Information Contact:

Ms Ruth E Schauer, Director
Bayonne Hospital School of Nursing
12 E 30th St
Bayonne, NJ 07002
(201) 339-9656

C E Gregory School of Nursing, Raritan Bay Medical Center
—Perth Amboy—

Full-Time Enrollments:	117	Evening Classes:	No
Part-Time Enrollments:	—	Weekend Classes:	No
Affiliation:	Private	Distance Learning:	No

NLN ACCREDITATION: Yes

Articulation: None

For Further Information Contact:

Miss C M McCormack, Director
C E Gregory School of Nursing, Raritan Bay Medical Center
530 New Brunswick Ave
Perth Amboy, NJ 08861
(908) 360-4190

Christ Hospital School of Nursing
—Jersey City—

Full-Time Enrollments:	86	Evening Classes:	Yes
Part-Time Enrollments:	62	Weekend Classes:	No
Affiliation:	Religious	Distance Learning:	No

NLN ACCREDITATION: Yes

Articulation: Diploma to Baccalaureate
RN to MSN

For Further Information Contact:

Ms Carol Fasano, Director
Christ Hospital School of Nursing
176 Palisade Ave
Jersey City, NJ 07306
(201) 795-8360

Elizabeth General Medical Center School of Nursing
—Elizabeth—

Full-Time Enrollments:	77	Evening Classes:	Yes
Part-Time Enrollments:	405	Weekend Classes:	Yes
Affiliation:	Private	Distance Learning:	No

NLN ACCREDITATION: Yes

Articulation: Diploma to Baccalaureate
LPN to Associate

For Further Information Contact:

Mrs Mary E Kelley, Dean
Elizabeth General Medical Center School of Nursing
925 E Jersey St
Elizabeth, NJ 07201
(908) 629-8144

DIPLOMA PROGRAMS

Helene Fuld School of Nursing in Camden County
—Blackwood—

Full-Time Enrollments:	244	Evening Classes:	Yes
Part-Time Enrollments:	62	Weekend Classes:	No
Affiliation:	Private	Distance Learning:	No

NLN ACCREDITATION: Yes

Articulation: Diploma to Baccalaureate

For Further Information Contact:

Dr Regina Mastrangelo, Dean
Helene Fuld School of Nursing in Camden County
Box 1669 College Dr
Blackwood, NJ 08012
(609) 374-0100

Helene Fuld School of Nursing of New Jersey
—Trenton—

Full-Time Enrollments:	10	Evening Classes:	No
Part-Time Enrollments:	154	Weekend Classes:	No
Affiliation:	Private	Distance Learning:	No

NLN ACCREDITATION: Yes

Articulation: None

For Further Information Contact:

Mrs Carol Hernandez, Dean
Helene Fuld School of Nursing of New Jersey
750 Brunswick Ave
Trenton, NJ 08638
(609) 394-3174

Holy Name Hospital School of Nursing
—Teaneck—

Full-Time Enrollments:	135	Evening Classes:	No
Part-Time Enrollments:	11	Weekend Classes:	No
Affiliation:	Religious	Distance Learning:	No

NLN ACCREDITATION: Yes

Articulation: Diploma to Baccalaureate

For Further Information Contact:

Sr Claire Tynan, Director
Holy Name Hospital School of Nursing
690 Teaneck Rd
Teaneck, NJ 07666
(201) 833-3007

Mercer Medical Center School of Nursing
—Trenton—

Full-Time Enrollments:	54	Evening Classes:	No
Part-Time Enrollments:	17	Weekend Classes:	No
Affiliation:	Public	Distance Learning:	No

NLN ACCREDITATION: Yes

Articulation: Diploma to Baccalaureate

For Further Information Contact:

Mrs Virginia Sternhagen, Director
Mercer Medical Center School of Nursing
446 Bellevue Ave, Box 1658
Trenton, NJ 08607
(609) 394-4050

Mountainside Hospital School of Nursing
—Montclair—

Full-Time Enrollments:	181	Evening Classes:	Yes
Part-Time Enrollments:	—	Weekend Classes:	No
Affiliation:	Private	Distance Learning:	No

NLN ACCREDITATION: Yes

Articulation: Diploma to Baccalaureate
RN to MSN

For Further Information Contact:

Mrs Louise DeBlois, Director
Mountainside Hospital School of Nursing
Bay & Highland Ave
Montclair, NJ 07042
(201) 429-6061

Muhlenberg Regional Medical Center School of Nursing
—Plainfield—

Full-Time Enrollments:	56	Evening Classes:	Yes
Part-Time Enrollments:	306	Weekend Classes:	—
Affiliation:	Public	Distance Learning:	—

NLN ACCREDITATION: Yes

Articulation: Diploma to Baccalaureate

For Further Information Contact:

Mrs Judith Mathews, Dean
Muhlenberg Regional Medical Center School of Nursing
Park Ave
Plainfield, NJ 07061
(908) 668-2418

Our Lady of Lourdes School of Nursing
—Camden—

Full-Time Enrollments:	50	Evening Classes:	No
Part-Time Enrollments:	46	Weekend Classes:	No
Affiliation:	Religious	Distance Learning:	No

NLN ACCREDITATION: Yes

Articulation: Diploma to Baccalaureate

For Further Information Contact:

Sr M J Francis Coyle, Dean
Our Lady of Lourdes School of Nursing
1565 Vesper Blvd
Camden, NJ 08103
(609) 757-3729

St Francis Hospital School of Nursing
—Jersey City—

Full-Time Enrollments:	65	Evening Classes:	No
Part-Time Enrollments:	9	Weekend Classes:	No
Affiliation:	Private	Distance Learning:	No

NLN ACCREDITATION: Yes

Articulation: Diploma to Baccalaureate

For Further Information Contact:

Ms Ruthanne Braddock, Director
St Francis Hospital School of Nursing
1 McWilliams Pl
Jersey City, NJ 07302
(201) 418-2200

St Francis Medical Center School of Nursing
—Trenton—

Full-Time Enrollments:	42	Evening Classes:	No
Part-Time Enrollments:	7	Weekend Classes:	No
Affiliation:	Private	Distance Learning:	No

NLN ACCREDITATION: Yes

Articulation: None

For Further Information Contact:

Ms Bonny Ross, Director
St Francis Medical Center School of Nursing
601 Hamilton Ave
Trenton, NJ 08629
(609) 599-5190

New York

Arnot-Ogden Medical Center
—Elmira—

Full-Time Enrollments:	42	Evening Classes:	No
Part-Time Enrollments:	7	Weekend Classes:	No
Affiliation:	Public	Distance Learning:	No

NLN ACCREDITATION: Yes

Articulation: Diploma to Baccalaureate

For Further Information Contact:

Mrs Lounell McGrady, Director
Arnot-Ogden Medical Center
600 Roe Ave
Elmira, NY 14905
(607) 737-4153

Memorial Hospital School of Nursing
—Albany—

Full-Time Enrollments:	27	Evening Classes:	Yes
Part-Time Enrollments:	50	Weekend Classes:	No
Affiliation:	Private	Distance Learning:	No

NLN ACCREDITATION: Yes

Articulation: Diploma to Baccalaureate

For Further Information Contact:

Mrs Janet Haebler, Director
Memorial Hospital School of Nursing
Northern Blvd
Albany, NY 12204
(518) 471-3262

St James Mercy Hospital School of Nursing
—Hornell—

Full-Time Enrollments:	—	Evening Classes:	—
Part-Time Enrollments:	—	Weekend Classes:	—
Affiliation:	Religious	Distance Learning:	—

NLN ACCREDITATION: Yes

Articulation: None

For Further Information Contact:

Ms Jean Bohomey, Director
St James Mercy Hospital School of Nursing
440 Monroe Ave
Hornell, NY 14843
(607) 324-0841

St Vincent's Hospital School of Nursing
—New York—

Full-Time Enrollments:	92	Evening Classes:	No
Part-Time Enrollments:	10	Weekend Classes:	No
Affiliation:	Religious	Distance Learning:	No

NLN ACCREDITATION: Yes

Articulation: Diploma to Baccalaureate

For Further Information Contact:

Sr Miriam Kevin Phillips, Director
St Vincent's Hospital School of Nursing
27 Christopher St
New York, NY 10014
(212) 604-8490

St Vincent's Medical Center of Richmond School of Nursing
—Staten Island—

Full-Time Enrollments:	—	Evening Classes:	—
Part-Time Enrollments:	—	Weekend Classes:	—
Affiliation:	Public	Distance Learning:	—

NLN ACCREDITATION: Yes

Articulation: —

For Further Information Contact:

Dr Roberta Marpet, Dean
St Vincent's Medical Center of Richmond School of
Nursing
2 Gridley Ave
Staten Island, NY 10303
(718) 876-1300

North Carolina

Mercy School of Nursing
—Charlotte—

Full-Time Enrollments:	30	Evening Classes:	No
Part-Time Enrollments:	87	Weekend Classes:	No
Affiliation:	Public	Distance Learning:	No

NLN ACCREDITATION: Yes

Articulation: Diploma to Baccalaureate

For Further Information Contact:

Dr Kay Smith, Director
Mercy School of Nursing
1921 Vail Ave
Charlotte, NC 28207
(704) 379-5840

Presbyterian Hospital School of Nursing
—Charlotte—

Full-Time Enrollments:	174	Evening Classes:	Yes
Part-Time Enrollments:	58	Weekend Classes:	Yes
Affiliation:	Private	Distance Learning:	No

NLN ACCREDITATION: Yes

Articulation: Diploma to Baccalaureate

For Further Information Contact:

Dr Judith Trexler, Director
Presbyterian Hospital School of Nursing
PO Box 33549
Charlotte, NC 28233
(704) 384-4143

Watts School of Nursing
—Durham—

Full-Time Enrollments:	108	Evening Classes:	No
Part-Time Enrollments:	—	Weekend Classes:	No
Affiliation:	Public	Distance Learning:	No

NLN ACCREDITATION: Yes

Articulation: Diploma to Baccalaureate

For Further Information Contact:

Dr Peggy Baker, Director
Watts School of Nursing
3643 N Roxboro St
Durham, NC 27704
(919) 470-7347

Ohio

Aultman Hospital School of Nursing
—Canton—

Full-Time Enrollments:	45	Evening Classes:	No
Part-Time Enrollments:	32	Weekend Classes:	No
Affiliation:	Private	Distance Learning:	No

NLN ACCREDITATION: Yes

Articulation: None

For Further Information Contact:

Mrs Joan Frey, Asst Vice President
Aultman Hospital School of Nursing
2614 6th St SW
Canton, OH 44710-1797
(330) 452-9911

Christ Hospital School of Nursing
—Cincinnati—

Full-Time Enrollments:	171	Evening Classes:	No
Part-Time Enrollments:	—	Weekend Classes:	No
Affiliation:	Private	Distance Learning:	No

NLN ACCREDITATION: Yes

Articulation: None

For Further Information Contact:

Ms Carol Dipilla, Asst Vice President
Christ Hospital School of Nursing
2139 Auburn Ave
Cincinnati, OH 45219-2988
(513) 369-3546

Fairview Hospital School of Nursing
—Cleveland—

Full-Time Enrollments:	134	Evening Classes:	No
Part-Time Enrollments:	—	Weekend Classes:	No
Affiliation:	Private	Distance Learning:	No

NLN ACCREDITATION: Yes

Articulation: Diploma to Associate
Diploma to Baccalaureate

For Further Information Contact:

Ms Patricia Rolince, Director
Fairview Hospital School of Nursing
18101 Lorain Ave
Cleveland, OH 44111-5656
(216) 476-7134

Good Samaritan Hospital School of Nursing
—Cincinnati—

Full-Time Enrollments:	127	Evening Classes:	Yes
Part-Time Enrollments:	109	Weekend Classes:	No
Affiliation:	Religious	Distance Learning:	No

NLN ACCREDITATION: Yes

Articulation: Diploma to Baccalaureate

For Further Information Contact:

Mr Morris Cohen, Director
Good Samaritan Hospital School of Nursing
375 Dixmyth Ave
Cincinnati, OH 45220-2489
(513) 872-2491

Mansfield General Hospital School of Nursing
—Mansfield—

Full-Time Enrollments:	47	Evening Classes:	No
Part-Time Enrollments:	30	Weekend Classes:	No
Affiliation:	Private	Distance Learning:	No

NLN ACCREDITATION: Yes

Articulation: Diploma to Baccalaureate

For Further Information Contact:

Mrs Nancy Collier, Director
Mansfield General Hospital School of Nursing
335 Glessner Ave
Mansfield, OH 44903-2265
(419) 526-8595

Meridia Huron School of Nursing
—Cleveland—

Full-Time Enrollments:	180	Evening Classes:	Yes
Part-Time Enrollments:	—	Weekend Classes:	Yes
Affiliation:	Private	Distance Learning:	No

NLN ACCREDITATION: Yes

Articulation: Diploma to Baccalaureate

For Further Information Contact:

Ms Kathleen Knittel, Director
Meridia Huron School of Nursing
13951 Terrace Rd
Cleveland, OH 44112-4399
(216) 761-7996

Providence Hospital School of Nursing
—Sandusky—

Full-Time Enrollments:	83	Evening Classes:	No
Part-Time Enrollments:	9	Weekend Classes:	No
Affiliation:	Religious	Distance Learning:	No

NLN ACCREDITATION: Yes

Articulation: None

For Further Information Contact:

Mrs Holly Price, Director
Providence Hospital School of Nursing
1912 Hayes Ave
Sandusky, OH 44870-4788
(419) 621-7111

St Vincent Medical Center School of Nursing
—Toledo—

Full-Time Enrollments:	140	Evening Classes:	No
Part-Time Enrollments:	22	Weekend Classes:	No
Affiliation:	Religious	Distance Learning:	No

NLN ACCREDITATION: Yes

Articulation: None

For Further Information Contact:

Mrs Elizabeth Cain, Director
St Vincent Medical Center School of Nursing
2201 Cherry St
Toledo, OH 43608-2695
(419) 251-4319

Summa St Thomas School of Nursing
—Akron—

Full-Time Enrollments:	108	Evening Classes:	No
Part-Time Enrollments:	—	Weekend Classes:	No
Affiliation:	Private	Distance Learning:	No

NLN ACCREDITATION: Yes

Articulation: None

For Further Information Contact:

Mrs Ruth Shiflett, Director
Summa St Thomas School of Nursing
41 Arch St
Akron, OH 44304
(330) 375-7560

The Community Hospital of Springfield
—Springfield—

Full-Time Enrollments:	71	Evening Classes:	No
Part-Time Enrollments:	4	Weekend Classes:	No
Affiliation:	Private	Distance Learning:	No

NLN ACCREDITATION: Yes

Articulation: None

For Further Information Contact:

Miss Marylin J Theurer, Director
The Community Hospital of Springfield
2615 E High St, PO Box 1228
Springfield, OH 45501-1228
(937) 328-8900

Trinity Health System School of Nursing
—Steubenville—

Full-Time Enrollments:	73	Evening Classes:	No
Part-Time Enrollments:	—	Weekend Classes:	No
Affiliation:	Religious	Distance Learning:	No

NLN ACCREDITATION: Yes

Articulation: None

For Further Information Contact:

Mr Roy J Karmosky, Director
Trinity Health System School of Nursing
380 Summit Ave
Steubenville, OH 43952-2699
(614) 283-7260

Pennsylvania

Abington Memorial Hospital School of Nursing
—Willow Grove—

Full-Time Enrollments:	50	Evening Classes:	No
Part-Time Enrollments:	—	Weekend Classes:	No
Affiliation:	Private	Distance Learning:	No

NLN ACCREDITATION: Yes

Articulation: Diploma to Baccalaureate

For Further Information Contact:

Mrs Dorothy Z Allison, Chair
Abington Memorial Hospital School of Nursing
2500 Maryland Rd Suite200
Willow Grove, PA 19090-1284
(215) 881-5500

Brandywine Hospital School of Nursing
—Coatesville—

Full-Time Enrollments:	54	Evening Classes:	No
Part-Time Enrollments:	17	Weekend Classes:	No
Affiliation:	Private	Distance Learning:	No

NLN ACCREDITATION: Yes

Articulation: Diploma to Baccalaureate

For Further Information Contact:

Mrs Colleen Meakim, Director
Brandywine Hospital School of Nursing
215 Reeceville Rd
Coatesville, PA 19320-1536
(610) 383-8206

Chester County Hospital School of Nursing
—West Chester—

Full-Time Enrollments:	85	Evening Classes:	No
Part-Time Enrollments:	—	Weekend Classes:	No
Affiliation:	Private	Distance Learning:	No

NLN ACCREDITATION: Yes

Articulation: Diploma to Baccalaureate

For Further Information Contact:

Mrs Dolores H Ott, Director
Chester County Hospital School of Nursing
701 E Marshall St
West Chester, PA 19380
(215) 431-5165

Citizens General Hospital School of Nursing
—New Kensington—

Full-Time Enrollments:	52	Evening Classes:	No
Part-Time Enrollments:	—	Weekend Classes:	No
Affiliation:	Private	Distance Learning:	No

NLN ACCREDITATION: Yes

Articulation: Diploma to Baccalaureate

For Further Information Contact:

Mrs Mary Lynne Rugh, Director
Citizens General Hospital School of Nursing
651 4th Ave
New Kensington, PA 15068
(412) 337-5090

Conemaugh Valley Mememorial Hospital School of Nursing
—Johnstown—

Full-Time Enrollments:	83	Evening Classes:	No
Part-Time Enrollments:	1	Weekend Classes:	No
Affiliation:	Public	Distance Learning:	No

NLN ACCREDITATION: Yes

Articulation: Diploma to Baccalaureate

For Further Information Contact:

Mrs L Pugliese, Director
Conemaugh Valley Mememorial Hospital School of
Nursing
1086 Franklin St
Johnstown, PA 15905
(814) 534-9118

Episcopal Hospital School of Nursing
—Philadelphia—

Full-Time Enrollments:	53	Evening Classes:	Yes
Part-Time Enrollments:	53	Weekend Classes:	Yes
Affiliation:	Private	Distance Learning:	—

NLN ACCREDITATION: Yes

Articulation: None

For Further Information Contact:

Mrs Beverly L Welhan, Director
Episcopal Hospital School of Nursing
100 East Lehigh Ave
Philadelphia, PA 19125
(215) 427-7468

Frankford Hospital School of Nursing
—Philadelphia—

Full-Time Enrollments:	500	Evening Classes:	No
Part-Time Enrollments:	—	Weekend Classes:	No
Affiliation:	Private	Distance Learning:	No

NLN ACCREDITATION: Yes

Articulation: Diploma to Baccalaureate

For Further Information Contact:

Dr Mary K Gilchrist, Dean
Frankford Hospital School of Nursing
4918 Penn St
Philadelphia, PA 19124
(215) 831-2362

Geisinger Medical Center School of Nursing
—Danville—

Full-Time Enrollments:	112	Evening Classes:	No
Part-Time Enrollments:	2	Weekend Classes:	No
Affiliation:	Private	Distance Learning:	No

NLN ACCREDITATION: Yes

Articulation: Diploma to Baccalaureate

For Further Information Contact:

Mrs Katherine Carter, Coordinator
Geisinger Medical Center School of Nursing
100 N Academy Ave
Danville, PA 17822-0403
(717) 271-6276

Germantown Hospital and Medical Center School of Nursing
—Philadelphia—

Full-Time Enrollments:	—	Evening Classes:	—
Part-Time Enrollments:	—	Weekend Classes:	—
Affiliation:	Public	Distance Learning:	—

NLN ACCREDITATION: Yes

Articulation: —

For Further Information Contact:

Mrs Mary Dorr, Director
Germantown Hospital and Medical Center School of Nursing
3 Penn Blvd
Philadelphia, PA 19144
(215) 951-8850

Jameson Memorial Hospital School of Nursing
—New Castle—

Full-Time Enrollments:	38	Evening Classes:	No
Part-Time Enrollments:	12	Weekend Classes:	No
Affiliation:	Private	Distance Learning:	No

NLN ACCREDITATION: Yes

Articulation: Diploma to Baccalaureate

For Further Information Contact:

Dr Joan P Byers, Director
Jameson Memorial Hospital School of Nursing
1211 Wilmington Ave
New Castle, PA 16105-2595
(412) 656-4052

Lancaster Institute for Health Education
—Lancaster—

Full-Time Enrollments:	254	Evening Classes:	No
Part-Time Enrollments:	34	Weekend Classes:	No
Affiliation:	Private	Distance Learning:	No

NLN ACCREDITATION: Yes

Articulation: Diploma to Baccalaureate

For Further Information Contact:

Dr Carol Hamer, Vice President
Lancaster Institute for Health Education
143 E Lemon St PO Box 3555
Lancaster, PA 17602
(717) 290-4913

Mercy Hospital School of Nursing
—Pittsburgh—

Full-Time Enrollments:	61	Evening Classes:	No
Part-Time Enrollments:	1	Weekend Classes:	No
Affiliation:	Religious	Distance Learning:	No

NLN ACCREDITATION: Yes

Articulation: None

For Further Information Contact:

Sr Carolyn Schallenberger, Director
Mercy Hospital School of Nursing
1401 Boulevard of the Allies
Pittsburgh, PA 15219
(412) 232-7940

Methodist Hospital School of Nursing
—Philadelphia—

Full-Time Enrollments:	97	Evening Classes:	No
Part-Time Enrollments:	—	Weekend Classes:	No
Affiliation:	Private	Distance Learning:	No

NLN ACCREDITATION: Yes

Articulation: Diploma to Baccalaureate

For Further Information Contact:

Mrs Robin Allen, Director
Methodist Hospital School of Nursing
2301 S Broad St
Philadelphia, PA 19148
(215) 952-9402

Northeastern Hospital School of Nursing
—Philadelphia—

Full-Time Enrollments:	60	Evening Classes:	No
Part-Time Enrollments:	—	Weekend Classes:	No
Affiliation:	Public	Distance Learning:	No

NLN ACCREDITATION: Yes

Articulation: Diploma to Baccalaureate

For Further Information Contact:

Ms Mary Wombwell, Director
Northeastern Hospital School of Nursing
2301 E Allegheny Ave
Philadelphia, PA 19134-4499
(215) 291-3135

Ohio Valley General Hospital School of Nursing
—McKees Rocks—

Full-Time Enrollments:	28	Evening Classes:	—
Part-Time Enrollments:	—	Weekend Classes:	—
Affiliation:	Private	Distance Learning:	—

NLN ACCREDITATION: Yes

Articulation: Diploma to Baccalaureate

For Further Information Contact:

Ms Susan E Woloshun, Director
Ohio Valley General Hospital School of Nursing
25 Heckel Rd
McKees Rocks, PA 15136
(412) 777-6255

Pottsville Hospital School of Nursing
—Pottsville—

Full-Time Enrollments:	83	Evening Classes:	No
Part-Time Enrollments:	20	Weekend Classes:	No
Affiliation:	Private	Distance Learning:	No

NLN ACCREDITATION: Yes

Articulation: Diploma to Baccalaureate

For Further Information Contact:

Mrs Angela Pasco, Director
Pottsville Hospital School of Nursing
Washington & Jackson Sts
Pottsville, PA 17901
(717) 621-5028

Reading Hospital School of Nursing
—West Reading—

Full-Time Enrollments:	160	Evening Classes:	No
Part-Time Enrollments:	6	Weekend Classes:	No
Affiliation:	Public	Distance Learning:	No

NLN ACCREDITATION: Yes

Articulation: Diploma to Baccalaureate

For Further Information Contact:

Miss Lorna Ramsay, Director
Reading Hospital School of Nursing
6th & Spruce Sts
West Reading, PA 19611
(610) 378-6331

Roxborough Memorial Hospital School of Nursing
—Philadelphia—

Full-Time Enrollments:	84	Evening Classes:	—
Part-Time Enrollments:	—	Weekend Classes:	—
Affiliation:	Private	Distance Learning:	—

NLN ACCREDITATION: Yes

Articulation: None

For Further Information Contact:

Mrs Mary G Simcox, Director
Roxborough Memorial Hospital School of Nursing
5800 Ridge Ave
Philadelphia, PA 19128
(215) 487-4591

Sewickley Valley Hospital School of Nursing
—Sewickley—

Full-Time Enrollments:	36	Evening Classes:	Yes
Part-Time Enrollments:	46	Weekend Classes:	Yes
Affiliation:	Private	Distance Learning:	No

NLN ACCREDITATION: Yes

Articulation: Diploma to Baccalaureate

For Further Information Contact:

Mrs Donna Wadding, Director
Sewickley Valley Hospital School of Nursing
720 Blackburn Rd
Sewickley, PA 15143
(412) 741-7300

Shadyside Hospital School of Nursing
—Pittsburgh—

Full-Time Enrollments:	73	Evening Classes:	Yes
Part-Time Enrollments:	85	Weekend Classes:	Yes
Affiliation:	Private	Distance Learning:	—

NLN ACCREDITATION: Yes

Articulation: Diploma to Baccalaureate

For Further Information Contact:

Dr Mary Aukerman, Director
Shadyside Hospital School of Nursing
5230 Centre Ave
Pittsburgh, PA 15232
(412) 623-2983

Sharon Regional Health System
—Sharon—

Full-Time Enrollments:	99	Evening Classes:	No
Part-Time Enrollments:	32	Weekend Classes:	No
Affiliation:	Private	Distance Learning:	No

NLN ACCREDITATION: Yes

Articulation: Diploma to Baccalaureate

For Further Information Contact:

Miss Jean Fobes, Director
Sharon Regional Health System
740 E State St
Sharon, PA 16146
(412) 983-3911

St Francis Hospital of New Castle School of Nursing
—New Castle—

Full-Time Enrollments:	63	Evening Classes:	No
Part-Time Enrollments:	—	Weekend Classes:	No
Affiliation:	Private	Distance Learning:	No

NLN ACCREDITATION: Yes

Articulation: Diploma to Baccalaureate

For Further Information Contact:

Mrs Gloria Minteer, Director
St Francis Hospital of New Castle School of Nursing
1100 S Mercer St
New Castle, PA 16101
(412) 656-6000

St Francis Medical Center School of Nursing
—Pittsburgh—

Full-Time Enrollments:	59	Evening Classes:	No
Part-Time Enrollments:	—	Weekend Classes:	No
Affiliation:	Public	Distance Learning:	No

NLN ACCREDITATION: Yes

Articulation: Diploma to Baccalaureate

For Further Information Contact:

Mrs Alexis Weber, Director
St Francis Medical Center School of Nursing
400 45th St
Pittsburgh, PA 15201-1198
(412) 622-4749

St Luke's Hospital School of Nursing
—Bethlehem—

Full-Time Enrollments:	89	Evening Classes:	Yes
Part-Time Enrollments:	64	Weekend Classes:	Yes
Affiliation:	Private	Distance Learning:	No

NLN ACCREDITATION: Yes

Articulation: Diploma to Baccalaureate

For Further Information Contact:

Dr Janet Sipple, Dean
St Luke's Hospital School of Nursing
801 Ostrum St
Bethlehem, PA 18015
(610) 954-3400

St Margaret Memorial Hospital School of Nursing
—Pittsburgh—

Full-Time Enrollments:	46	Evening Classes:	No
Part-Time Enrollments:	—	Weekend Classes:	No
Affiliation:	Private	Distance Learning:	No

NLN ACCREDITATION: Yes

Articulation: Diploma to Baccalaureate

For Further Information Contact:

Dr Ann D Ciak, Director
St Margaret Memorial Hospital School of Nursing
815 Freeport Rd
Pittsburgh, PA 15215-3399
(412) 784-4980

St Vincent Health Center School of Nursing
—Erie—

Full-Time Enrollments:	135	Evening Classes:	No
Part-Time Enrollments:	—	Weekend Classes:	No
Affiliation:	Religious	Distance Learning:	No

NLN ACCREDITATION: Yes

Articulation: None

For Further Information Contact:

Mrs Joyce Boxer, Director
St Vincent Health Center School of Nursing
148 West 21 St Box 740
Erie, PA 16544
(814) 452-5675

Washington Hospital School of Nursing
—Washington—

Full-Time Enrollments:	113	Evening Classes:	—
Part-Time Enrollments:	—	Weekend Classes:	—
Affiliation:	Public	Distance Learning:	—

NLN ACCREDITATION: Yes

Articulation: None

For Further Information Contact:

Ms Barbara Rodebaugh, Director
Washington Hospital School of Nursing
155 Wilson Ave
Washington, PA 15301-3398
(412) 223-3172

Western Pennsylvania Hospital School of Nursing
—Pittsburgh—

Full-Time Enrollments:	72	Evening Classes:	No
Part-Time Enrollments:	—	Weekend Classes:	No
Affiliation:	Private	Distance Learning:	No

NLN ACCREDITATION: Yes

Articulation: Diploma to Baccalaureate

For Further Information Contact:

Mrs Nancy Cobb, Director
Western Pennsylvania Hospital School of Nursing
4900 Friendship Ave
Pittsburgh, PA 15224
(412) 578-5531

Rhode Island

St Joseph Hospital School of Nursing
—N Providence—

Full-Time Enrollments:	105	Evening Classes:	No
Part-Time Enrollments:	—	Weekend Classes:	No
Affiliation:	Religious	Distance Learning:	No

NLN ACCREDITATION: Yes

Articulation: Diploma to Baccalaureate

For Further Information Contact:

Ms Elizabeth DeCosta, Director
St Joseph Hospital School of Nursing
200 High Service Ave
N Providence, RI 02904
(401) 456-3050

Tennessee

Baptist Memorial Hospital School of Nursing
—Memphis—

Full-Time Enrollments:	53	Evening Classes:	No
Part-Time Enrollments:	—	Weekend Classes:	No
Affiliation:	Religious	Distance Learning:	No

NLN ACCREDITATION: Yes

Articulation: Diploma to Baccalaureate

For Further Information Contact:

Ms Denese Shumaker, Director
Baptist Memorial Hospital School of Nursing
Monroe Ave
Memphis, TN 38104
(901) 227-4447

Fort Sanders School of Nursing
—Knoxville—

Full-Time Enrollments:	73	Evening Classes:	No
Part-Time Enrollments:	—	Weekend Classes:	No
Affiliation:	Private	Distance Learning:	No

NLN ACCREDITATION: Yes

Articulation: None

For Further Information Contact:

Dr Margaret Heins, Director
Fort Sanders School of Nursing
1915 White Ave
Knoxville, TN 37916
(423) 541-1290

Methodist Hospital School of Nursing
—Memphis—

Full-Time Enrollments:	153	Evening Classes:	No
Part-Time Enrollments:	93	Weekend Classes:	No
Affiliation:	Private	Distance Learning:	No

NLN ACCREDITATION: Yes

Articulation: None

For Further Information Contact:

Ms Elizabeth Clarke, Asst Vice President
Methodist Hospital School of Nursing
251 S Claybrook
Memphis, TN 38104
(901) 726-8525

St Joseph Hospital School of Nursing
—Memphis—

Full-Time Enrollments:	101	**Evening Classes:**	Yes
Part-Time Enrollments:	38	**Weekend Classes:**	Yes
Affiliation:	Religious	**Distance Learning:**	—

NLN ACCREDITATION: Yes

Articulation: None

For Further Information Contact:

Miss Ann Warblow, Director
St Joseph Hospital School of Nursing
204 Overton Ave
Memphis, TN 38105
(901) 577-2955

Texas

Baptist Memorial Healthcare System
—San Antonio—

Full-Time Enrollments:	132	**Evening Classes:**	No
Part-Time Enrollments:	—	**Weekend Classes:**	No
Affiliation:	Religious	**Distance Learning:**	No

NLN ACCREDITATION: Yes

Articulation: None

For Further Information Contact:

Dr Judith Vallery, Director
Baptist Memorial Healthcare System
111 Dallas St
San Antonio, TX 78205-1230
(210) 302-2053

Methodist Hospital School of Nursing
—Lubbock—

Full-Time Enrollments:	206	**Evening Classes:**	No
Part-Time Enrollments:	—	**Weekend Classes:**	No
Affiliation:	Religious	**Distance Learning:**	No

NLN ACCREDITATION: Yes

Articulation: None

For Further Information Contact:

Mrs Irene S Wilson, Dean
Methodist Hospital School of Nursing
2002 Miami Ave
Lubbock, TX 79410
(806) 797-0955

Virginia

Bon Secous- De Paul Medical Center
—Norfolk—

Full-Time Enrollments:	48	**Evening Classes:**	No
Part-Time Enrollments:	46	**Weekend Classes:**	No
Affiliation:	Religious	**Distance Learning:**	No

NLN ACCREDITATION: Yes

Articulation: None

For Further Information Contact:

Mrs Rose Saunders, Director
Bon Secous- De Paul Medical Center
150 Kingsley Ln
Norfolk, VA 23505
(757) 889-5131

Danville Region Medical Center-School of Nursing
—Danville—

Full-Time Enrollments:	71	**Evening Classes:**	No
Part-Time Enrollments:	—	**Weekend Classes:**	No
Affiliation:	Private	**Distance Learning:**	No

NLN ACCREDITATION: Yes

Articulation: None

For Further Information Contact:

Dr Darnell H Cockram, Director
Danville Region Medical Center-School of Nursing
142 South Main St
Danville, VA 24541
(804) 799-4510

Louise Obici School of Nursing
—Suffolk—

Full-Time Enrollments:	81	**Evening Classes:**	No
Part-Time Enrollments:	—	**Weekend Classes:**	No
Affiliation:	Private	**Distance Learning:**	No

NLN ACCREDITATION: Yes

Articulation: None

For Further Information Contact:

Mrs Sondra Statzer, Director
Louise Obici School of Nursing
PO Box 1100
Suffolk, VA 23439-1100
(757) 934-4742

Lynchburg General Hospital School of Nursing
—Lynchburg—

Full-Time Enrollments:	97	Evening Classes:	No
Part-Time Enrollments:	27	Weekend Classes:	No
Affiliation:	Private	Distance Learning:	No

NLN ACCREDITATION: Yes

Articulation: None

For Further Information Contact:

Mrs Patricia J Uzsoy, Director
Lynchburg General Hospital School of Nursing
1901 Tate Springs Rd
Lynchburg, VA 24501
(804) 947-3070

Richmond Memorial Hospital School of Nursing
—Richmond—

Full-Time Enrollments:	68	Evening Classes:	No
Part-Time Enrollments:	8	Weekend Classes:	No
Affiliation:	Private	Distance Learning:	No

NLN ACCREDITATION: Yes

Articulation: Diploma to Baccalaureate

For Further Information Contact:

Miss Cynia Katsorelos, Director
Richmond Memorial Hospital School of Nursing
1300 Westwood Ave
Richmond, VA 23227
(804) 254-6293

Riverside School of Professional Nursing
—Newport News—

Full-Time Enrollments:	182	Evening Classes:	Yes
Part-Time Enrollments:	2	Weekend Classes:	Yes
Affiliation:	Private	Distance Learning:	No

NLN ACCREDITATION: Yes

Articulation: None

For Further Information Contact:

Mrs Mary A Ford, Director
Riverside School of Professional Nursing
500 J Clyde Morris Blvd
Newport News, VA 23601
(804) 594-2700

Sentara Norfolk General Hospital School of Nursing
—Norfolk—

Full-Time Enrollments:	60	Evening Classes:	No
Part-Time Enrollments:	—	Weekend Classes:	No
Affiliation:	Private	Distance Learning:	No

NLN ACCREDITATION: Yes

Articulation: None

For Further Information Contact:

Mrs Shelly G Vinson, Director
Sentara Norfolk General Hospital School of Nursing
600 Gresham Dr
Norfolk, VA 23507
(757) 668-2900

Southside Regional Medical Center School of Nursing
—Petersburg—

Full-Time Enrollments:	121	Evening Classes:	No
Part-Time Enrollments:	—	Weekend Classes:	No
Affiliation:	Private	Distance Learning:	No

NLN ACCREDITATION: Yes

Articulation: None

For Further Information Contact:

Dr Clementine S Pollok, Vice President
Southside Regional Medical Center School of Nursing
801 S Adams St
Petersburg, VA 23803
(804) 862-5801

West Virginia

St Mary's Hospital School of Nursing
—Huntington—

Full-Time Enrollments:	2	Evening Classes:	No
Part-Time Enrollments:	2	Weekend Classes:	No
Affiliation:	Religious	Distance Learning:	No

NLN ACCREDITATION: Yes

Articulation: None

For Further Information Contact:

Mrs Barbara Stevens, Director
St Mary's Hospital School of Nursing
2900 First Ave
Huntington, WV 25702
(304) 526-1415

Wisconsin

Milwaukee County Medical Complex School
of Nursing
—Milwaukee—

Full-Time Enrollments:	57	**Evening Classes:**	No
Part-Time Enrollments:	—	**Weekend Classes:**	No
Affiliation:	Public	**Distance Learning:**	No

NLN ACCREDITATION: Yes

Articulation: None

For Further Information Contact:

Ms P Loesing Haslbeck, Director
Milwaukee County Medical Complex School of Nursing
1025 N Broadway
Milwaukee, WI 53202-3109
(414) 277-4522

Section 4
Baccalaureate Degree Programs Designed Exclusively for RNs by State

BS PROGRAMS FOR RNs

Alabama

Oakwood College
—Huntsville—

Full-Time Enrollments:	—	Evening Classes:	No
Part-Time Enrollments:	1	Weekend Classes:	No
Affiliation:	Religious	Distance Learning:	No

NLN ACCREDITATION: No

Articulation: Associate to Baccalaureate
LPN to Associate

For Further Information Contact:

Mrs Selena P Simons, Chair
Oakwood College
Oakwood Rd, NW
Huntsville, AL 35896
(205) 726-7287

Arizona

University of Phoenix (19 Campuses-Incl: CO,CA,UT,NM,HI)
—Phoenix—

Full-Time Enrollments:	2100	Evening Classes:	Yes
Part-Time Enrollments:	—	Weekend Classes:	Yes
Affiliation:	Private	Distance Learning:	Yes

NLN ACCREDITATION: Yes

Articulation: Associate to Baccalaureate
Diploma to Baccalaureate
RN to MSN

For Further Information Contact:

Dr Sandra W Pepicello, Exec Director
University of Phoenix (19 Campuses-Incl:
CO,CA,UT,NM,HI)
4615 E Elwood St
Phoenix, AZ 85040
(602) 966-9577

California

California State University at Fullerton
—Fullerton—

Full-Time Enrollments:	29	Evening Classes:	Yes
Part-Time Enrollments:	146	Weekend Classes:	No
Affiliation:	Public	Distance Learning:	Yes

NLN ACCREDITATION: Yes

Articulation: Associate to Baccalaureate

For Further Information Contact:

Dr Judith Ramirez, Acting Head
California State University at Fullerton
Fullerton, CA 92634
(714) 278-2255

California State University-Dominguez Hills
—Carson—

Full-Time Enrollments:	131	Evening Classes:	Yes
Part-Time Enrollments:	1278	Weekend Classes:	Yes
Affiliation:	Public	Distance Learning:	Yes

NLN ACCREDITATION: Yes

Articulation: Associate to Baccalaureate

For Further Information Contact:

Dr Laura Inouye, Acting Director
California State University-Dominguez Hills
1000 E Victoria St
Carson, CA 90747
(310) 243-2002

California State University-Stanislaus
—Turlock—

Full-Time Enrollments:	18	Evening Classes:	Yes
Part-Time Enrollments:	66	Weekend Classes:	—
Affiliation:	Public	Distance Learning:	—

NLN ACCREDITATION: Yes

Articulation: Associate to Baccalaureate

For Further Information Contact:

Dr June Boffman, Chair
California State University-Stanislaus
801 W Monte Vista
Turlock, CA 95380
(209) 667-3141

Holy Names College
—Oakiand—

Full-Time Enrollments:	10	Evening Classes:	Yes
Part-Time Enrollments:	162	Weekend Classes:	Yes
Affiliation:	Religious	Distance Learning:	Yes

NLN ACCREDITATION: Yes

Articulation: Associate to Baccalaureate
Diploma to Baccalaureate

For Further Information Contact:

Dr Arlene Sargent, Chair
Holy Names College
3500 Mountain Blvd
Oakland, CA 94619
(510) 436-1024

National University
—San Diego—

Full-Time Enrollments:	—	Evening Classes:	—
Part-Time Enrollments:	—	Weekend Classes:	—
Affiliation:		Distance Learning:	—

NLN ACCREDITATION: Yes

Articulation: None

For Further Information Contact:

Dr Susan Harris, Chair
National University
4121 Camino Del Rio South
San Diego, CA 92108
(619) 642-8344

Pacific Union College
—Los Angeles—

Full-Time Enrollments:	—	Evening Classes:	—
Part-Time Enrollments:	—	Weekend Classes:	—
Affiliation:	Religious	Distance Learning:	—

NLN ACCREDITATION: Yes

Articulation: None

For Further Information Contact:

Dr Lenoa Jones, Director
Pacific Union College
1720 Cesar Chavez Ave
Los Angeles, CA 90033
(213) 268-5000

Sonoma State University
—Rohnert Park—

Full-Time Enrollments:	33	Evening Classes:	No
Part-Time Enrollments:	39	Weekend Classes:	No
Affiliation:	Public	Distance Learning:	No

NLN ACCREDITATION: Yes

Articulation: Associate to Baccalaureate

For Further Information Contact:

Dr Janice Hitchcock, Acting Chair
Sonoma State University
1801 E Cotati Ave
Rohnert Park, CA 94928
(707) 664-2466

University of San Diego
—San Diego—

Full-Time Enrollments:	—	Evening Classes:	—
Part-Time Enrollments:	—	Weekend Classes:	—
Affiliation:	Religious	Distance Learning:	—

NLN ACCREDITATION: Yes

Articulation: None

For Further Information Contact:

Dr Janet Rodgers, Dean
University of San Diego
Alcala Park
San Diego, CA 92110
(619) 260-4550

Colorado

Metropolitan State College
—Denver—

Full-Time Enrollments:	75	Evening Classes:	Yes
Part-Time Enrollments:	201	Weekend Classes:	Yes
Affiliation:	Public	Distance Learning:	Yes

NLN ACCREDITATION: Yes

Articulation: Associate to Baccalaureate
              Diploma to Baccalaureate

For Further Information Contact:

Dr Joseph Sandoval, Interim Chair
Metropolitan State College
Box 173362
Denver, CO 80217-3362
(303) 556-3136

Connecticut

Central Connecticut State University
—New Britain—

Full-Time Enrollments:	25	Evening Classes:	Yes
Part-Time Enrollments:	335	Weekend Classes:	Yes
Affiliation:	Public	Distance Learning:	Yes

NLN ACCREDITATION: Yes

Articulation: Associate to Baccalaureate

For Further Information Contact:

Dr Judith Hriceniak, Chair
Central Connecticut State University
1615 Stanley St
New Britain, CT 06050
(860) 827-7116

Sacred Heart University
—Fairfield—

Full-Time Enrollments:	4	Evening Classes:	Yes
Part-Time Enrollments:	88	Weekend Classes:	No
Affiliation:	Private	Distance Learning:	No

NLN ACCREDITATION: Yes

Articulation: Associate to Baccalaureate
Diploma to Baccalaureate
RN to MSN

For Further Information Contact:

Dr Anne Barker, Director
Sacred Heart University
5151 Park Ave
Fairfield, CT 06432-1023
(203) 371-7715

University of Hartford
—West Hartford—

Full-Time Enrollments:	—	Evening Classes:	Yes
Part-Time Enrollments:	78	Weekend Classes:	Yes
Affiliation:	Private	Distance Learning:	—

NLN ACCREDITATION: Yes

Articulation: Associate to Baccalaureate
Diploma to Baccalaureate

For Further Information Contact:

Dr Barbara Witt, Chair
University of Hartford
200 Bloomfield Ave
West Hartford, CT 06117
(860) 768-4213

Delaware

University of Delaware
—Newark—

Full-Time Enrollments:	—	Evening Classes:	Yes
Part-Time Enrollments:	195	Weekend Classes:	Yes
Affiliation:	Private	Distance Learning:	Yes

NLN ACCREDITATION: Yes

Articulation: None

For Further Information Contact:

Dr Madeline Lambrecht, Director
University of Delaware
Newark, DE 19716
(302) 831-4444

Wilmington College
—New Castle—

Full-Time Enrollments:	32	Evening Classes:	Yes
Part-Time Enrollments:	164	Weekend Classes:	Yes
Affiliation:	Private	Distance Learning:	No

NLN ACCREDITATION: Yes

Articulation: None

For Further Information Contact:

Dr Betty Caffo, Chair
Wilmington College
New Castle, DE 19720
(302) 328-9401

Florida

Florida Southern College
—Lakeland—

Full-Time Enrollments:	14	Evening Classes:	Yes
Part-Time Enrollments:	183	Weekend Classes:	—
Affiliation:	Religious	Distance Learning:	—

NLN ACCREDITATION: No

Articulation: Associate to Baccalaureate

For Further Information Contact:

Miss Janet Ross, Chair
Florida Southern College
111 Lake Hollingsworth Dr
Lakeland, FL 33801-5698
(941) 680-4306

Lynn University
—Boca Raton—

Full-Time Enrollments:	22	Evening Classes:	Yes
Part-Time Enrollments:	69	Weekend Classes:	Yes
Affiliation:	Private	Distance Learning:	—

NLN ACCREDITATION:

Articulation: None

For Further Information Contact:

Dr Joan Scialli, Director
Lynn University
3601 N Military Trail
Boca Raton, FL 33441-5598
(407) 994-0770

University of Tampa
—Tampa—

Full-Time Enrollments: 13   Evening Classes: Yes
Part-Time Enrollments: 119   Weekend Classes: Yes
Affiliation: Private   Distance Learning: Yes
    NLN ACCREDITATION: Yes

Articulation: Associate to Baccalaureate

For Further Information Contact:

Dr Nancy Ross, Director
University of Tampa
Tampa, FL 33606
(813) 253-6223

University of West Florida
—Pensacola—

Full-Time Enrollments: 2   Evening Classes: Yes
Part-Time Enrollments: 86   Weekend Classes: Yes
Affiliation: Public   Distance Learning: —
    NLN ACCREDITATION: Yes

Articulation: Associate to Baccalaureate

For Further Information Contact:

Dr Marilyn Lamborn, Chair
University of West Florida
Pensacola, FL 32514-5751
(904) 474-3321

Georgia

Clayton State College and State University
—Morrow—

Full-Time Enrollments: —   Evening Classes: —
Part-Time Enrollments: —   Weekend Classes: —
Affiliation: Public   Distance Learning: —
    NLN ACCREDITATION: Yes

Articulation: None

For Further Information Contact:

Dr Linda F Samson, Dean
Clayton State College and State University
School of Hlth Sciences
Morrow, GA 30260
(770) 961-3430

Georgia Southwestern State University
—Americus—

Full-Time Enrollments: 36   Evening Classes: Yes
Part-Time Enrollments: 32   Weekend Classes: No
Affiliation: Public   Distance Learning: No
    NLN ACCREDITATION: Yes

Articulation: Associate to Baccalaureate
Diploma to Baccalaureate

For Further Information Contact:

Dr Martha S Buhler, Chair
Georgia Southwestern State University
Wheatley St
Americus, GA 31709
(912) 928-1270

North Georgia College & State University
—Dahlonega—

Full-Time Enrollments: 23   Evening Classes: Yes
Part-Time Enrollments: 24   Weekend Classes: No
Affiliation: Public   Distance Learning: No
    NLN ACCREDITATION: Yes

Articulation: Associate to Baccalaureate
Diploma to Baccalaureate
LPN to Associate

For Further Information Contact:

Dr Linda Roberts-Betsch, Head
North Georgia College & State University
Dahlonega, GA 30597
(706) 864-1930

State University of West Georgia
—Carrollton—

Full-Time Enrollments: 16   Evening Classes: Yes
Part-Time Enrollments: 81   Weekend Classes: No
Affiliation: Public   Distance Learning: Yes
    NLN ACCREDITATION: Yes

Articulation: Associate to Baccalaureate

For Further Information Contact:

Dr Jeanette C Bernhardt, Chair
State University of West Georgia
Carrollton, GA 30118-4500
(770) 836-6552

Thomas College
—Thomasville—

Full-Time Enrollments:	—	Evening Classes:	Yes
Part-Time Enrollments:	4	Weekend Classes:	—
Affiliation:	Private	Distance Learning:	—

NLN ACCREDITATION: No

Articulation: Associate to Baccalaureate

For Further Information Contact:

Dr Rebecca Stephens, Chair
Thomas College
1501 Millpond Rd
Thomasville, GA 31792-7499
(912) 226-1621

Illinois

Barat College-Chicago Medical School
—North Chicago—

Full-Time Enrollments:	—	Evening Classes:	Yes
Part-Time Enrollments:	42	Weekend Classes:	—
Affiliation:	Private	Distance Learning:	—

NLN ACCREDITATION: Yes

Articulation: Associate to Baccalaureate

For Further Information Contact:

Dr Sandra Salloway, Chair
Barat College-Chicago Medical School
3333 North Green Rd
North Chicago, IL 60064
(847) 578-3324

Benedictine University
—Lisle—

Full-Time Enrollments:	25	Evening Classes:	Yes
Part-Time Enrollments:	29	Weekend Classes:	Yes
Affiliation:	Religious	Distance Learning:	No

NLN ACCREDITATION: Yes

Articulation: Associate to Baccalaureate

For Further Information Contact:

Dr Michele Young, Chair
Benedictine University
5700 College Rd
Lisle, IL 60532
(630) 829-6582

De Paul University
—Chicago—

Full-Time Enrollments:	7	Evening Classes:	Yes
Part-Time Enrollments:	25	Weekend Classes:	Yes
Affiliation:	Religious	Distance Learning:	Yes

NLN ACCREDITATION: Yes

Articulation: Associate to Baccalaureate

For Further Information Contact:

Dr Susan Poslusny, Chair
De Paul University
802 Bolder Ave
Chicago, IL 60614
(773) 325-7281

Franklin University
—Columbus—

Full-Time Enrollments:	7	Evening Classes:	Yes
Part-Time Enrollments:	193	Weekend Classes:	No
Affiliation:	Private	Distance Learning:	Yes

NLN ACCREDITATION: Yes

Articulation: Associate to Baccalaureate

For Further Information Contact:

Dr Louise Gallaway, Chair
Franklin University
201 South Grant
Columbus, OH 43215
(614) 341-6318

Governors State University
—University Park—

Full-Time Enrollments:	50	Evening Classes:	Yes
Part-Time Enrollments:	45	Weekend Classes:	No
Affiliation:	Public	Distance Learning:	Yes

NLN ACCREDITATION: Yes

Articulation: Associate to Baccalaureate
Diploma to Baccalaureate
RN to MSN

For Further Information Contact:

Dr Annic L Lawrence, Chair
Governors State University
Div of Nsg
University Park, IL 60466
(708) 534-5000

McKendree College
—Lebanon—

Full-Time Enrollments:	313	Evening Classes:	Yes
Part-Time Enrollments:	21	Weekend Classes:	Yes
Affiliation:	Private	Distance Learning:	—

NLN ACCREDITATION: Yes

Articulation: Associate to Baccalaureate

For Further Information Contact:

Dr Karen Muench, Chair
McKendree College
701 College Rd
Lebanon, IL 62254
(618) 537-4481

University of Illinois at Springfield
—Springfield—

Full-Time Enrollments:	15	Evening Classes:	Yes
Part-Time Enrollments:	127	Weekend Classes:	No
Affiliation:	Public	Distance Learning:	Yes

NLN ACCREDITATION: Yes

Articulation: None

For Further Information Contact:

Dr Margie Williams, Director
University of Illinois at Springfield
Shepherd Rd
Springfield, IL 62794-9293
(217) 786-7531

Indiana

Indiana University-Purdue University at Fort Wayne
—Fort Wayne—

Full-Time Enrollments:	8	Evening Classes:	Yes
Part-Time Enrollments:	126	Weekend Classes:	Yes
Affiliation:	Public	Distance Learning:	Yes

NLN ACCREDITATION: Yes

Articulation: Associate to Baccalaureate
LPN to Associate

For Further Information Contact:

Dr Elaine W Cowen, Chair
Indiana University-Purdue University at Fort Wayne
2101 Coliseum Blvd E
Fort Wayne, IN 46805
(219) 481-6816

Lutheran College
—Fort Wayne—

Full-Time Enrollments:	3	Evening Classes:	Yes
Part-Time Enrollments:	52	Weekend Classes:	—
Affiliation:	Religious	Distance Learning:	—

NLN ACCREDITATION: Yes

Articulation: None

For Further Information Contact:

Ms Vicky Kirkton, Associate Dean
Lutheran College
3024 Fairfield Ave
Fort Wayne, IN 46807-1695
(219) 458-2475

Purdue University-Calumet Campus
—Hammond—

Full-Time Enrollments:	8	Evening Classes:	Yes
Part-Time Enrollments:	112	Weekend Classes:	No
Affiliation:	Public	Distance Learning:	No

NLN ACCREDITATION: Yes

Articulation: None

For Further Information Contact:

Miss Gail Wegner, Coordinator
Purdue University-Calumet Campus
Hammond, IN 46323
(219) 989-2820

Saint Joseph's College
—Rensselaer—

Full-Time Enrollments:	13	Evening Classes:	Yes
Part-Time Enrollments:	2	Weekend Classes:	No
Affiliation:	Religious	Distance Learning:	—

NLN ACCREDITATION: No

Articulation: Diploma to Baccalaureate

For Further Information Contact:

Mrs Judith A Jezierski, Chair
Saint Joseph's College
PO Box 849
Rensselaer, IN 47978
(219) 866-6202

Iowa

Drake University
—Des Moines—

Full-Time Enrollments:	—	Evening Classes:	Yes
Part-Time Enrollments:	92	Weekend Classes:	Yes
Affiliation:	Private	Distance Learning:	Yes

NLN ACCREDITATION: Yes

Articulation: Associate to Baccalaureate
Diploma to Baccalaureate

For Further Information Contact:

Dr Linda H Brady, Chair
Drake University
452 Olin Hall
Des Moines, IA 50311
(515) 271-2830

Mercy College of Health Science
—Des Moines—

Full-Time Enrollments:	—	Evening Classes:	Yes
Part-Time Enrollments:	40	Weekend Classes:	No
Affiliation:	Private	Distance Learning:	No

NLN ACCREDITATION: 0

Articulation: Associate to Baccalaureate

For Further Information Contact:

Dr Mary Kelly, Director
Mercy College of Health Science
928 6th Ave
Des Moines, IA 50309
(515) 247-3180

University of Dubuque
—Dubuque—

Full-Time Enrollments:	2	Evening Classes:	—
Part-Time Enrollments:	6	Weekend Classes:	—
Affiliation:	Private	Distance Learning:	—

NLN ACCREDITATION: Yes

Articulation: None

For Further Information Contact:

Ms Virginia Cruz, Chair
University of Dubuque
2050 Univ Ave
Dubuque, IA 52001
(319) 589-3504

Kansas

Kansas Newman College
—Wichita—

Full-Time Enrollments:	5	Evening Classes:	Yes
Part-Time Enrollments:	73	Weekend Classes:	No
Affiliation:	Religious	Distance Learning:	Yes

NLN ACCREDITATION: Yes

Articulation: Associate to Baccalaureate
Diploma to Baccalaureate
LPN to Associate

For Further Information Contact:

Dr Joan Felts, Chair
Kansas Newman College
3100 McCormick Ave
Wichita, KS 67213
(316) 942-4291

Kansas Wesleyan University
—Salina—

Full-Time Enrollments:	7	Evening Classes:	Yes
Part-Time Enrollments:	20	Weekend Classes:	No
Affiliation:	Religious	Distance Learning:	No

NLN ACCREDITATION: Yes

Articulation: Associate to Baccalaureate
Diploma to Baccalaureate

For Further Information Contact:

Dr Patricia Kissell, Director
Kansas Wesleyan University
100 Claflin
Salina, KS 67402
(913) 827-5541

Kentucky

Kentucky Wesleyan College
—Owensboro—

Full-Time Enrollments:	4	Evening Classes:	Yes
Part-Time Enrollments:	11	Weekend Classes:	No
Affiliation:	Religious	Distance Learning:	No

NLN ACCREDITATION: No

Articulation: None

For Further Information Contact:

Dr Elizabeth G Johnson, Chair
Kentucky Wesleyan College
3000 Frederick St Box 1039
Owensboro, KY 42302-1039
(502) 926-3111

Midway College
—Midway—

Full-Time Enrollments:	8	Evening Classes:	Yes
Part-Time Enrollments:	40	Weekend Classes:	Yes
Affiliation:	Religious	Distance Learning:	Yes

NLN ACCREDITATION: Yes

Articulation: Associate to Baccalaureate

For Further Information Contact:

Ms Barbara Clark, Chair
Midway College
Midway, KY 40347
(606) 846-5336

Northern Kentucky University
—Highland Heights—

Full-Time Enrollments:	31	Evening Classes:	Yes
Part-Time Enrollments:	51	Weekend Classes:	—
Affiliation:	Public	Distance Learning:	—

NLN ACCREDITATION: Yes

Articulation: Associate to Baccalaureate

For Further Information Contact:

Dr Mary Jeremy Buckman, Chair
Northern Kentucky University
Highland Heights, KY 41076
(606) 572-5248

Louisiana

Loyola University of New Orleans
—New Orleans—

Full-Time Enrollments:	5	Evening Classes:	Yes
Part-Time Enrollments:	279	Weekend Classes:	Yes
Affiliation:	Religious	Distance Learning:	Yes

NLN ACCREDITATION: Yes

Articulation: Associate to Baccalaureate

For Further Information Contact:

Dr Billie Ann Wilson, Chair
Loyola University of New Orleans
6363 St Charles Ave
New Orleans, LA 70118
(504) 865-3142

Maine

University of New England
—Biddeford—

Full-Time Enrollments:	2	Evening Classes:	No
Part-Time Enrollments:	13	Weekend Classes:	No
Affiliation:	Private	Distance Learning:	No

NLN ACCREDITATION: No

Articulation: Associate to Baccalaureate

For Further Information Contact:

Ms Barbara Teague, Chair
University of New England
Eleven Hills Beach Rd
Biddeford, ME 04005
(207) 283-0171

Maryland

Bowie State University
—Bowie—

Full-Time Enrollments:	5	Evening Classes:	Yes
Part-Time Enrollments:	74	Weekend Classes:	No
Affiliation:	Public	Distance Learning:	No

NLN ACCREDITATION: Yes

Articulation: Associate to Baccalaureate
Diploma to Baccalaureate
RN to MSN

For Further Information Contact:

Dr Eleanor Walker, Chair
Bowie State University
Dept of Nursing
Bowie, MD 20715
(301) 464-7273

College of Notre Dame of Maryland
—Baltimore—

Full-Time Enrollments:	—	Evening Classes:	Yes
Part-Time Enrollments:	323	Weekend Classes:	Yes
Affiliation:	Religious	Distance Learning:	No

NLN ACCREDITATION: Yes

Articulation: Associate to Baccalaureate

For Further Information Contact:

Dr Sandra Dunnington, Chair
College of Notre Dame of Maryland
4701 N Charles St
Baltimore, MD 21210
(410) 532-5509

Massachusetts

Anna Maria College
—Paxton—

Full-Time Enrollments:	1	Evening Classes:	Yes
Part-Time Enrollments:	87	Weekend Classes:	Yes
Affiliation:	Religious	Distance Learning:	No

NLN ACCREDITATION: Yes

Articulation: Associate to Baccalaureate
Diploma to Baccalaureate

For Further Information Contact:

Ms Evelyn D Murphy, Chair
Anna Maria College
Paxton, MA 01612
(508) 849-3352

Atlantic Union College
—South Lancaster—

Full-Time Enrollments:	12	Evening Classes:	Yes
Part-Time Enrollments:	149	Weekend Classes:	No
Affiliation:	Religious	Distance Learning:	—

NLN ACCREDITATION: Yes

Articulation: Associate to Baccalaureate

For Further Information Contact:

Mrs Vera B Davis, Chair
Atlantic Union College
South Lancaster, MA 01561
(508) 368-2400

Emmanuel College
—Boston—

Full-Time Enrollments:	—	Evening Classes:	Yes
Part-Time Enrollments:	120	Weekend Classes:	Yes
Affiliation:	Religious	Distance Learning:	Yes

NLN ACCREDITATION: Yes

Articulation: Associate to Baccalaureate
Diploma to Baccalaureate

For Further Information Contact:

Dr Joan Riley, Chair
Emmanuel College
400 The Fenway
Boston, MA 02115
(617) 735-9935

Endicott College
—Beverly—

Full-Time Enrollments:	4	Evening Classes:	Yes
Part-Time Enrollments:	2	Weekend Classes:	No
Affiliation:	Private	Distance Learning:	No

NLN ACCREDITATION: No

Articulation: Associate to Baccalaureate

For Further Information Contact:

Dr Sherry Merrow, Associate Dean
Endicott College
376 Hale St
Beverly, MA 01915
(508) 927-0585

Framingham State College
—Framingham—

Full-Time Enrollments:	8	Evening Classes:	Yes
Part-Time Enrollments:	68	Weekend Classes:	—
Affiliation:	Public	Distance Learning:	—

NLN ACCREDITATION: Yes

Articulation: Associate to Baccalaureate
Diploma to Baccalaureate

For Further Information Contact:

Dr Dolores Rojas-Torti, Chair
Framingham State College
100 State St
Framingham, MA 07101
(508) 626-4715

Massachusetts College of Pharmacy & Allied Health Science
—Boston—

Full-Time Enrollments:	11	Evening Classes:	Yes
Part-Time Enrollments:	40	Weekend Classes:	Yes
Affiliation:	Private	Distance Learning:	No

NLN ACCREDITATION: Yes

Articulation: Associate to Baccalaureate

For Further Information Contact:

Dr Donna Trainor, Director
Massachusetts College of Pharmacy & Allied Health
Science
179 Longwood Ave
Boston, MA 02115
(617) 732-2863

Regis College
—Weston—

Full-Time Enrollments:	8	Evening Classes:	Yes
Part-Time Enrollments:	119	Weekend Classes:	Yes
Affiliation:	Religious	Distance Learning:	—

NLN ACCREDITATION: Yes

Articulation: Associate to Baccalaureate
Diploma to Baccalaureate

For Further Information Contact:

Dr Amy Anderson, Chair
Regis College
235 Wellesley St
Weston, MA 02193
(617) 893-1820

Michigan

Ferris State University
—Big Rapids—

Full-Time Enrollments:	9	Evening Classes:	Yes
Part-Time Enrollments:	233	Weekend Classes:	—
Affiliation:	Public	Distance Learning:	Yes

NLN ACCREDITATION: Yes

Articulation: Associate to Baccalaureate
Diploma to Baccalaureate

For Further Information Contact:

Dr Sally K Johnson, Head
Ferris State University
Birkam Hlth Center Rm 210
Big Rapids, MI 49307-2295
(616) 592-2267

University of Michigan
—Flint—

Full-Time Enrollments:	—	Evening Classes:	Yes
Part-Time Enrollments:	39	Weekend Classes:	No
Affiliation:	Public	Distance Learning:	No

NLN ACCREDITATION: Yes

Articulation: None

For Further Information Contact:

Dr Ellen Woodman, Director
University of Michigan
303 E Kearsley St
Flint, MI 48502-2186
(810) 762-3420

Minnesota

Augsburg College
—Minneapolis—

Full-Time Enrollments:	—	Evening Classes:	Yes
Part-Time Enrollments:	46	Weekend Classes:	Yes
Affiliation:	Religious	Distance Learning:	No

NLN ACCREDITATION: Yes

Articulation: Associate to Baccalaureate

For Further Information Contact:

Dr Beverly Nilsson, Dept Chair
Augsburg College
2211 Riverside Ave S
Minneapolis, MN 55454
(612) 330-1211

Bemidji State University
—Bemidji—

Full-Time Enrollments:	—	Evening Classes:	Yes
Part-Time Enrollments:	70	Weekend Classes:	No
Affiliation:	Public	Distance Learning:	Yes

NLN ACCREDITATION: Yes

Articulation: Associate to Baccalaureate

For Further Information Contact:

Dr Ranae Womack, Chair
Bemidji State University
1500 Birchmont Dr
Bemidji, MN 56601
(218) 755-3860

Metropolitan State University
—St Paul—

Full-Time Enrollments:	25	Evening Classes:	Yes
Part-Time Enrollments:	229	Weekend Classes:	Yes
Affiliation:	Public	Distance Learning:	Yes

NLN ACCREDITATION: Yes

Articulation: Associate to Baccalaureate

For Further Information Contact:

Dr Marilyn Molen, Dean
Metropolitan State University
700 E Seventh St
St Paul, MN 55106-5000
(612) 772-7714

Moorhead State University
—Moorhead—

Full-Time Enrollments:	39	Evening Classes:	Yes
Part-Time Enrollments:	40	Weekend Classes:	Yes
Affiliation:	Public	Distance Learning:	Yes

NLN ACCREDITATION: Yes

Articulation: Associate to Baccalaureate

For Further Information Contact:

Dr Rhoda T Hooper, Director
Moorhead State University
Nursing Dept
Moorhead, MN 56560
(218) 236-4698

Mississippi

Mississippi University for Women-Tupelo
—Tupelo—

Full-Time Enrollments:	30	Evening Classes:	—
Part-Time Enrollments:	—	Weekend Classes:	—
Affiliation:	Public	Distance Learning:	—

NLN ACCREDITATION: Yes

Articulation: None

For Further Information Contact:

Ms Kathy McShane, Coordinator
Mississippi University for Women-Tupelo
655 Eason Blvd
Tupelo, MS 38801
(601) 329-7299

Missouri

Central Methodist College
—Fayette—

Full-Time Enrollments:	20	Evening Classes:	Yes
Part-Time Enrollments:	25	Weekend Classes:	No
Affiliation:	Religious	Distance Learning:	Yes

NLN ACCREDITATION: No

Articulation: Associate to Baccalaureate
Diploma to Baccalaureate

For Further Information Contact:

Dr Shirley J Peterson, Chair
Central Methodist College
Fayette, MO 65248
(816) 248-3391

Drury College
—Springfield—

Full-Time Enrollments:	—	Evening Classes:	—
Part-Time Enrollments:	—	Weekend Classes:	—
Affiliation:	Private	Distance Learning:	—

NLN ACCREDITATION: No

Articulation: None

For Further Information Contact:

Dr Barbara Wing, Nsg Advisor
Drury College
900 N Benton St
Springfield, MO 65802
(417) 865-8731

Hannibal-La Grange College
—Hannibal—

Full-Time Enrollments:	8	Evening Classes:	Yes
Part-Time Enrollments:	22	Weekend Classes:	Yes
Affiliation:	Religious	Distance Learning:	No

NLN ACCREDITATION: No

Articulation: Associate to Baccalaureate
Diploma to Baccalaureate

For Further Information Contact:

Ms Jane Johnson, Interim Director
Hannibal-La Grange College
2800 Palmyra Rd
Hannibal, MO 63401
(314) 221-3675

Jewish Hospital College of Nursing
—St Louis—

Full-Time Enrollments:	30	Evening Classes:	Yes
Part-Time Enrollments:	83	Weekend Classes:	Yes
Affiliation:	Private	Distance Learning:	No

NLN ACCREDITATION: Yes

Articulation: Associate to Baccalaureate

For Further Information Contact:

Dr Sandra Jones, Director
Jewish Hospital College of Nursing
306 S Kings Highway
St Louis, MO 63110
(314) 454-8416

Lincoln University
—Jefferson City—

Full-Time Enrollments:	2	Evening Classes:	Yes
Part-Time Enrollments:	46	Weekend Classes:	No
Affiliation:	Public	Distance Learning:	No

NLN ACCREDITATION: 0

Articulation: None

For Further Information Contact:

Mrs Linda Bickel, Dept Head
Lincoln University
Nsg Science Dept
Jefferson City, MO 65102-0029
(573) 681-5421

Southwest Baptist University
—Springfield—

Full-Time Enrollments:	238	Evening Classes:	Yes
Part-Time Enrollments:	11	Weekend Classes:	No
Affiliation:	Private	Distance Learning:	No

NLN ACCREDITATION: Yes

Articulation: None

For Further Information Contact:

Dr Marilyn Meinert, Chair
Southwest Baptist University
4431 Freemont
Springfield, MO 65804
(417) 841-5049

Southwest Missouri State University
—Springfield—

Full-Time Enrollments:	10	Evening Classes:	Yes
Part-Time Enrollments:	75	Weekend Classes:	No
Affiliation:	Public	Distance Learning:	Yes

NLN ACCREDITATION: Yes

Articulation: None

For Further Information Contact:

Dr Alex Trombetta, Acting Dept Head
Southwest Missouri State University
901 S National
Springfield, MO 65804
(417) 836-5310

University of Missouri-Kansas City
—Kansas City—

Full-Time Enrollments:	4	Evening Classes:	Yes
Part-Time Enrollments:	66	Weekend Classes:	Yes
Affiliation:	Public	Distance Learning:	Yes

NLN ACCREDITATION: Yes

Articulation: Associate to Baccalaureate
RN to MSN

For Further Information Contact:

Dr Nancy Mills, Dean
University of Missouri-Kansas City
5100 Rockville Rd
Kansas City, MO 64110
(816) 235-1740

University of Missouri-St Louis
—St Louis—

Full-Time Enrollments:	16	Evening Classes:	Yes
Part-Time Enrollments:	158	Weekend Classes:	Yes
Affiliation:	Public	Distance Learning:	Yes

NLN ACCREDITATION: Yes

Articulation: Associate to Baccalaureate
Diploma to Baccalaureate

For Further Information Contact:

Dr Shirley A Martin, Dean
University of Missouri-St Louis
8001 Natural Bridge
St Louis, MO 63121
(314) 516-6067

Webster University
—St Louis—

Full-Time Enrollments:	21	Evening Classes:	Yes
Part-Time Enrollments:	354	Weekend Classes:	Yes
Affiliation:	Private	Distance Learning:	No

NLN ACCREDITATION: Yes

Articulation: None

For Further Information Contact:

Dr Janice I Hooper, Chair
Webster University
470 E Lockwood
St Louis, MO 63119
(314) 968-7688

Montana

Montana State University-Northern
—Havre—

Full-Time Enrollments:	14	Evening Classes:	No
Part-Time Enrollments:	12	Weekend Classes:	No
Affiliation:	Public	Distance Learning:	No

NLN ACCREDITATION: Yes

Articulation: Associate to Baccalaureate
LPN to Baccalaureate
LPN to Associate

For Further Information Contact:

Dr Jackie Swanson, Chair
Montana State University-Northern
Havre, MT 59501
(406) 265-4196

Nebraska

College of St Mary
—Omaha—

Full-Time Enrollments:	15	Evening Classes:	Yes
Part-Time Enrollments:	56	Weekend Classes:	Yes
Affiliation:	Private	Distance Learning:	—

NLN ACCREDITATION: Yes

Articulation: Associate to Baccalaureate

For Further Information Contact:

Dr Mary E Partusch, Director
College of St Mary
72nd and Mercy Rd
Omaha, NE 68124
(402) 399-2653

Nebraska Wesleyan University
—Lincoln—

Full-Time Enrollments:	—	Evening Classes:	—
Part-Time Enrollments:	—	Weekend Classes:	—
Affiliation:	Religious	Distance Learning:	—

NLN ACCREDITATION: Yes

Articulation: None

For Further Information Contact:

Dr Patricia J Morin, Chair
Nebraska Wesleyan University
5000 Saint Paul
Lincoln, NE 68504
(402) 465-2333

New Hampshire

Rivier College/St Joseph Hospital
—Nashua—

Full-Time Enrollments:	14	Evening Classes:	Yes
Part-Time Enrollments:	177	Weekend Classes:	Yes
Affiliation:	Religious	Distance Learning:	No

NLN ACCREDITATION: Yes

Articulation: LPN to Associate

For Further Information Contact:

Dr Judith Haywood, Dean
Rivier College/St Joseph Hospital
420 S Main St
Nashua, NH 03063
(603) 888-1311

New Jersey

College of St Elizabeth
—Morristown—

Full-Time Enrollments:	2	Evening Classes:	Yes
Part-Time Enrollments:	150	Weekend Classes:	Yes
Affiliation:	Religious	Distance Learning:	No

NLN ACCREDITATION: Yes

Articulation: Associate to Baccalaureate
Diploma to Baccalaureate

For Further Information Contact:

Sr Janet Lehmann, Chair
College of St Elizabeth
2 Convent Rd
Morristown, NJ 07960
(201) 292-6330

Felician College
—Lodi—

Full-Time Enrollments:	4	Evening Classes:	Yes
Part-Time Enrollments:	64	Weekend Classes:	Yes
Affiliation:	Religious	Distance Learning:	No

NLN ACCREDITATION: Yes

Articulation: LPN to Associate
RN to MSN

For Further Information Contact:

Dr Rona F Levin, Director
Felician College
South Main St
Lodi, NJ 07644
(201) 778-1190

Jersey City State College
—Jersey City—

Full-Time Enrollments:	24	Evening Classes:	Yes
Part-Time Enrollments:	277	Weekend Classes:	Yes
Affiliation:	Public	Distance Learning:	Yes

NLN ACCREDITATION: Yes

Articulation: Diploma to Baccalaureate

For Further Information Contact:

Dr Eileen Gardner, Chair
Jersey City State College
2039 Kennedy Blvd
Jersey City, NJ 07305
(201) 200-3157

Kean College of New Jersey
—Union—

Full-Time Enrollments:	10	Evening Classes:	Yes
Part-Time Enrollments:	260	Weekend Classes:	No
Affiliation:	Public	Distance Learning:	No

NLN ACCREDITATION: Yes

Articulation: Associate to Baccalaureate
Diploma to Baccalaureate

For Further Information Contact:

Dr Virginia Fitzsimons, Chair
Kean College of New Jersey
Morris Ave
Union, NJ 07083
(908) 527-2608

Monmouth University
—West Long Branch—

Full-Time Enrollments:	4	Evening Classes:	Yes
Part-Time Enrollments:	138	Weekend Classes:	No
Affiliation:	Private	Distance Learning:	No

NLN ACCREDITATION: Yes

Articulation: Associate to Baccalaureate
Diploma to Baccalaureate

For Further Information Contact:

Dr Emily Tompkins, Chair
Monmouth University
West Long Branch, NJ 07764
(908) 571-3443

Ramapo College/University of Medicine & Dentistry
—Mahwah—

Full-Time Enrollments:	—	Evening Classes:	Yes
Part-Time Enrollments:	290	Weekend Classes:	No
Affiliation:	Public	Distance Learning:	Yes

NLN ACCREDITATION: Yes

Articulation: Associate to Baccalaureate
Diploma to Baccalaureate
RN to MSN

For Further Information Contact:

Dr Kathleen Burke, Coordinator
Ramapo College/University of Medicine & Dentistry
505 Ramapo Valley Rd
Mahwah, NJ 07430-1680
(201) 529-7749

Richard Stockton State College
—Pomona—

Full-Time Enrollments:	21	Evening Classes:	Yes
Part-Time Enrollments:	84	Weekend Classes:	No
Affiliation:	Public	Distance Learning:	No

NLN ACCREDITATION: Yes

Articulation: Associate to Baccalaureate
Diploma to Associate

For Further Information Contact:

Dr Linda Aaronson, Coordinator
Richard Stockton State College
Jim Leeds Rd
Pomona, NJ 08240
(609) 652-4250

Saint Peter's College
—Jersey City—

Full-Time Enrollments:	11	Evening Classes:	Yes
Part-Time Enrollments:	192	Weekend Classes:	Yes
Affiliation:	Religious	Distance Learning:	No

NLN ACCREDITATION: Yes

Articulation: Associate to Baccalaureate
Diploma to Baccalaureate

For Further Information Contact:

Dr Doris L Collins, Chair
Saint Peter's College
Jersey City, NJ 07306
(201) 915-9412

Thomas Edison State College
—Trenton—

Full-Time Enrollments:	—	Evening Classes:	—
Part-Time Enrollments:	259	Weekend Classes:	Yes
Affiliation:	Public	Distance Learning:	—

NLN ACCREDITATION: Yes

Articulation: Associate to Baccalaureate

For Further Information Contact:

Dr Dolores Brown Hall, Associate Dean
Thomas Edison State College
101 W State St
Trenton, NJ 08625-1176
(609) 633-6460

New Mexico

Eastern New Mexico University
—Portales—

Full-Time Enrollments:	12	Evening Classes:	Yes
Part-Time Enrollments:	70	Weekend Classes:	Yes
Affiliation:	Public	Distance Learning:	Yes

NLN ACCREDITATION: Yes

Articulation: None

For Further Information Contact:

Dr Ginny Guido, Chair
Eastern New Mexico University
Station #12
Portales, NM 88130
(505) 562-2403

New York

Adelphi University School of Nursing
—Garden City—

Full-Time Enrollments:	7	Evening Classes:	Yes
Part-Time Enrollments:	89	Weekend Classes:	No
Affiliation:	Private	Distance Learning:	No

NLN ACCREDITATION: Yes

Articulation: None

For Further Information Contact:

Dr Caryle Wolahan, Dean
Adelphi University School of Nursing
Box 516
Garden City, NY 11530
(516) 877-4524

College of Staten Island
—Staten Island—

Full-Time Enrollments:	25	Evening Classes:	Yes
Part-Time Enrollments:	202	Weekend Classes:	Yes
Affiliation:	Public	Distance Learning:	—

NLN ACCREDITATION: Yes

Articulation: Associate to Baccalaureate
Diploma to Baccalaureate

For Further Information Contact:

Dr Louise M Malarkey, Chair
College of Staten Island
2800 Victory Blvd
Staten Island, NY 10314
(718) 390-7516

Daemen College
—Amherst—

Full-Time Enrollments:	43	Evening Classes:	Yes
Part-Time Enrollments:	333	Weekend Classes:	Yes
Affiliation:	Private	Distance Learning:	Yes

NLN ACCREDITATION: Yes

Articulation: Associate to Baccalaureate
Diploma to Baccalaureate

For Further Information Contact:

Dr Mary Lou Rusin, Chair
Daemen College
4380 Main St
Amherst, NY 14226
(716) 839-3600

Long Island University C W Post Campus
—Brookville—

Full-Time Enrollments:	—	Evening Classes:	Yes
Part-Time Enrollments:	178	Weekend Classes:	Yes
Affiliation:	Private	Distance Learning:	No

NLN ACCREDITATION: Yes

Articulation: Associate to Baccalaureate

For Further Information Contact:

Dr Theodora Grauer, Chair
Long Island University C W Post Campus
Brookville, NY 11548
(516) 299-2320

Medgar Evers College of CUNY
—Brooklyn—

Full-Time Enrollments:	2	Evening Classes:	Yes
Part-Time Enrollments:	101	Weekend Classes:	No
Affiliation:	Public	Distance Learning:	—

NLN ACCREDITATION: Yes

Articulation: Associate to Baccalaureate
Diploma to Baccalaureate
LPN to Associate

For Further Information Contact:

Dr Bertie M Gilmore, Director
Medgar Evers College of CUNY
1150 Carroll St
Brooklyn, NY 11225
(718) 270-6441

Mercy College
—Dobbs Ferry—

Full-Time Enrollments:	20	Evening Classes:	—
Part-Time Enrollments:	150	Weekend Classes:	—
Affiliation:	Private	Distance Learning:	—

NLN ACCREDITATION: Yes

Articulation: None

For Further Information Contact:

Dr J Mae Pepper, Chair
Mercy College
555 Broadway
Dobbs Ferry, NY 10522
(914) 674-9331

Nazareth College
—Rochester—

Full-Time Enrollments:	2	Evening Classes:	Yes
Part-Time Enrollments:	181	Weekend Classes:	No
Affiliation:	Private	Distance Learning:	Yes

NLN ACCREDITATION: Yes

Articulation: Associate to Baccalaureate

For Further Information Contact:

Dr Margaret M Andrews, Chair
Nazareth College
4245 East Ave
Rochester, NY 14618
(716) 586-2525

Pace University
—New York—

Full-Time Enrollments:	18	Evening Classes:	Yes
Part-Time Enrollments:	177	Weekend Classes:	No
Affiliation:	Private	Distance Learning:	No

NLN ACCREDITATION: Yes

Articulation: Associate to Baccalaureate
RN to MSN

For Further Information Contact:

Dr Susan Gordon, Chair
Pace University
41 Park Row
New York, NY 10038
(212) 346-1716

Pace University
—Pleasantville—

Full-Time Enrollments:	9	Evening Classes:	Yes
Part-Time Enrollments:	57	Weekend Classes:	No
Affiliation:	Private	Distance Learning:	No

NLN ACCREDITATION: Yes

Articulation: Associate to Baccalaureate

For Further Information Contact:

Dr Susan Gordon, Chair
Pace University
861 Bedford Rd Rm L3-14
Pleasantville, NY 10570
(914) 773-3373

SUNY College at New Paltz
—New Paltz—

Full-Time Enrollments:	9	Evening Classes:	Yes
Part-Time Enrollments:	187	Weekend Classes:	Yes
Affiliation:	Public	Distance Learning:	Yes

NLN ACCREDITATION: Yes

Articulation: Associate to Baccalaureate

For Further Information Contact:

Dr Ide Katims, Director
SUNY College at New Paltz
Dept of Nsg VLC 205
New Paltz, NY 12561
(914) 257-2922

SUNY Hlth Science Center at Syracuse
—Syracuse—

Full-Time Enrollments:	26	Evening Classes:	Yes
Part-Time Enrollments:	128	Weekend Classes:	No
Affiliation:	Public	Distance Learning:	No

NLN ACCREDITATION: Yes

Articulation: Associate to Baccalaureate
Diploma to Baccalaureate
RN to MSN

For Further Information Contact:

Dr M Janice Nelson, Dean
SUNY Hlth Science Center at Syracuse
750 East Adams St
Syracuse, NY 13210
(315) 464-4276

SUNY Institute of Technology
—Utica—

Full-Time Enrollments:	93	Evening Classes:	Yes
Part-Time Enrollments:	305	Weekend Classes:	Yes
Affiliation:	Public	Distance Learning:	No

NLN ACCREDITATION: Yes

Articulation: Associate to Baccalaureate
Diploma to Baccalaureate

For Further Information Contact:

Dr Elizabeth Kellogg Walker, Dean
SUNY Institute of Technology
PO Box 3050 Marcy Campus
Utica, NY 13504-3050
(315) 792-7295

Saint Joseph's College (2 Campuses)
—Brooklyn—

Full-Time Enrollments:	43	Evening Classes:	Yes
Part-Time Enrollments:	276	Weekend Classes:	Yes
Affiliation:	Private	Distance Learning:	—

NLN ACCREDITATION: Yes

Articulation: None

For Further Information Contact:

Dr Audrey Conley, Director
Saint Joseph's College (2 Campuses)
245 Clinton Ave
Brooklyn, NY 11205
(718) 622-4690

York College
—Jamaica—

Full-Time Enrollments:	4	Evening Classes:	Yes
Part-Time Enrollments:	43	Weekend Classes:	Yes
Affiliation:	Public	Distance Learning:	—

NLN ACCREDITATION: Yes

Articulation: Associate to Baccalaureate

For Further Information Contact:

Dr Pearl Bailey, Director
York College
Science Bldg Rm 110
Jamaica, NY 11451
(718) 262-2054

North Carolina

Gardner-Webb University
—Boiling Springs—

Full-Time Enrollments:	44	Evening Classes:	Yes
Part-Time Enrollments:	168	Weekend Classes:	—
Affiliation:	Religious	Distance Learning:	Yes

NLN ACCREDITATION: Yes

Articulation: Associate to Baccalaureate

For Further Information Contact:

Dr Shirley P Toney, Dean
Gardner-Webb University
PO Box 268
Boiling Springs, NC 28017
(704) 434-4366

Pembroke State University
—Pembroke—

Full-Time Enrollments:	—	Evening Classes:	Yes
Part-Time Enrollments:	64	Weekend Classes:	No
Affiliation:	Public	Distance Learning:	Yes

NLN ACCREDITATION: No

Articulation: None

For Further Information Contact:

Dr Margaret Opitz, Director
Pembroke State University
Pembroke, NC 28372-1512
(910) 521-6526

North Dakota

Dickinson State University
—Dickinson—

Full-Time Enrollments:	32	Evening Classes:	Yes
Part-Time Enrollments:	26	Weekend Classes:	No
Affiliation:	Public	Distance Learning:	No

NLN ACCREDITATION: Yes

Articulation: Associate to Baccalaureate
Diploma to Baccalaureate
LPN to Associate

For Further Information Contact:

Dr Sandra Affeldt, Chair
Dickinson State University
Dickinson, ND 58601
(701) 227-2172

Ohio

Ashland University
—Ashland—

Full-Time Enrollments:	2	Evening Classes:	Yes
Part-Time Enrollments:	79	Weekend Classes:	Yes
Affiliation:	Religious	Distance Learning:	—

NLN ACCREDITATION: Yes

Articulation: Associate to Baccalaureate
Diploma to Baccalaureate

For Further Information Contact:

Dr Ella Kick, Chair
Ashland University
Dept of Nursing
Ashland, OH 44805
(419) 289-5242

Case Western Reserve University/F P Bolton
—Cleveland—

Full-Time Enrollments:	3	Evening Classes:	Yes
Part-Time Enrollments:	16	Weekend Classes:	—
Affiliation:		Distance Learning:	Yes

NLN ACCREDITATION: Yes

Articulation: None

For Further Information Contact:

Dr Joyce Fitzpatrick, Dean
Case Western Reserve University/F P Bolton
10900 Euclid Ave
Cleveland, OH 44106-4904
(216) 368-2545

Franklin University
—Columbus—

Full-Time Enrollments:	7	Evening Classes:	—
Part-Time Enrollments:	193	Weekend Classes:	—
Affiliation:		Distance Learning:	—

NLN ACCREDITATION: Yes

Articulation: None

For Further Information Contact:

Dr Lousie Gallaway, Chair
Franklin University
201 S Grant Ave
Columbus, OH 43215
(614) 341-6318

Miami University
—Oxford—

Full-Time Enrollments:	25	Evening Classes:	Yes
Part-Time Enrollments:	78	Weekend Classes:	No
Affiliation:	Public	Distance Learning:	Yes

NLN ACCREDITATION: Yes

Articulation: None

For Further Information Contact:

Dr Eugenia Mills, Chair
Miami University
221 Kreger Hall
Oxford, OH 45056
(513) 863-8833

Ohio University
—Athens—

Full-Time Enrollments:	—	Evening Classes:	—
Part-Time Enrollments:	—	Weekend Classes:	—
Affiliation:	Public	Distance Learning:	—

NLN ACCREDITATION: Yes

Articulation: None

For Further Information Contact:

Dr K Rose-Grippa, Director
Ohio University
312 McCracken Hall
Athens, OH 45701
(614) 593-4494

Walsh University College Nursing Program
—North Canton—

Full-Time Enrollments:	2	Evening Classes:	Yes
Part-Time Enrollments:	22	Weekend Classes:	No
Affiliation:	Religious	Distance Learning:	No

NLN ACCREDITATION: Yes

Articulation: Associate to Baccalaureate

For Further Information Contact:

Dr Joyce Soehnlen, Interim Chair
Walsh University College Nursing Program
2020 Easton St NW
North Canton, OH 44720
(330) 499-7090

Xavier University
—Cincinnati—

Full-Time Enrollments:	34	Evening Classes:	Yes
Part-Time Enrollments:	55	Weekend Classes:	No
Affiliation:	Religious	Distance Learning:	No

NLN ACCREDITATION: Yes

Articulation: None

For Further Information Contact:

Dr Evelyn Lutz, Interim Chair
Xavier University
3800 Victory Parkway
Cincinnati, OH 45207-1092
(513) 745-3815

Oklahoma

Northeastern State University
—Tahlequah—

Full-Time Enrollments:	2	Evening Classes:	Yes
Part-Time Enrollments:	22	Weekend Classes:	No
Affiliation:	Public	Distance Learning:	No

NLN ACCREDITATION: Yes

Articulation: Associate to Baccalaureate

For Further Information Contact:

Dr Joyce Van Nostrand, Head
Northeastern State University
Dept of Nursing
Tahlequah, OK 74464
(918) 456-5511

Pennsylvania

Allegheny University of the Health Sciences
—Philadelphia—

Full-Time Enrollments:	81	Evening Classes:	Yes
Part-Time Enrollments:	239	Weekend Classes:	Yes
Affiliation:	Private	Distance Learning:	No

NLN ACCREDITATION: Yes

Articulation: Associate to Baccalaureate
Diploma to Baccalaureate

For Further Information Contact:

Dr Gloria Donnelly, Dean
Allegheny University of the Health Sciences
MS 501 Broad & Vine
Philadelphia, PA 19102
(215) 762-7149

Alvernia College
—Reading—

Full-Time Enrollments:	4	Evening Classes:	Yes
Part-Time Enrollments:	42	Weekend Classes:	No
Affiliation:	Religious	Distance Learning:	No

NLN ACCREDITATION: No

Articulation: None

For Further Information Contact:

Dr Deborah Castellucci, Chair
Alvernia College
400 St Bernardine St
Reading, PA 19607
(610) 796-8256

California University of Pennsylvania
—California—

Full-Time Enrollments:	10	Evening Classes:	Yes
Part-Time Enrollments:	46	Weekend Classes:	Yes
Affiliation:	Public	Distance Learning:	No

NLN ACCREDITATION: Yes

Articulation: Associate to Baccalaureate
Diploma to Baccalaureate

For Further Information Contact:

Dr Margaret A Marcinek, Chair
California University of Pennsylvania
California, PA 15419
(412) 938-5739

Clarion University of Pennsylvania
—Oil City—

Full-Time Enrollments:	25	Evening Classes:	Yes
Part-Time Enrollments:	131	Weekend Classes:	No
Affiliation:	Public	Distance Learning:	Yes

NLN ACCREDITATION: Yes

Articulation: Associate to Baccalaureate
Diploma to Baccalaureate

For Further Information Contact:

Dr T Audean Duespohl, Dean
Clarion University of Pennsylvania
1801 W First St
Oil City, PA 16301
(814) 677-6107

Eastern College
—St Davids—

Full-Time Enrollments:	3	Evening Classes:	Yes
Part-Time Enrollments:	136	Weekend Classes:	Yes
Affiliation:	Religious	Distance Learning:	No

NLN ACCREDITATION: Yes

Articulation: Associate to Baccalaureate
Diploma to Baccalaureate

For Further Information Contact:

Dr Sara Wuthnow, Chair
Eastern College
Fairview Dr
St Davids, PA 19087
(610) 341-5896

Gwynedd Mercy College
—Gwynedd Valley—

Full-Time Enrollments:	20	Evening Classes:	—
Part-Time Enrollments:	170	Weekend Classes:	—
Affiliation:	Religious	Distance Learning:	—

NLN ACCREDITATION: Yes

Articulation: None

For Further Information Contact:

Dr Mary Dressler, Dean
Gwynedd Mercy College
Sumneytown Pike
Gwynedd Valley, PA 19437
(215) 641-5501

Immaculata College
—Immaculata—

Full-Time Enrollments:	5	Evening Classes:	Yes
Part-Time Enrollments:	96	Weekend Classes:	Yes
Affiliation:	Religious	Distance Learning:	No

NLN ACCREDITATION: Yes

Articulation: Associate to Baccalaureate
Diploma to Baccalaureate

For Further Information Contact:

Dr Elizabeth F Wagoner, Chair
Immaculata College
Immaculata, PA 19345
(610) 647-4400

Kutztown University
—Kutztown—

Full-Time Enrollments:	12	Evening Classes:	Yes
Part-Time Enrollments:	190	Weekend Classes:	No
Affiliation:	Public	Distance Learning:	No

NLN ACCREDITATION: Yes

Articulation: Diploma to Baccalaureate

For Further Information Contact:

Mrs Vera Brancato, Chair
Kutztown University
Kutztown, PA 19530
(610) 683-4330

La Roche College
—Pittsburgh—

Full-Time Enrollments:	7	Evening Classes:	—
Part-Time Enrollments:	147	Weekend Classes:	—
Affiliation:	Private	Distance Learning:	—

NLN ACCREDITATION: Yes

Articulation: None

For Further Information Contact:

Dr Kathleen Sullivan, Chair
La Roche College
9000 Babcock Blvd
Pittsburgh, PA 15237
(412) 367-9300

La Salle University
—Philadelphia—

Full-Time Enrollments:	2	Evening Classes:	Yes
Part-Time Enrollments:	285	Weekend Classes:	Yes
Affiliation:	Private	Distance Learning:	No

NLN ACCREDITATION: Yes

Articulation: Associate to Baccalaureate
Diploma to Baccalaureate

For Further Information Contact:

Dr Cynthia Capers, Interim Dean
La Salle University
20th & Olney Ave
Philadelphia, PA 19141
(215) 951-1430

Millersville University
—Millersville—

Full-Time Enrollments:	26	Evening Classes:	Yes
Part-Time Enrollments:	135	Weekend Classes:	Yes
Affiliation:	Public	Distance Learning:	No

NLN ACCREDITATION: Yes

Articulation: Associate to Baccalaureate
Diploma to Baccalaureate

For Further Information Contact:

Dr Carol Y Phillips, Chair
Millersville University
Millersville, PA 17551
(717) 872-3416

Slippery Rock University
—Slippery Rock—

Full-Time Enrollments:	17	Evening Classes:	Yes
Part-Time Enrollments:	117	Weekend Classes:	No
Affiliation:	Public	Distance Learning:	No

NLN ACCREDITATION: Yes

Articulation: Associate to Baccalaureate
Diploma to Baccalaureate

For Further Information Contact:

Mrs Ruth Leo, Chair
Slippery Rock University
Behavioral Science Bldg 119
Slippery Rock, PA 16057
(412) 738-2324

University of Pittsburgh
—Bradford—

Full-Time Enrollments:	2	Evening Classes:	Yes
Part-Time Enrollments:	23	Weekend Classes:	No
Affiliation:	Public	Distance Learning:	No

NLN ACCREDITATION: Yes

Articulation: Associate to Baccalaureate
Diploma to Baccalaureate
LPN to Associate

For Further Information Contact:

Ms Lisa Fiorentino, Director
University of Pittsburgh
300 Campus Dr
Bradford, PA 16701
(814) 362-7640

Widener University
—Chester—

Full-Time Enrollments:	—	Evening Classes:	Yes
Part-Time Enrollments:	139	Weekend Classes:	Yes
Affiliation:	Private	Distance Learning:	Yes

NLN ACCREDITATION: Yes

Articulation: None

For Further Information Contact:

Dr Marguerite Barbiere, Dean
Widener University
One University Place
Chester, PA 19013-5792
(610) 499-4213

South Carolina

University of South Carolina
—Aiken—

Full-Time Enrollments:	19	Evening Classes:	Yes
Part-Time Enrollments:	88	Weekend Classes:	No
Affiliation:	Public	Distance Learning:	No

NLN ACCREDITATION: Yes

Articulation: Associate to Baccalaureate
LPN to Associate

For Further Information Contact:

Dr Trudy Groves, Head
University of South Carolina
171 Univ Parkway
Aiken, SC 29801
(803) 648-6851

South Dakota

Presentation College
—Aberdeen—

Full-Time Enrollments:	9	Evening Classes:	—
Part-Time Enrollments:	12	Weekend Classes:	—
Affiliation:	Religious	Distance Learning:	No

NLN ACCREDITATION: Yes

Articulation: Associate to Baccalaureate
Diploma to Baccalaureate

For Further Information Contact:

Mr Thomas Stenvig, Chair
Presentation College
1500 North Main St
Aberdeen, SD 57401
(605) 229-8472

Tennessee

Aguinas College
—Nashville—

Full-Time Enrollments:	—	Evening Classes:	—
Part-Time Enrollments:	—	Weekend Classes:	—
Affiliation:	Religious	Distance Learning:	—

NLN ACCREDITATION: No

Articulation: None

For Further Information Contact:

Mrs Peggy Daniel, Director
Aguinas College
4210 Harding Rd
Nashville, TN 37205
(615) 297-2008

Lincoln Memorial University
—Harrogate—

Full-Time Enrollments:	2	Evening Classes:	Yes
Part-Time Enrollments:	22	Weekend Classes:	No
Affiliation:	Private	Distance Learning:	No

NLN ACCREDITATION: Yes

Articulation: Associate to Baccalaureate

For Further Information Contact:

Dr Elisa Barr, Coordinator
Lincoln Memorial University
Div of Nursing
Harrogate, TN 37752
(423) 869-3611

Southern College of Seventh-Day Adventists
—Collegedale—

Full-Time Enrollments:	20	Evening Classes:	Yes
Part-Time Enrollments:	124	Weekend Classes:	No
Affiliation:	Religious	Distance Learning:	Yes

NLN ACCREDITATION: Yes

Articulation: Associate to Baccalaureate
Diploma to Baccalaureate

For Further Information Contact:

Mrs Katie A Lamb, Chair
Southern College of Seventh-Day Adventists
Collegedale, TN 37315
(423) 238-2942

Texas

Abilene Inter Collegiate School
—Abeline—

Full-Time Enrollments:	2	Evening Classes:	No
Part-Time Enrollments:	—	Weekend Classes:	No
Affiliation:	Religious	Distance Learning:	No

NLN ACCREDITATION: Yes

Articulation: Associate to Baccalaureate
Diploma to Baccalaureate

For Further Information Contact:

Dr Corine Bonnet, Dean
Abilene Inter Collegiate School
2149 Hickory
Abeline, TX 79601
(915) 672-2441

Angelo State University
—San Angelo—

Full-Time Enrollments:	10	Evening Classes:	Yes
Part-Time Enrollments:	56	Weekend Classes:	No
Affiliation:	Public	Distance Learning:	No

NLN ACCREDITATION: Yes

Articulation: Associate to Baccalaureate
Diploma to Baccalaureate
LPN to Associate

For Further Information Contact:

Dr Leslie Mayrand, Head
Angelo State University
PO Box 10902 ASU
San Angelo, TX 76909
(915) 942-2224

Lubbock Christian College
—Lubbock—

Full-Time Enrollments:	12	Evening Classes:	Yes
Part-Time Enrollments:	—	Weekend Classes:	—
Affiliation:	Religious	Distance Learning:	—

NLN ACCREDITATION: Yes

Articulation: None

For Further Information Contact:

Ms Beverly Byers, Interim Director
Lubbock Christian College
5601 19th St
Lubbock, TX 79407
(806) 796-8800

Southwestern Adventist University
—Keene—

Full-Time Enrollments:	13	Evening Classes:	No
Part-Time Enrollments:	6	Weekend Classes:	No
Affiliation:	Religious	Distance Learning:	No

NLN ACCREDITATION: Yes

Articulation: Associate to Baccalaureate
LPN to Associate

For Further Information Contact:

Dr Catherine Turner, Chair
Southwestern Adventist University
PO Box 58
Keene, TX 76059
(817) 645-3921

Texas A&M International University
—Loredo—

Full-Time Enrollments:	16	Evening Classes:	—
Part-Time Enrollments:	29	Weekend Classes:	—
Affiliation:	Private	Distance Learning:	—

NLN ACCREDITATION:

Articulation: None

For Further Information Contact:

Dr Susan S Baker, Interim Director
Texas A&M International University
5201 University Blvd
Loredo, TX 78041
(210) 326-2450

The University of Texas
—Brownsville—

Full-Time Enrollments:	16	Evening Classes:	Yes
Part-Time Enrollments:	10	Weekend Classes:	—
Affiliation:	Public	Distance Learning:	—

NLN ACCREDITATION:

Articulation: Associate to Baccalaureate

For Further Information Contact:

Dr Katherine Dougherty, Director
The University of Texas
80 Fort Brown
Brownsville, TX 78520
(210) 544-8270

Utah

Weber State University
—Ogden—

Full-Time Enrollments:	195	Evening Classes:	Yes
Part-Time Enrollments:	14	Weekend Classes:	No
Affiliation:	Public	Distance Learning:	Yes

NLN ACCREDITATION: Yes

Articulation: Associate to Baccalaureate
LPN to Baccalaureate
LPN to Associate

For Further Information Contact:

Dr Gerry Hansen, Director
Weber State University
3750 Harrison Blvd, 1602
Ogden, UT 84408-3912
(801) 626-6122

Vermont

Norwich University
—Northfield—

Full-Time Enrollments:	22	Evening Classes:	—
Part-Time Enrollments:	88	Weekend Classes:	—
Affiliation:	Private	Distance Learning:	—

NLN ACCREDITATION: Yes

Articulation: None

For Further Information Contact:

Dr Linda Ellis, Director
Norwich University
Div of Nursing
Northfield, VT 05663
(802) 485-2600

Southern Vermont College
—Bennington—

Full-Time Enrollments:	—	Evening Classes:	Yes
Part-Time Enrollments:	32	Weekend Classes:	No
Affiliation:	Private	Distance Learning:	Yes

NLN ACCREDITATION: No

Articulation: Associate to Baccalaureate

For Further Information Contact:

Ms Wendy LaFage, Director
Southern Vermont College
Bennington, VT 05201
(802) 447-8681

Virginia

CHRV College of Health Sciences
—Roanoke—

Full-Time Enrollments:	43	Evening Classes:	Yes
Part-Time Enrollments:	12	Weekend Classes:	No
Affiliation:	Private	Distance Learning:	No

NLN ACCREDITATION: No

Articulation: Associate to Baccalaureate
LPN to Associate

For Further Information Contact:

Dr Rebecca Clark, Director
CHRV College of Health Sciences
PO Box 13186
Roanoke, VA 24031
(540) 985-8208

Clinch Valley College
—Wise—

Full-Time Enrollments:	9	Evening Classes:	Yes
Part-Time Enrollments:	49	Weekend Classes:	No
Affiliation:	Public	Distance Learning:	No

NLN ACCREDITATION: Yes

Articulation: Associate to Baccalaureate

For Further Information Contact:

Dr Betty Johnson, Chair
Clinch Valley College
One College Ave
Wise, VA 24293
(540) 328-0275

Marymount University School of Nursing
—Arlington—

Full-Time Enrollments:	17	Evening Classes:	Yes
Part-Time Enrollments:	7	Weekend Classes:	No
Affiliation:	Religious	Distance Learning:	No

NLN ACCREDITATION: Yes

Articulation: Associate to Baccalaureate
LPN to Associate

For Further Information Contact:

Dr Shirley Jarecki, Acting Dean
Marymount University School of Nursing
2807 North Glebe Rd
Arlington, VA 22207
(703) 284-1581

Norfolk State University
—Norfolk—

Full-Time Enrollments:	529	Evening Classes:	—
Part-Time Enrollments:	87	Weekend Classes:	—
Affiliation:	Public	Distance Learning:	—

NLN ACCREDITATION: Yes

Articulation: None

For Further Information Contact:

Ms Candace Rogers, Acting Dept Head
Norfolk State University
2401 Corprew Ave
Norfolk, VA 23504
(804) 683-9014

Shenandoah College
—Winchester—

Full-Time Enrollments:	24	Evening Classes:	Yes
Part-Time Enrollments:	37	Weekend Classes:	Yes
Affiliation:	Religious	Distance Learning:	Yes

NLN ACCREDITATION: Yes

Articulation: Associate to Baccalaureate
Diploma to Baccalaureate
LPN to Associate

For Further Information Contact:

Dr Pamela Webber, Chair
Shenandoah College
203 S Cameron St
Winchester, VA 22601
(540) 665-0960

BS PROGRAMS FOR RNs

Washington

Gonzaga University
—Spokane—

Full-Time Enrollments:	—	Evening Classes:	—
Part-Time Enrollments:	—	Weekend Classes:	—
Affiliation:	Religious	Distance Learning:	—

NLN ACCREDITATION: Yes

Articulation: None

For Further Information Contact:

Dr Gail Ray, Chair
Gonzaga University
502 East Boone
Spokane, WA 99258
(509) 328-4220

St Martin College
—Olympia—

Full-Time Enrollments:	4	Evening Classes:	Yes
Part-Time Enrollments:	32	Weekend Classes:	Yes
Affiliation:	Religious	Distance Learning:	No

NLN ACCREDITATION: Yes

Articulation: Associate to Baccalaureate

For Further Information Contact:

Dr Marilyn L de Give, Chair
St Martin College
Olympia, WA 98503
(206) 438-4330

West Virginia

Bluefield State College
—Bluefield—

Full-Time Enrollments:	54	Evening Classes:	Yes
Part-Time Enrollments:	—	Weekend Classes:	—
Affiliation:	Public	Distance Learning:	Yes

NLN ACCREDITATION: Yes

Articulation: Associate to Baccalaureate

For Further Information Contact:

Ms Beth Pritchett, Director
Bluefield State College
219 Rock St
Bluefield, WV 24701
(304) 327-4139

Fairmont State College
—Fairmont—

Full-Time Enrollments:	6	Evening Classes:	Yes
Part-Time Enrollments:	69	Weekend Classes:	No
Affiliation:	Public	Distance Learning:	No

NLN ACCREDITATION: No

Articulation: LPN to Associate

For Further Information Contact:

Dr Deborah M Kisner, Director
Fairmont State College
Fairmont, WV 26554
(304) 367-4767

Wisconsin

University of Wisconsin-Green Bay
—Green Bay—

Full-Time Enrollments:	—	Evening Classes:	Yes
Part-Time Enrollments:	148	Weekend Classes:	No
Affiliation:	Public	Distance Learning:	Yes

NLN ACCREDITATION: Yes

Articulation: Associate to Baccalaureate
Diploma to Baccalaureate

For Further Information Contact:

Dr Jane Muhl, Chair
University of Wisconsin-Green Bay
2420 Nicolet Dr
Green Bay, WI 54311-7001
(414) 465-2826

Glossary of Terms

Articulation. The process of advancing from one degree program in nursing to another, that is, practical or diploma to associate, bachelor and master's degree.

Certification. A process by which a non-governmental agency, based upon specific standards, validates an individual nurse's qualifications and knowledge for practice in a defined area of nursing.

Clinical Nurse Specialist (CNS). A registered nurse, who through a formal post-basic education program, continuing education courses and/or clinical experiences has developed expertise within a specialty area of nursing practice.

Continuing Education. A formal, post-licensure, non-academic credit educational program designed to increase knowledge and/or skills in health care. Such programs may include workshops, institutes, clinical conferences, staff development courses, and individual studies.

Graduate Nurse (GN). An individual who has graduated from a state-approved program prepared for initial licensure as a registered nurse or licensed practical/vocational nurse.

Licensed Practical/Vocational Nurse (LPN/VN). An individual who holds a current license to practice within the scope of practical or vocational nursing in a state of the United States.

Licensure. A method of qualifying an individual to practice a profession within a state by passing an exam, and meeting other state requirements.

National League for Nursing (NLN). The national organization that accredits nursing education programs and whose membership includes health care agencies as well as nurses and non-nurses involved in the improvement of health care.

National Council for Licensure Exam (NCLEX). The exam required for licensure as a practical or registered nurse. (NCLEX-RN and NCLEX-PN).

Nurse Practice Act. The individual state's legal definition of the scope of nursing practice.

Nurse Practitioner (NP). A registered nurse educated and certified beyond a baccalaureate degree, usually a master's level and qualified to practice in an expanded role. Some specific areas of practice include family, adult, pediatric and midwifery. The scope of practice is usually determined by individual states.

Registered Nurse (RN). An individual who holds a current license to practice professional nursing within a state.

State Board of Nursing. The agency in each state that exercises legal control over nursing schools, curricula, and licensure of individual nurses within that state.